2003
YEAR BOOK OF
VASCULAR SURGERY®

The 2003 Year Book Series

Year Book of Allergy, Asthma, and Clinical Immunology™: Drs Rosenwasser, Boguniewicz, Milgrom, Routes, and Spahn

Year Book of Anesthesiology and Pain Management™: Drs Chestnut, Abram, Black, Lang, Roizen, Trankina, and Wood

Year Book of Cardiology®: Drs Gersh, Graham, Kaplan, and Waldo

Year Book of Critical Care Medicine®: Drs Dellinger, Parrillo, Balk, Bekes, Roberts, and Ross

Year Book of Dentistry®: Drs Zakariasen, Boghosian, Dederich, Hatcher, Horswell, and McIntyre

Year Book of Dermatology and Dermatologic Surgery™: Drs Thiers and Lang

Year Book of Diagnostic Radiology®: Drs Osborn, Birdwell, Dalinka, Groskin, Maynard, Oestreich, Pentecost, and Ros

Year Book of Emergency Medicine®: Drs Burdick, Cone, Cydulka, Hamilton, Kassutto, and Niemann

Year Book of Endocrinology®: Drs Mazzaferri, Becker, Horton, Kannan, Kennedy, Kreisberg, Meikle, Molitch, Osei, Poehlman, and Rogol

Year Book of Family Practice®: Drs Bowman, Apgar, Dexter, Gilchrist, Neill, and Scherger

Year Book of Gastroenterology™: Drs Lichtenstein, Dempsey, Ginsberg, Katzka, Kochman, Morris, Nunes, Rosato, and Stein

Year Book of Hand Surgery®: Drs Berger and Ladd

Year Book of Medicine®: Drs Barkin, Frishman, Klahr, Loehrer, Mazzaferri, Phillips, and Pillinger

Year Book of Neonatal and Perinatal Medicine®: Drs Fanaroff, Maisels, and Stevenson

Year Book of Neurology and Neurosurgery®: Drs Bradley, Gibbs, and Verma

Year Book of Nuclear Medicine®: Drs Gottschalk, Blaufox, Coleman, Strauss, and Zubal

Year Book of Obstetrics, Gynecology, and Women's Health®: Drs Mishell, Kirschbaum, and Miller

Year Book of Oncology®: Drs Loehrer, Arceci, Glatstein, Gordon, Johnson, Morrow, and Thigpen

Year Book of Ophthalmology®: Drs Rapuano, Cohen, Eagle, Grossman, Myers, Nelson, Penne, Regillo, Sergott, Shields, and Tipperman

Year Book of Orthopedics®: Drs Morrey, Beauchamp, Peterson, Swiontkowski, Trigg, and Yaszemski

Year Book of Otolaryngology-Head and Neck Surgery®: Drs Paparella, Keefe, and Otto

Year Book of Pathology and Laboratory Medicine®: Drs Raab, Grzybicki, Bejarano, Bissell, Silverman, and Stanley

Year Book of Pediatrics®: Dr Stockman

Year Book of Plastic and Aesthetic Surgery™: Drs Miller, Bartlett, Garner, McKinney, Ruberg, Salisbury, and Smith

Year Book of Psychiatry and Applied Mental Health®: Drs Talbott, Ballenger, Frances, Jensen, Markowitz, Meltzer, and Simpson

Year Book of Pulmonary Disease®: Drs Phillips, Anstead, Barker, Berger, Dunlap, and Maurer

Year Book of Rheumatology, Arthritis, and Musculoskeletal Disease™: Drs Panush, Hadler, Hellmann, Hochberg, Lahita, and LeRoy

Year Book of Sports Medicine®: Drs Shephard, Alexander, Cantu, Kohrt, Nieman, and Shrier

Year Book of Surgery®: Drs Copeland, Bland, Cerfolio, Daly, Eberlein, Howard, Luce, Mozingo, and Seeger

Year Book of Urology®: Drs Andriole and Coplen

Year Book of Vascular Surgery®: Dr Moneta

2003

The Year Book of
VASCULAR
SURGERY®

Editor-in-Chief
Gregory L. Moneta, MD
*Professor of Surgery, Chief of Vascular Surgery, Oregon Health Sciences
University, Oregon Health and Science University Hospital, Portland VA
Medical Center, Portland, Oregon*

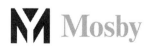 Mosby

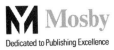

Dedicated to Publishing Excellence

Vice President, Continuity Publishing: Glen P. Campbell
Developmental Editor: Beth Martz
Senior Manager, Continuity Production: Idelle L. Winer
Senior Production Editor: Pat Costigan
Composition Specialist: Betty Dockins
Illustrations and Permissions Coordinator: Kimberly E. Hulett

Printed in the United States of America
Composition by Thomas Technology Solutions, Inc.
Printing/binding by Sheridan Books, Inc

Editorial Office:
Elsevier
The Curtis Center
Suite 300
Independence Square West
Philadelphia, PA 19106

International Standard Serial Number: 0749-4041
International Standard Book Number: 0-323-02066-6

Contributors

Jon S. Matsumura, MD

Assistant Professor of Surgery, Northwestern University; Chief, Vascular Surgery, VA Chicago Health Care System—Lakeside Division, Chicago, Illinois

Michael S. Conte, MD

Assistant Professor of Surgery, Harvard Medical School; Associate Surgeon, Brigham and Women's Hospital, Boston, Massachusetts

Lloyd M. Taylor, Jr, MD

Professor of Surgery, Oregon Health and Sciences University, Oregon Health and Science University Hospital, Portland, Oregon

Michael T. Watkins, MD

Director, Vascular Surgery Research Laboratories, Harvard Medical School; Associate Visiting Surgeon, Massachusetts General Hospital, Boston, Massachusetts

Table of Contents

Journals Represented

Mosby and its editors survey approximately 500 journals for its abstract and commentary publications. From these journals, the editors select the articles to be abstracted. Journals represented in this YEAR BOOK are listed below.

American Journal of Cardiology
American Journal of Epidemiology
American Journal of Kidney Diseases
American Journal of Medicine
American Journal of Neuroradiology
American Journal of Obstetrics and Gynecology
American Journal of Physiology
American Journal of Roentgenology
American Journal of Surgery
American Surgeon
Anaesthesia and Intensive Care
Anesthesia and Analgesia
Anesthesiology
Annals of Internal Medicine
Annals of Neurology
Annals of Plastic Surgery
Annals of Surgery
Annals of Thoracic Surgery
Annals of Vascular Surgery
Archives of Neurology
Archives of Surgery
British Journal of Obstetrics and Gynaecology
British Journal of Surgery
British Medical Journal
Cardiovascular Surgery
Circulation
Critical Care Medicine
Diabetes Care
Diabetic Medicine
Digestive Diseases and Sciences
European Journal of Surgery
European Journal of Vascular Surgery
European Journal of Vascular and Endovascular Surgery
Hepatology
Injury
Journal of Bone and Joint Surgery (American Volume)
Journal of Clinical Neuroscience
Journal of Computer Assisted Tomography
Journal of Human Hypertension
Journal of Internal Medicine
Journal of Investigative Dermatology
Journal of Neurosurgery
Journal of Neurosurgery: Spine
Journal of Pathology
Journal of Pediatrics
Journal of Rheumatology
Journal of Surgical Research

Journal of Thoracic and Cardiovascular Surgery
Journal of Ultrasound in Medicine
Journal of Vascular Surgery
Journal of the American College of Cardiology
Journal of the American College of Surgeons
Journal of the American Medical Association
Journal of the American Society of Nephrology
Kidney International
Lancet
Mayo Clinic Proceedings
Medical Care
Medicine
Medicine and Science in Sports and Exercise
Nephrology, Dialysis, Transplantation
Neurology
Neurosurgery
New England Journal of Medicine
Obstetrics and Gynecology
Radiology
Spine
Stroke
Surgery
Surgical Neurology
Texas Heart Institute Journal
Transplantation Proceedings
World Journal of Surgery

STANDARD ABBREVIATIONS

The following terms are abbreviated in this edition: acquired immunodeficiency syndrome (AIDS), cardiopulmonary resuscitation (CPR), central nervous system (CNS), cerebrospinal fluid (CSF), computed tomography (CT), deoxyribonucleic acid (DNA), electrocardiography (ECG), health maintenance organization (HMO), human immunodeficiency virus (HIV), intensive care unit (ICU), intramuscular (IM), intravenous (IV), magnetic resonance (MR) imaging (MRI), ribonucleic acid (RNA), and ultrasound (US).

NOTE

The YEAR BOOK OF VASCULAR SURGERY® is a literature survey service providing abstracts of articles published in the professional literature. Every effort is made to assure the accuracy of the information presented in these pages. Neither the editors nor the publisher of the YEAR BOOK OF VASCULAR SURGERY® can be responsible for errors in the original materials. The editors' comments are their own opinions. Mention of specific products within this publication does not constitute endorsement.

To facilitate the use of the YEAR BOOK OF VASCULAR SURGERY® as a reference tool, all illustrations and tables included in this publication are now identified as they appear in the original article. This change is meant to help the reader recognize that any illustration or table appearing in the YEAR BOOK OF VASCULAR SURGERY® may be only one of many in the original article. For this reason, figure and table numbers will often appear to be out of sequence within the YEAR BOOK OF VASCULAR SURGERY®.

Introduction

This, the 2003 YEAR BOOK OF VASCULAR SURGERY, marks my first crack at being the primary editor of anything. It is a job I certainly did not request, and it required a bit of, although not much, arm-twisting for me to accept. Given this job became available only as a consequence of the death of my partner, mentor, and friend, Dr John Porter, I would have preferred not to have had it. I have not tried to replicate Dr Porter. To try and do so would be a mistake. The Camel Dung Award has been retired. There are no comments in this introduction on the status of health care in America or perceived evils of HMOs or managed care. However, after years of association, there is probably some Dr Porter in me, and some of it, for good or bad, comes out now and then. I admit the editorship grew on me during the course of the year. It certainly gave me something to do on the airplane, on Sunday afternoons, and most other spare moments that came along. On the positive side, there is no better way to keep up with developments in the care of patients with vascular disease and in basic vascular research than to serve as editor of the YEAR BOOK OF VASCULAR SURGERY. I examined thousands of articles for possible inclusion in the YEAR BOOK. Only a few hundred could be chosen. I accept responsibility both for those chosen and those left out. I also accept responsibility for all the comments that accompany the abstracts, including those of my guest commentators. Articles were included to reflect the depth and broad base of what constitutes vascular surgery. These articles were also included because I believed they had the potential to influence, either immediately or in the future, the care of patients with vascular disease. It was not necessary for me to agree with the article or even for me personally to be particularly interested in the subject. Cost effectiveness and decision analysis studies bore me to tears. However, they seem to be important, and so some are in this edition of the YEAR BOOK.

I have defined rather broadly what influences care. I admit to being a bit conservative, although I almost always vote Democratic. I believe well-conducted, major, multicenter, randomized trials that address critical clinical questions will or should influence care. Who can doubt that the Department of Veterans Affairs cooperative study comparing surveillance versus immediate repair of small abdominal aortic aneurysms (the ADAM trial) is an important publication? This study, combined with the British small aneurysm trial, has to make any reasonable surgeon think twice about the merits of repairing asymptomatic infrarenal abdominal aortic aneurysms smaller than 5.5 cm in diameter. This year's YEAR BOOK also highlights randomized trials addressing insulin therapy, transfusion thresholds, and frequency of dialysis in critically ill patients. A comparison of warfarin versus aspirin in the prevention of recurrent ischemic stroke is included, and trials of propranolol therapy in patients with abdominal aortic aneurysms and drug-releasing stents in coronary angioplasty are also included. An important new anticoagulant, fondaparinux, may have significant advantages over low molecular weight heparins in prevention of venous thromboembolism and has undergone extensive evaluation in orthopedic patients. Nonsteroidal anti-inflammatory agents may adversely impact the benefits of aspirin therapy in patients with arterial disease.

All vascular surgeons, rightly or wrongly, consider themselves experts. Like it or not, some are more expert than others. (I have always found it amusing that a surgeon will agree Brett Favre is a better quarterback than some rookie third-stringer while remaining reluctant to admit some other surgeon may be a better surgeon than themselves.) Given the fact that expertise, knowledge, and experience vary among surgeons, I have chosen to include some articles only because they address an interesting question and come from individuals I consider experts, or at least enthusiasts. Frequently, these reports are not great science. They are often just case series, certainly not level-1 evidence for anything. Dr Porter may have found some of them worthy of a Camel Dung Award. Nevertheless, I believe readers of the YEAR BOOK OF VASCULAR SURGERY will find it interesting to hear how Hazim Safi or Joe Coselli fare with thoracoabdominal aneurysm repair. The Brigham surgeons have a huge series of infrainguinal vein bypass grafts originating distal to the common femoral artery. There is absolutely no science in the article, but it is interesting to see how well these grafts work. Bill Hiatt knows more about drug therapy of claudication than almost anyone. His comments on medical treatment of peripheral arterial disease and claudication should be of interest to us all. The American Heart Association has published guidelines on perioperative cardiac evaluation in noncardiac surgical patients. We should all be curious as to what these experts believe constitutes reasonable preoperative cardiac evaluation.

The Albany group has accumulated an experience of nearly 500 renal artery prosthetic grafts. How in the world anyone can find indications for that many renal artery bypasses in one center is beyond me. Nevertheless, regardless of indications, some insights must have been gained doing that many procedures, and so I have included their report in the YEAR BOOK. Similarly, stents are flying into iliac veins in Mississippi at a rate I never believed would be possible. We need to consider whether these surgeons may be onto something most of us have never considered.

Politics, practice patterns, and objective evaluation of everyday surgical results are always of interest. I have included a number of such articles, as they certainly are thought-provoking and perhaps, to some of us, even threatening. In this year's YEAR BOOK, we find across-the-board poor results from mesenteric and renal artery bypass as well as thoracoabdominal aneurysm repair. Even some more frequently performed procedures have better results when performed in higher-volume centers. We are not as good as our European colleagues in providing autogenous dialysis access. Race, gender, and patient social strata influence our treatment decisions. I think one of the purposes of the YEAR BOOK is to highlight our success, but an equally important purpose is to hint at where we can do better.

The endovascular tidal wave rolls on. Despite my predecessor's clear doubts about the merits of endovascular therapy and the role of vascular surgeons in performing catheter-based procedures, there is no going back. Right now, the endovascular movement has a life of its own. Endovascular topics dominate regional, national, and international vascular surgical meetings. Patients want it, surgeons want to incorporate it into their practice, and endovascular training is mandated as a component of vascular surgical training. Whether endovascular therapy currently works better than open therapy doesn't really matter. What matters is that, in some cases, it is as good as open therapy and in others it may someday be equal or better. Despite the doubts of Dr Porter and the whining and protestations of some interventional radiologists, for better or worse, endovascular therapy has become a part of vascular surgery. In the parlance of a current best seller, "They moved the cheese." There is a whole lot of endovascular in the 2003 YEAR BOOK OF VASCULAR SURGERY.

I personally do not do bench or animal research. The only rat operation I ever participated in was removing a mammary tumor from my youngest daughter's pet. Basic research, however, is critically important. I know most readers of the YEAR BOOK are also not well-versed in basic science techniques and may find that much of the first section of this book has little immediate relevance to their clinical practice. However, all of us should at least be aware of bench and animal research relevant to clinical vascular surgery. I have relied more heavily on guest commentators in Chapter 1 of the YEAR BOOK than did Dr Porter. (Dr Porter wasn't a bench researcher either, but he was a very good professor and seemed, at least on our Sunday morning fishing trips, to believe that being a professor made you an authority on everything from entomology to particle physics.) For future editions of the YEAR BOOK, I invite readers well-versed in basic science to suggest articles for the "Basic Considerations" part of the YEAR BOOK. All suggestions will be appreciated and carefully considered.

The YEAR BOOK is not created in a vacuum. My office manager Barbara McNamee; Heather Morin, who has for years coordinated YEAR BOOK activities in our office; and the excellent staff at Saunders/Elsevier keep me so organized it hurts. My comments that accompany the abstracts were written only by me. The comments, however, are not just me. They reflect the input of years of conversations with colleagues internationally, nationally, and locally, as well as those with the attending surgeons and physicians and surgical residents of the Oregon Health and Science University. To everyone who has influenced my thoughts, especially Drs Porter and Strandness, I offer my profound appreciation. I hope you enjoy and learn from the book.

Gregory L. Moneta, MD
Editor-in-Chief

1 Basic Considerations

Cyclooxygenase Inhibitors and the Antiplatelet Effects of Aspirin
Catella-Lawson F, Reilly MP, Kapoor SC, et al (Univ of Pennsylvania, Philadelphia)
N Engl J Med 345:1809-1817, 2001
1-1

Objective.—Many patients with arthritis and vascular disease may take both nonsteroidal anti-inflammatory drugs (NSAIDs) and low-dose aspirin. There is the potential for competitive interaction between these medications, but it is unknown whether such interactions actually occur. The existence and implications of interactions between NSAIDs and aspirin were studied.

FIGURE 2

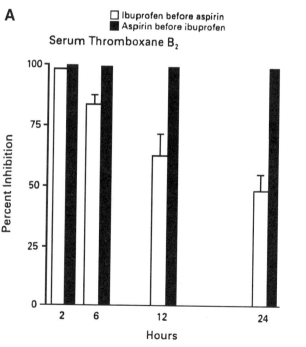

(*Continued*)

FIGURE 2 (cont.)

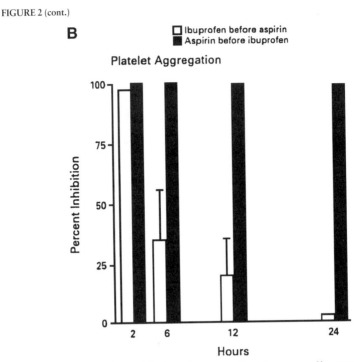

B

☐ Ibuprofen before aspirin
■ Aspirin before ibuprofen

Platelet Aggregation

Hours

FIGURE 2.—Mean inhibition of platelet cyclooxygenase-1 activity, as assessed by measurement of serum thromboxane B₂ (**Panel A**) and inhibition of platelet aggregation (**Panel B**) in subjects taking ibuprofen before aspirin or aspirin before ibuprofen on day 6 of prolonged dosing. The baseline level of serum thromboxane B₂ was 473 ± 92 ng/mL when ibuprofen was administered before aspirin and 503 ± 57 ng/mL when aspirin was administered before ibuprofen. The *I bars* represent SEs. At 24 hours, $P < .001$ for both comparisons between ibuprofen-before-aspirin and aspirin-before-ibuprofen. All times are hours after the administration of the first study drug. (Reprinted by permission of *The New England Journal of Medicine* from Catella-Lawson F, Reilly MP, Kapoor SC, et al: Cyclooxygenase inhibitors and the antiplatelet effects of aspirin. *N Engl J Med* 345:1809-1817, 2001. Copyright 2001, Massachusetts Medical Society. All rights reserved.)

Methods.—Various combinations of drugs were administered to healthy adults for 6 days each as follows: aspirin, 81 mg every morning, given 2 hours before ibuprofen, 400 mg every morning; ibuprofen given 2 hours before aspirin, at the same doses; aspirin given 2 hours before acetaminophen, 1000 mg every morning; acetaminophen given 2 hours before aspirin; aspirin given 2 hours before rofecoxib (a cyclooxygenase-2 inhibitor), 25 mg every morning; rofecoxib given 2 hours before aspirin; enteric coated aspirin given 2 hours before ibuprofen, 400 mg 3 times a day; and enteric coated aspirin given 2 hours before delayed-release diclofenac, 75 mg twice daily. The presence of pharmacodynamic interactions between aspirin and NSAIDs was evaluated under all these conditions.

Results.—By day 6, research subjects taking aspirin before a single daily dose of any of the other drugs showed significant inhibition of serum thromboxane B₂—a marker of platelet cyclooxygenase–1 activity—and of platelet aggregation (Fig 2). The same effect was noted when the cyclooxygenase–2 inhibitor rofecoxib or acetaminophen was taken before aspirin. However, taking a single dose of ibuprofen before aspirin or taking multiple doses of ibuprofen blocked the aspirin-induced inhibition of serum thromboxane B_2 and platelet aggregation. Giving rofecoxib, acetaminophen, or diclofenac concomitantly with aspirin did not alter the pharmacodynamic effects of the latter drug.

Conclusions.—Giving ibuprofen concomitantly with aspirin interferes with aspirin's platelet-inhibiting effect. This interaction does not occur with rofecoxib, acetaminophen, or diclofenac. The results suggest that ibuprofen may reduce the cardioprotective benefits of daily aspirin therapy. The mechanism of these effects seems to involve competitive inhibition of the acetylation site in platelet cyclooxygenase–1.

▶ Aspirins and NSAIDs both act through inhibition of cyclooxygenase-dependent thromboxane A_2 production, with aspirin providing irreversible inhibition and NSAIDs impairing cyclooxygenase only for a portion of the dosing period. Nevertheless, it appears the drugs compete to inhibit cyclooxygenase production such that when NSAIDs are given before aspirin, the ability of aspirin to permanently block platelet aggregation is essentially nullified. These data have significant implications for all our patients on aspirin therapy. Patients should be instructed to take their aspirin dose at least 2 hours before an NSAID if they hope to achieve the cardiovascular benefits of aspirin therapy.

G. L. Moneta, MD

Cerebrovascular Events in Patients With Significant Stenosis of the Carotid Artery Are Associated With Hyperhomocysteinemia and Platelet Antigen-1 (Leu33Pro) Polymorphism

Streifler JY, Rosenberg N, Chetrit A, et al (Rabin Med Ctr, Petach-Tikva, Israel; Tel Aviv Univ, Israel)

Stroke 32:2753-2758, 2001

1–2

Background.—The risk factors for atherosclerosis of the carotid arteries are well recognized, but little is known about what factors may trigger thromboembolic events. Potential triggering factors were evaluated in a group of symptomatic and asymptomatic patients with carotid atherosclerosis.

Methods.—The study included 153 patients with 50% or greater carotid stenosis: 67 with ipsilateral ischemic events (mean age, 69.5 years) and 86 asymptomatic patients (mean age, 73.7 years). The 2 groups were comparable in their major stroke risk factors. Patients underwent measurement of plasma levels of various thrombophilic factors, platelet glycoprotein polymorphisms, and homocysteine.

Findings.—Hyperhomocysteinemia was found in 34.3% of symptomatic patients, compared with 12.8% of asymptomatic patients. The rates of human platelet antigen (HPA)-1a/b were 38.8% and 20.9%, respectively. These were the only 2 significant differences between the groups. Both remained significant on multivariate analysis, with odds ratios of 4.07 for hyperhomocysteinemia and 3.4 for HPA-1a/b.

Conclusion.—Among patients with significant carotid stenosis, plasma homocysteine and HPA-1a/b are independently associated with cerebral ischemic events. Pending confirmation in future studies, efforts to reduce hyperhomocysteinemia may reduce the risk of cerebrovascular events in patients with carotid atherosclerosis.

▶ Since the Asymptomatic Carotid Atherosclerosis Study established that it is necessary to perform about 20 carotid endarterectomies for asymptomatic stenosis in order to prevent 1 stroke, everyone would like to find some factor or factors which reliably identify patients with asymptomatic stenosis who are truly at risk for stroke. This article adds another possible pair of factors—hyperhomocysteinemia and platelet antigen-1 (Leu33Pro) polymorphism—to some already known—other hypercoagulable states, diabetes, soft plaque. It will take more information than can be gained from 153 patients to confirm the authors' suspicions, but the goal is a worthy one. Stay tuned.

L. M. Taylor, Jr, MD

C-Reactive Protein Is an Independent Predictor of the Rate of Increase in Early Carotid Atherosclerosis
Hashimoto H, Kitagawa K, Hougaku H, et al (Osaka Univ, Japan)
Circulation 104:63-67, 2001
1–3

Background.—It is now thought that an inflammatory response is a component in the development of atherosclerosis. Several circulating markers of inflammation have been studied as potential predictors of the presence of cardiovascular disease and the risk of future cardiovascular events. Of these potential markers, high-sensitivity C-reactive protein (hs-CRP) has the most consistent relationship to the risk of cardiovascular events in a variety of clinical settings. hs-CRP has been shown to be predictive of cardiovascular disease in healthy men and women, in selected high-risk patients with traditional risk factors, and in patients with cardiovascular disease. The ability of hs-CRP to predict the risk of cardiovascular disease is independent of the effects of traditional risk factors, and hs-CRP in combination with the total/high-density lipoprotein (HDL) cholesterol ratio is more strongly predictive of cardiovascular disease than either factor alone. Previously there had been no longitudinal studies of the relationships between the development of atherosclerotic lesions and hs-CRP concentrations. Whether increased hs-CRP concentrations result in the development of atherosclerosis was investigated.

Methods.—The study group included 179 patients (age, 40-79 years) who were treated at 1 institution for the traditional risk factors for cardiovascular disease. The patients had no evidence of advanced carotid atherosclerosis at the time of baseline examination. Patients underwent repeated US evaluation of the carotid arteries for 35 ± 10 months, and blood samples were col-

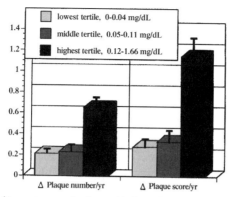

FIGURE 3.—Annual increasing rate of early carotid atherosclerosis according to tertiles of hs-CRP concentration. *Bars* represent means, and *lines* represent SEM. ΔPN/year and ΔPS/year in highest tertile of baseline hs-CRP concentration were significantly higher than those in middle or lowest tertiles ($P < .05$), respectively. (Courtesy of Hashimoto H, Kitigawa K, Hougake H, et al: C-reactive protein is an independent predictor of the rate of increase in early carotid atherosclerosis. *Circulation* 104:63-67, 2001.)

lected for measurement of hs-CRP. Plaque number and plaque score were calculated on the basis of focal intima-media thickening (≥ 1.1 mm representing plaque). The formula Δvalue/year = (last value − baseline value)/ number of follow-up years was used to estimate the development of atherosclerosis.

Results.—Multivariate linear regression analysis indicated that the log-transformed value for hs-CRP concentration was not related to baseline plaque number or plaque score but was related to Δplaque number/year and Δplaque score/year, independently of the effect of traditional risk factors (Fig 3).

Conclusions.—The hs-CRP concentration is a marker of carotid atherosclerotic activity, rather than the extent of atherosclerosis, in the early stages of carotid atherosclerosis.

▶ The correlation of elevated C-reactive protein with the rate of development of atherosclerosis suggests inflammation is inherent to the atherosclerotic process. What causes this inflammation or if the inflammation is merely the result of increasing atherosclerosis is unclear. (See also Abstract 1–4.)

G. L. Moneta, MD

C-Reactive Protein Levels and Viable *Chlamydia pneumoniae* in Carotid Artery Atherosclerosis

Johnston SC, Messina LM, Browner WS, et al (Univ of California, San Francisco; California Pacific Med Ctr Research Inst, San Francisco; Children's Hosp of Oakland Research Inst, Calif)
Stroke 32:2748-2752, 2001 1–4

Background.—C-reactive protein is a sensitive indicator of both acute and chronic inflammation. An elevated serum level of C-reactive protein is a predictor of long-term risk of coronary artery disease and stroke and is an independent predictor of the risk for cardiovascular events in patients with coronary artery disease. Chronic infection of blood vessels with *Chlamydia pneumoniae* could result in elevation of C-reactive protein levels and may contribute to the instability or progression of atherosclerotic plaques. Studies of the potential association between C-reactive protein and serologic evidence of *C pneumoniae* have been contradictory. Whether chronic infection with *C pneumoniae* is responsible for systemic inflammation was studied by an evaluation of the association between serum C-reactive protein levels and infection of carotid artery atherosclerotic plaque with viable *C pneumoniae*.

Methods.—There were 48 endarterectomy samples obtained from 46 patients scheduled for endarterectomy for carotid artery stenosis. Plaques were then tested for *C pneumoniae* mRNA (which indicates viability) as well as for DNA by polymerase chain reaction (PCR).

Results.—Of 48 samples studied, 18 were infected with viable *C pneumoniae* as indicated by isolated chlamydial mRNA. Serum C-reactive protein levels were higher in samples with viable *C pneumoniae* than in samples without infection (median, 8 mg/L vs undetectable). Multivariate models indicated that the only independent predictor of the presence of viable *C pneumoniae* was a detectable C-reactive protein level.

Conclusions.—A significant number of carotid artery atherosclerotic plaques contain viable *C pneumoniae*, which are associated with increased levels of serum C-reactive protein. These findings might explain the link between an elevated level of C-reactive protein and the risk of cardiovascular disease and stroke.

▶ Infection, particularly infection with *Chlamydia pneumoniae*, is enjoying a resurgence of interest as a possible important etiologic factor in the generation of an atherosclerotic plaque. In this study, C-reactive protein, known to be a predictor of stroke and coronary artery disease, was associated with the presence of viable *Chlamydia* in carotid plaques removed at the time of carotid endarterectomy. Of course, studies such as this raise the "chicken and egg" question. Is the *C pneumoniae* there because it caused the atherosclerosis, or is it there because the plaque provided a suitable environment for adherence and growth?

G. L. Moneta, MD

Human Vascular Smooth Muscle Cells of Diabetic Origin Exhibit Increased Proliferation, Adhesion, and Migration
Faries PL, Rohan DI, Takahara H, et al (Harvard Med School, Boston)
J Vasc Surg 33:601-607, 2001   1–5

Background.—From 20 to 25 million persons in the United States are affected with diabetes mellitus, at an estimated annual cost of more than $50 billion. Diabetes has been established as an independent risk factor for atherosclerosis. Patients with diabetes mellitus have progressive macrovascular atherosclerosis, and intimal hyperplastic restenosis develops with greater frequency than in nondiabetic patients. This suggests vascular smooth muscle cells (VSMCs) behave in a phenotypically different and more aggressive way in patients with diabetes than in patients without diabetes. The in vitro rates of proliferation, adhesion, and migration of human VSMCs in these 2 populations were compared.

Methods.—Vascular biopsy specimens were obtained at surgery from 23 diabetic and 15 nondiabetic patients with extensive lower extremity atherosclerosis. The patients ranged in age from 61 to 78 years. All of the patients with diabetes had type 2 diabetes mellitus. Cells obtained from the biopsy specimens were assayed for their proliferative capacity with total DNA fluorescence photometry and for adhesion and migration with a modified Boyden chamber.

Results.—The average duration of diabetes was 11.6 ± 4.1 years, and the average number of diabetic complications was 2.8 ± 0.7 per patient. Complications included retinopathy, neuropathy, nephropathy, and coronary artery disease. Abnormal morphology was seen in VSMCs from patients with diabetes, with loss of the normal hill-and-valley configuration. VSMCs obtained from patients with diabetes also demonstrated significantly increased proliferation and greater adhesion compared with VSMCs of nondiabetic origin.

Conclusions.—Significantly increased rates of proliferation, adhesion, and migration were observed in diabetic VSMCs compared with nondiabetic VSMCs, along with abnormal cell culture morphology, which is suggestive of abnormal contact inhibition. These findings are consistent with the increased rates of infragenicular atherosclerosis and restenosis observed in patients with diabetes. The promotion of atherosclerosis and hyperplasia seems to be intrinsic to the diabetes mellitus VSMC phenotype and is a factor for consideration in the development of therapies to limit atherosclerosis and intimal hyperplasia in patients with diabetes mellitus.

▶ This article seeks to provide an understanding of why atherosclerosis and intimal hyperplasia appear to have greater clinical prevalence and severity in patients with diabetes. The authors compare well-established phenotypic measures of vascular smooth muscle cellular adhesion, migration, and proliferation in cells procured from patients with and without diabetes. Diabetics were found significantly different from nondiabetics in all indices. Since matrix synthesis appears to be a long-term component of the constrictive remodeling associated with vascular injury, it's surprising that this characteristic was not investigated. This article leads the way to try and understand these differences from a proteomic and genomic perspective. Furthermore, it would be interesting to know if arteries and veins are different in patients with and without diabetes. Excellent work like this often asks more questions than it answers but does provide considerable "food for thought."

M. T. Watkins, MD

Inhibition of Inducible Nitric Oxide Synthase Limits Nitric Oxide Production and Experimental Aneurysm Expansion

Johanning JM, Franklin DP, Han DC, et al (Geisinger Med Ctr, Danville, Pa)

J Vasc Surg 33:579-586, 2001   1–6

Background.—Nitric oxide (NO), which is often cited for its protective role, is also capable of generating toxic metabolites that are known to degrade elastin. Abdominal aortic aneurysms (AAAs) and inducible nitric oxide synthase (iNOS) have been associated with inflammatory states, but the expression of iNOS and the role of NO during the development of AAA have not been investigated. There is indirect evidence to suggest that NO may play a role in the pathogenesis of aneurysm. The expression of iNOS, NO production, and the effects of selective inhibition of iNOS by aminoguanidine in experimental AAAs were examined.

Methods.—This study used an intra-aortic elastase infusion model in which control rats were given intra-aortic saline infusion and postoperative intraperitoneal saline injections (group 1). Three other groups were given intra-aortic elastase infusion to induce aneurysm formation. The rats in group 2 were treated with postoperative intraperitoneal injections of saline solution, group 3 rats were given aminoguanidine postoperatively, and rats in group 4 were given aminoguanidine both preoperatively and postoperatively. The aortic diameter and the plasma nitrite/nitrate levels were measured on the day of surgery and again on postoperative day 7. Aortas were harvested for biochemical and histologic analysis on postoperative day 7.

Results.—The infusion of elastase produced AAAs with significant iNOS and nitrite/nitrate production compared with controls. Aneurysm size was significantly reduced by the selective inhibition of iNOS with aminoguanidine in elastase-infused aortas compared with elastase infusion alone. Rats treated with aminoguanidine showed suppression of iNOS expression and plasma nitrite/nitrate production that was not significantly different from that of the control group. Elastase-infused groups had equivalent inflammatory infiltrates on histologic evaluation.

Conclusions.—In experimental AAA, the expression of iNOS is induced and plasma nitrite/nitrate levels are increased. The inhibition of iNOS with aminoguanidine limits production of NO and expression of iNOS, which results in a significant limitation of aneurysmal expansion.

▶ The role of NO in both physiologic and pathologic vascular remodeling is an area of intense investigation. In particular, a putative role for NO in the pathogenesis of aneurysms had been suggested by several investigators. These authors examined the role of one of the NO producing enzymes, iNOS, in the rat model of elastase perfusion of the abdominal aorta. This model produces dramatic acute inflammation and rapid aneurysm growth within days. Their findings suggest an association between iNOS activity and aneurysm development in this model. The translation of the findings in this model to AAA disease in humans remains far less clear, and much further study is required to determine if local NO dysregulation is the "chicken or the egg" in the pathogenesis of AAA.

M. S. Conte, MD

Comparison of Efficacy and Safety of Atorvastatin (10 mg) With Simvastatin (10 mg) at Six Weeks

Kafonek S, for the ASSET Investigators (Pfizer Inc, New York; et al)
Am J Cardiol 87:554-559, 2001   1–7

Background.—In patients with primary hypercholesterolemia, atorvastatin achieves low-density lipoprotein (LDL) cholesterol reductions similar to those of simvastatin and other statin drugs, with similar safety. Data from a larger trial were used to analyze the 6-week outcomes of atorvastatin and simvastatin in patients with mixed dyslipidemia, with or without diabetes.

Methods.—The multicenter open-label trial included 1424 patients with mixed dyslipidemia, including a triglyceride level of 200 to 600 mg/dL. They were randomly assigned to receive atorvastatin or simvastatin, both at a dose of 10 mg/d.

Results.—After 6 weeks, LDL cholesterol was reduced by about 37% from baseline in the atorvastatin group, compared with 30% in the sim-

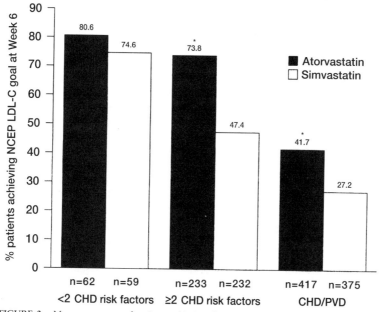

FIGURE 2.—Mean percentage of patients achieving their National Cholesterol Education Program (*NCEP*) low-density lipoprotein (*LDL*) cholesterol (C) goal by coronary heart disease (*CHD*) risk category after 6 weeks of treatment with 10-mg once-daily doses of atorvastatin or simvastatin. *Abbreviation: PVD*, Peripheral vascular disease. (Reprinted from *American Journal of Cardiology* courtesy of Kafonek S, for the ASSET Investigators: Comparison of efficacy and safety of atorvastatin (10 mg) with simvastatin (10 mg) at six weeks. *Am J Cardiol* 87:554-559, 2001. Copyright 2001, by permission from Excerpta Medica Inc.)

vastatin group. Simvastatin also achieved greater reductions in total cholesterol (28% vs 22%), triglycerides (22% vs 16%), LDL to high-density lipoprotein (HDL) cholesterol ratio (41% vs 34%), and apoliprotein B (28% vs 21%). Both treatments yielded approximately a 7% increase in HDL cholesterol. Fifty-six percent of the atorvastatin patients achieved LDL cholesterol target levels, compared with 38% of the simvastatin group (Fig 2). The rate of treatment-related adverse effects was under 6% in both groups, with most being mild to moderate. The efficacy and safety results were similar in diabetic and nondiabetic patients.

Conclusion.—In patients with mixed dyslipidemia, atorvastatin appears to be more effective in reducing lipid levels compared with simvastatin. Like the other statin drugs, both medications are safe and well tolerated.

▶ It would be nice to say "a statin is a statin is a statin," but it appears statins are not all the same. If all statins are not created equal, why not use the one that is most effective in lowering lipid levels provided, of course, side effects are not increased with the more effective drug.

G. L. Moneta, MD

Enhancement of Neointima Formation With Tissue-Type Plasminogen Activator

Hilfiker PR, Waugh JM, Li-Hawkins JJ, et al (Stanford Univ, Calif; Baylor College of Medicine, Houston; Univ of Texas, Dallas)
J Vasc Surg 33:821-828, 2001   1–8

Background.—Clinically significant restenosis occurs within 6 months in 40% of patients undergoing balloon angioplasty. Indirect evidence suggests that tissue plasminogen activator (tPA) either limits or does not alter restenosis. However, tPA enhances the invasiveness of a tumor through matrix remodeling, and a number of elements of degraded matrix enhance mitogenesis of smooth muscle cells. Because tPA is commonly used and exhibits functions that may to some degree both limit and enhance neointima formation in vivo, a study was conducted to evaluate the effects of tPA on neointima formation by using either local adenoviral-mediated overexpression of tPA or systemic infusion of recombinant tPA in combination with mechanical overdilation of rabbit common femoral arteries.

Methods.—In New Zealand white rabbits, the left common femoral artery was transfected in situ with either an adenoviral-construct–expressing tPA or a viral (adenoviral-construct–expressing β-galactosidase) or nonviral (buffer) control after balloon angioplasty injury. Artery segments were harvested at 7 and 28 days from each group and examined for intima-to-media ratio, smooth muscle cell proliferation, extracellular matrix, and inflammatory response. Thrombus formation was evaluated after 3 days. In the second experiment, rabbits underwent mechanical dilation followed by buffer treatment or systemic tPA infusion. Treated artery segments were then harvested after 7 or 28 days and processed for evaluation of the intima-to-media

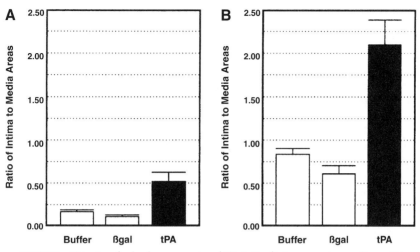

FIGURE 1.—I/M ratios after local overexpression of tPA. Ratio of intima area n-to n-media area 7 days (a) or 28 days (b) after balloon dilation and delivery of PBS, Adv/RSV-(gal, or Adv/RSV-tPA. Values represent mean plus standard error of 3 randomly selected cross sections per vessel. *Abbreviation: tPA,* Tissue plasminogen activator. (Courtesy of Hilfiker PR, Waugh JM, Li-Hawkins JJ, et al: Enhancement of neointima formation with tissue-type plasminogen activator. *J Vasc Surg* 33:821-828, 2001.)

ratio and classwide histochemical determination of collagenous extracellular matrix and collagen content.

Results.—Overexpression of tPA was associated with dramatic increases in both rate and degree of neointima formation (Fig 1). Local overexpression of tPA results in substantial early matrix degradation but no increases in local inflammation or in smooth muscle proliferation. In this model, the systemic infusion of tPA resulted in early and late enhancement of neointima formation with significant early collagenous matrix degradation. Systemic infusion did not attain the degree of neointima formation observed in association with overexpression.

Conclusions.—Tissue plasminogen activator enhances neointima formation in a rabbit model of angioplasty, and there is evidence that this effect is dose-dependent. Early matrix degradation is followed by changes in rates of proliferation and is a key component in this neointima formation despite several antirestenotic actions, including decreased thrombus and macrophage recruitment in this model.

▶ The data in this article provide scientific rationale for paying attention to the long-term versus initial success rates when using tPA for thrombolytic therapy in patients with vascular disease. These authors provide data to show that tPA promotes matrix accumulation in injured arteries. There is a mismatch in the timing and degree of the progression of neointima hyperplasia when compared with indices of smooth muscle cellular proliferation. tPA was found to increase vascular neointima with the use of both clinical systemic infusion and an experimental overexpression protocol. These findings suggest that tPA can modulate matrix remodeling independent of its thrombolytic properties. The data also suggest tPA may promote injury in a long-term manner, independent of its thrombolytic potential. This plot will only thicken!

M. T. Watkins, MD

Comparative Effects of Aging in Men and Women on the Properties of the Arterial Tree

Smulyan H, Asmar RG, Rudnicki A, et al (State Univ of New York, Syracuse; Institut Cardiovasculaire, Paris; Covance, Malmaison, France; et al)
J Am Coll Cardiol 37:1374-1380, 2001   1–9

Background.—Both sexes show stiffening of the arterial tree with age, although the factors affecting this process differ for women and men. One important factor is hormonal status, but a wide range of other variables may be relevant as well. Nonhormonal factors affecting the arterial tree, including their relationship with pulse pressure, were compared between the sexes at different ages.

Methods.—The study included 347 men and 183 women divided into 4 age groups as follows: 40 years or less, 41 to 47 years, 48 to 54 years, and 55 years or older. Variables assessed included brachial artery blood pressure, aortic pulse wave velocity; B-mode US and wave form analysis of the common carotid artery (CCA), with its conversion to the aortic waveform; echocardiographic measurement of left ventricular dimensions and flow values; and calculated measures such as CCA compliance and distensibility, systemic compliance, stroke volume, and peripheral resistance.

Results.—Across age quartiles, heart rate was higher and blood pressure lower in women than in men. Among women, however, pulse pressure was lower in the younger age group and higher in the older age group. Common carotid artery diameter, compliance, and systemic compliance were influenced by body size and therefore lower in women. In contrast, there was no difference in measurements related to arterial wall properties, such as distensibility of the CCA and aorta. Both sexes had similar aging-related increases in aortic pulse wave velocity. However, pulse wave velocity affected pulse pressure to a greater extent than blood pressure for women, but the opposite was true for men.

Conclusion.—Women show a greater increase in pulsatility as they age, compared with men. This phenomenon reflects women's smaller body size and arteries and is unaffected by hormonal changes associated with menopause.

▶ With respect to the conclusion in the abstract, is it pulsatility or volatility?

G. L. Moneta, MD

Basic Science Curriculum in Vascular Surgery Residency

Sidawy AN, Sumpio B, Clowes AW, et al (George Washington Univ, Washington, DC; Georgetown Univ, Washington, DC; Yale Univ, New Haven, Conn; et al)

J Vasc Surg 33:854-860, 2001

1–10

Background.—An understanding of the basic science that forms the basis of disease processes is a hallmark of modern medical education. The leadership of the Association of Program Directors in Vascular Surgery (APDVS) recognized the importance of this basic science teaching to surgical education and appointed a panel to gather the opinions of program directors regarding basic science teaching in vascular residencies and to gather information on the performance of vascular residents on the basic science items on the Vascular Surgery Qualifying Examination (VQE). The panel was also charged with using the data gathered to make recommendations for the integration of basic science teaching into vascular residencies. Those findings and resulting recommendations were summarized.

Methods.—A questionnaire was distributed to program directors attending the 1999 annual fall meeting of the APDVS. The 12-item questionnaire was designed to gather opinions regarding what basic science should be taught, the appropriate content of the course, and who should teach. Information was also gathered from the American Board of Surgery regarding the basic science content in the vascular surgery item pool of the VQE.

Results.—The questionnaire was completed by 53 (64%) program directors. Only 2 program directors believed that their residents were better prepared to answer basic science questions, but the results of the VQE indicated that the examinees as a group do not perform differently on basic science items than on clinical management questions. Only 15% of the program directors use a specific method to monitor the learning process of their residents. Most (75%) of the program directors who responded to the questionnaire indicated that they believed themselves to be capable of teaching basic science to residents. Nearly half of the respondents indicated that they believed a basic science curriculum should be comprehensive and not limited to clinically relevant information. However, a review of the VQE content outline and the vascular surgery unit of the surgical resident curriculum showed great emphasis on clinically relevant basic science information.

Conclusions.—The APDVS recommendations for basic science curriculum in vascular surgery residency state that a basic science curriculum should be comprehensive but clinically relevant and completely integrated into the clinical curriculum. The panel supports the use of teaching conferences that are problem-based with a faculty member functioning as the resource person and with specific goals set for the conferences. The panel also suggests the development of a Web site to provide interactive training and the ability of program directors to provide feedback and monitor the progress of their residents.

▶ This article provides a concise history detailing the fusion of medical education with science. The fundamental rationale for providing basic science as an important part of the vascular fellowship is convincingly described. Concise and practical recommendations are made on how to integrate basic science into the vascular surgery curriculum. This article provides a structural outline for all program directors in vascular surgery.

M. T. Watkins, MD

Impact of Infectious Burden on Extent and Long-term Prognosis of Atherosclerosis
Espinola-Klein C, for the AtheroGene Investigators (Johannes Gutenberg Univ, Mainz, Germany; et al)
Circulation 105:15-21, 2002   1–11

Introduction.—Inflammatory mechanisms are suspected in the pathogenesis of atherosclerosis. Earlier investigations have reported a link between elevated inflammatory markers and the development of atherosclerosis. Many trials have revealed associations between atherosclerosis and various pathogens. A total of 572 patients undergoing coronary angiography, along with carotid duplex sonography and Doppler sonography in the peripheral arteries, were examined to determine (1) if there is an association between the extent of atherosclerosis and persistent infections with various bacterial or viral pathogens, (2) if there is a correlation between the extent of atherosclerosis and the number of infectious pathogens to which an individual has been exposed, and (3) if a previous infection with multiple pathogens has any influence on adverse outcome in patients with extended atherosclerosis in various vascular regions.

Methods.—The 572 patients underwent measurements of immunoglobulin (Ig) G or IgA antibodies to herpes simplex virus 1 and 2, cytomegalovirus, Epstein-Barr virus, *Hemophilus influenzae*, *Chlamydia pneumoniae*, *Mycoplasma pneumoniae*, and *Helicobacter pylori*. The extent of atherosclerosis was ascertained by coronary angiography, carotid duplex sonography, and assessment of the ankle-arm index.

Results.—Elevated IgA antibodies against *C pneumoniae* ($P < .01$) and IgG antibodies against *H pylori* ($P < .02$), cytomegalovirus ($P < .05$), and herpes simplex virus 2 ($P < .01$) were correlated with advanced atherosclerosis (r2 vascular regions), adjusted for age, sex, cardiovascular risk factors, and highly sensitive C-reactive protein. Infectious burden divided into 0 to 3, 4 to 5, and 6 to 8 seropositivities was significantly correlated with advanced atherosclerosis; OR 1.8 (95% CI, 1.2-2.6) for 4 to 5 ($P < .01$) and OR 2.5 (95% CI, 1.2-5.1) for 6 to 8 seropositivities ($P < .02$) (adjusted). At a mean follow-up of 3.2 years, the cardiovascular mortality rate was 7.0% for patients with advanced atherosclerosis and seropositive for 0 to 3 pathogens versus 20.0% for those seropositive for 6 to 8 pathogens.

Conclusion.—Infectious agents appear to be involved in the development of atherosclerosis. A significant correlation was observed between infectious burden and the extent of atherosclerosis. The risk for future death was increased by the number of infectious pathogens, particularly in persons with advanced atherosclerosis.

▶ An infectious etiology of atherosclerosis is an intriguing possibility. The "chicken and egg" question still applies (see Abstract 1–4).

G. L. Moneta, MD

Functional Outcome of New Blood Vessel Growth Into Ischemic Skeletal Muscle
Lee SL, Pevec WC, Carlsen RC (Univ of California, Davis, Sacramento)
J Vasc Surg 34:1096-1102, 2001   1–12

Introduction.—The development of new blood vessels into ischemic muscle can be induced with the administration of angiogenic growth factors and the transfer of well-vascularized tissues. The functional importance of these new vessels is not known. The ability of the transfer of vascularized muscle and the local infusion of basic fibroblast growth tissue (bFGF) to synergistically improve contractile function of ischemic skeletal muscle was examined in an animal model of hindlimb ischemia.

Methods.—Twenty-six New Zealand white rabbits were placed in 1 of 4 groups. An ischemic hindlimb was produced in each animal by ligating the right common iliac artery. Six rabbits in the flap + bFGF group underwent transposition of a contralateral rectus muscle flap onto the thigh; bFGF 3 ng/h was continuously infused at the flap-thigh interface. A similar muscle flap was created for the 6 animals in the flap group; carrier solution was infused at the interface. For the 6 animals in the bFGF alone group, no muscle flap was created; rather, bFGF 3 ng/h was infused into the external iliac artery of the ischemic limb. In the control group of 8 rabbits, carrier solution was infused into the external iliac artery; there was no flap and no bFGF. One week later, the soleus muscle was isolated and stimulated. Maximum twitch tension, the fatigue index (force of contraction after 2 minutes of continuous stimulation/initial force of contraction), maximum recovery, and the number of limbs recovered (limbs that achieved a force of contraction during the recovery period of more than 75% of the force of the initial contraction at the beginning of continuous stimulation) were noted. Blood vessel density was ascertained by immunostaining the soleus muscle with the use of anti–α-antibody.

Results.—All the values were indexed to the contralateral nonoperated, normal limb. The flap + bFGF group had significant improvement compared with controls in maximum twitch tension (mean, 1.07 vs 0.63; $P <$ .05), maximum recovery (mean, 0.94 vs 0.58; $P <$ .05), and the number of limbs recovered (5/5 vs 0/6; $P < .05$). This improved function was associated with increased vessel density (flap + bFGF group, 1.44 vs control group, 0.72; $P < .05$).

Conclusion.—Reperfusion of an ischemic limb with a well-vascularized muscle flap and local bFGF infusion stimulated increased blood vessel density in distal ischemic muscle. The increase in vascularity was correlated with restoration of otherwise impaired muscle function. Improved function was observed within 1 week. A transposed muscle flap supplied a functional blood supply to the site of maximum ischemia. This approach may be useful in salvaging otherwise nonreconstructible ischemic limbs.

▶ These authors have used an interesting model in which a free flap is placed to an acutely ischemic hindlimb. There is evidence from this group and others that local vascular connections develop between a vascularized flap and surrounding ischemic tissue, thereby improving local perfusion. In this study, they demonstrate that the addition of local infusion of an angiogenic cytokine, basic fibroblast growth factor, to the free flap resulted in increased vessel density and contractile function of distal ischemic muscle. The work is interesting but the clinical implications remain unclear in that patients with severe distal ischemia would likely require a bypass graft to support a free flap in the first place; hence, the added value of the flap alone for the treatment of ischemia is nebulous.

M. S. Conte, MD

Apolipoprotein J/Clusterin Is Induced in Vascular Smooth Muscle Cells After Vascular Injury

Miyata M, Biro S, Kaieda H, et al (Kagoshima Univ, Japan)
Circulation 104:1407-1412, 2001   1–13

Introduction.—Intimal thickening and constrictive remodeling are important components in the process of restenosis after percutaneous transluminal angioplasty. Smooth muscle cells (SMCs) have a key role in this phenomenon. The ability to understand how this occurs may help in the development of a new strategy for the treatment of restenosis after angioplasty. Restenosis may involve cascades of autocrine and paracrine cytokine and growth factor signaling after vascular injury; there may be a master gene that controls this mechanism. Differential hybridization was used in a rabbit aorta model after balloon injury to identify mRNA with increased levels of expression to initiate identification of the genes involved in vascular restenosis.

Findings.—Six cDNA clones were upregulated after injury after applying a differential hybridization method to a model of the balloon-injured rabbit aorta. Northern blot demonstrated that 5 genes, and not apolipoprotein J (apoJ)/clusterin, were constitutively expressed in noninjured aorta and upregulated after balloon injury. The ApoJ mRNA was not identified in the noninjured control aorta and started to be expressed at 6 hours after injury.

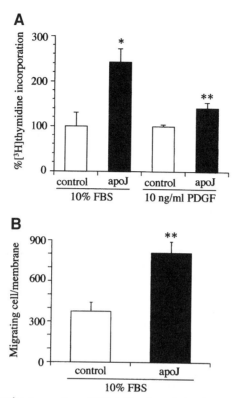

FIGURE 6.—Effects of apoJ expression on SMC proliferation and migration. **A,** Proliferation assay: after starvation, with 0.1% fetal bovine serum (FBS) for 48 hours, SMCs were stimulated by 10% FBS or 10 ng/mL platelet-derived growth factor (PDGF). On 10% FBS or 10 ng/mL PDGF medium, [³H]thymidine incorporation in apoJ-transfected SMCs *(solid bar)* was significantly higher than that in SMCs transfected with plasmid vector *(control, open bar)*. Results are presented as percentage increase from each control. **B,** Migration assay: number of migrating apoJ-transfected SMCs induced by 10% FBS was significantly higher than in control. All experiments were performed in quadruplicate, and each experiment was repeated 4 times. Values are mean ± SD. *P < .005, **P < .001 vs control. (Courtesy of Miyata M, Biro S, Kaieda H, et al: Apolipoprotein J/clusterin is induced in vascular smooth muscle cells after vascular injury. *Circulation* 104:1407-1412, 2001.)

It reached a peak level at 24 hours (a 48-fold increase), gradually diminished, then returned to the control level at 24 weeks. Western blot and immunohistochemistry showed no expression of apoJ protein in the noninjured aorta, expression of apoJ at 2 days after balloon injury, and a peak level (a 55-fold increase) at 2 to 8 weeks. This expression of apoJ was sustained until 24 weeks after injury. In situ hybridization demonstrated that apoJ mRNA was expressed in SMCs of media 2 days after injury and in SMCs of media and neointima at 2 weeks. To assess the function of apoJ, stably transfected rabbit SMCs were produced. The expression of apoJ activated proliferation and migration of SMCs (Fig 6).

Conclusion.—ApoJ is dramatically induced in media and neointima after vascular injury, indicating that apoJ facilitates restenosis after angioplasty.

▶ This experimental study used a powerful technique, differential hybridization, to identify genes that were induced after balloon injury of the rabbit aorta. Six up regulated genes were identified, of which apoJ was the most strongly induced. ApoJ has important properties in cell-cell interactions and migration, and others have identified apoJ in association with anastomotic intimal hyperplasia. These authors now demonstrate sustained upregulation of apoJ in medial and intimal SMC out to 24 weeks after injury, and also demonstrate a strong increase in SMC migration and proliferation in vitro associated with up regulation of apoJ. There is now considerable evidence that apoJ plays a role in the regulation of SMC behavior in the vascular injury response.

M. S. Conte, MD

Influence of Pravastatin on Lipoproteins, and on Endothelial, Platelet, and Inflammatory Markers in Subjects With Peripheral Artery Disease
Blann AD, Gurney D, Hughes E, et al (City Hosp, Birmingham, England; Sandwell Gen Hosp, Lyndon, West Bromwich, UK)
Am J Cardiol 88:89-92, 2001   1–14

Background.—Among patients with peripheral artery disease, the treatment of hypercholesterolemia with pravastatin was hypothesized to also reduce levels of plasma markers for platelet activity, endothelial cell function, and inflammation. The validity of this hypothesis was tested.

Methods.—The patients evaluated had peripheral artery disease and hypercholesterolemia (total cholesterol levels of 5.5-7.5 mmol/L, or 201-290 mg/mL). Each patient received either placebo (n = 15) or pravastatin (n = 17) in a daily dose of 40 mg during 4 months. A control group of 32 healthy subjects was used for comparison. Assessments included measurements of total cholesterol, high-density lipoprotein, triglycerides, von Willebrand factor, soluble intercellular adhesion molecule-1 (sICAM-1), soluble P-selectin, lipoprotein(a), and C-reactive protein (CRP).

Results.—After 2 months of pravastatin therapy, sICAM-1 fell significantly, and significant reductions in total and low-density lipoprotein cholesterol, sICAM-1, CRP, and von Willebrand factor occurred after 4 months. CRP showed the most significant reduction (45%). None of the patients taking placebo showed any significant changes.

Conclusions.—Reductions in von Willebrand factor, sICAM-1, total cholesterol, low-density lipoprotein cholesterol, and CRP occurred with pravastatin therapy in patients with peripheral artery disease. The most significant reduction was in CRP, an average decrease of 45%, indicating a significant anti-inflammatory effect for pravastatin. Thus, pravastatin exerts a positive effect on endothelial function and reduces inflammation among these patients.

▶ Statins, at least the one provided by the drug company that sponsored this research, would appear to have mechanisms of action other than lowering lipid levels. Their effects on endothelial function and levels of inflammation may be as important as their lipid-lowering effects. I suspect we will eventually see pharmaceutical companies trying to target these individual effects of the statins and maximize them with the targeted drugs.

G. L. Moneta, MD

Impaired Angiogenesis in the Remnant Kidney Model: II. Vascular Endothelial Growth Factor Administration Reduces Renal Fibrosis and Stabilizes Renal Function

Kang D-H, Hughes J, Mazzali M, et al (Univ of Washington, Seattle; Scios Inc, Sunnyvale, Calif)
J Am Soc Nephrol 12:1448-1457, 2001   1–15

Introduction.—Both experimental and human progressive renal disease are linked to capillary loss and a decrease in renal vascular endothelial growth factor (VEGF) expression. It is not known if replacement of VEGF could maintain the microvasculature and thus slow progression. Reported is evidence that VEGF administration in the remnant kidney stimulates endothelial proliferation, maintains capillary density, decreases renal interstitial fibrosis, and stabilizes renal function and that these effects occur independently of effects on systemic blood pressure or proteinuria.

Findings.—Male Sprague-Dawley rats used in the remnant kidney model underwent administration of VEGF 50 μg/kg twice daily between 4 and 8 weeks after surgery. The animals were euthanized at 8 weeks for histologic

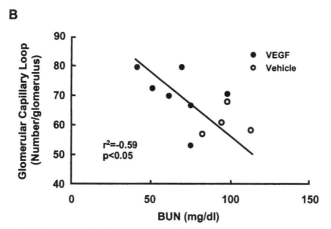

FIGURE 3.—B, There was a significant inverse correlation between the number of glomerular capillary loops and blood urea nitrogen levels in the remnant kidney rats. Data are expressed as mean ± SD. (Courtesy of Kang D-H, Hughes J, Mazzali M, et al: Impaired angiogenesis in the remnant kidney model: II. Vascular endothelial growth factor administration reduces renal fibrosis and stabilizes renal function. *J Am Soc Nephrol* 12:1448-1457, 2001.)

examination. During administration of VEGF in 7 animals or vehicle in 6 others, systemic blood pressure was similar in both groups. Treatment with VEGF resulted in improved renal function and lower mortality rates compared with controls. Renal histologic analyses verified a 3.5-fold increase in glomerular endothelial cell proliferation (0.14 vs 0.04 proliferating endothelial cells/glomerulus; $P < .05$, VEGF vs vehicle), a 2-fold increase in peritubular capillary endothelial cell proliferation (1.60 vs 0.78 cells/mm^2; $P < .01$, VEGF vs vehicle), a 3-fold reduction in peritubular capillary rarefaction ($P < .01$), and a 2-fold increase in endothelial nitric oxide synthase expression ($P < .05$) in the VEGF-treated group; an 8-fold increase in urinary nitrate/nitrite levels ($P < .05$) was also observed. The difference in glomerulosclerosis scores did not reach statistical significance (0.67 vs 1.22 VEGF vs vehicle; range, 0-4; $P =$ NS), yet VEGF-treated animals had less interstitial collagen type III deposition (9.32% vs 17.45%; $P < .01$, VEGF vs vehicle) and diminished tubular epithelial cell injury, as demonstrated by osteopontin expression (5.57% vs 1.60%; $P < .01$, VEGF vs vehicle). A significant inverse association was seen between the number of glomerular capillary loops and blood urea nitrogen levels (Fig 3).

Conclusion.—Treatment with VEGF decreases fibrosis and stabilizes renal function in the remnant kidney model. The use of angiogenic factors may be helpful in treating kidney disease.

▶ This is an interesting study in which the authors used a rat model of progressive nephropathy and examined the influence of systemic administration of the angiogenic cytokine VEGF. VEGF treatment resulted in improved renal function and histologic markers consistent with preserved glomerular vessel density. This highlights the potential importance of VEGF and other angiogenic molecules for maintenance and survival of existing microvascular structures, in addition to new vessel growth. Further work will be important to define the role of these cytokines for the amelioration of a host of chronic end-organ conditions marked by progressive microvascular dysfunction.

M. S. Conte, MD

Altered Ubiquitin/Proteasome Expression in Anastomotic Intimal Hyperplasia

Stone DH, Sivamurthy N, Contreras MA, et al (Harvard Med School, Boston)
J Vasc Surg 34:1016-1022, 2001   1–16

Introduction.—Anastomotic intimal hyperplasia continues to be a leading cause of delayed prosthetic arterial graft failure. Earlier trials have shown altered proteasome gene expression at the anastomoses in an expanded polytetrafluoroethylene canine carotid model. This method is technically limited because of a lack of available hyperplastic tissue at earlier time periods after arterial injury. Microarray technology offers a new and highly sensitive approach for assaying gene expression that requires only 5 to 10 µg of specimen and is therefore more useful in determining the early molecular events after arterial injury. Differential gene expression at 48 hours and 14 days after grafting was examined in mongrel dogs after prosthetic arterial grafting.

Methods.—Expanded polytetrafluoroethylene grafts (6-mm diameter) were implanted into 9 25-kg dogs. The normal intervening carotid artery acted as control. At 48 hours and 14 days, RNA was extracted from the perianastomotic tissue and compared with RNA from controls. Messenger RNA was hybridized to microarray genomes used to screen for differential gene expression.

Results.—Two 26S proteasomal genes (26S proteasomal subunit p55 [0.26], and 26S proteasomal subunit p40.5 [0.13]) and 5 ubiquitin pathway genes were significantly underexpressed at 48 hours among hundreds of significantly expressed clones. Among the underexpressed ubiquitin genes were ubiquitin (0.31), Nedd-4–like ubiquitin-protein ligase (0.30), ubiquitin conjugating enzyme UbcH2 (0.25), putative ubiquitin C-terminal hydrolase UHX1 (0.11), and ubiquitin-conjugating enzyme UbcH7 (0.12). Six ubiquitin genes were underexpressed on day 14 and 17 26S proteasome genes were significantly downregulated.

Conclusion.—Reduced expression of the ubiquitin/proteasome pathway 48 hours after graft implantation and similarly decreased expression patterns were observed after 14 days. This early and ongoing underexpression after arterial bypass may produce altered cell cycle control and matrix protein signaling, adding to the unregulated proliferation of smooth muscle cells and extracellular matrix in anastomotic intimal hyperplasia after prosthetic arterial grafting.

▶ These authors used state-of-the-art micro array chip technology to examine alterations in gene expression in the anastomotic zones of a prosthetic bypass in canines. Previous work had suggested that function of the proteasome, an essential cellular housekeeping system involved in virtually all major cellular processes, was dysregulated in hyperplastic tissue. In this study, they extend those observations by demonstrating persistent decreases in expression of several proteasome related genes after prosthetic grafting. Given the diverse functions of the proteasome, much additional work will be required to directly connect these observations to specific changes in vascular cell phenotype.

M. S. Conte, MD

Activities of Arginase I and II Are Limiting for Endothelial Cell Proliferation
Li H, Meininger CJ, Kelly KA, et al (Texas A&M Univ, College Station; Univ of Pittsburgh, Pa)
Am J Physiol 282:R64-R69, 2002　　　　　　　　　　　　　　　　1–17

Background.—Polyamines are known to be essential for cell proliferation. Whether arginase I or II activities, through production of ornithine for polyamine synthesis, limit proliferation of endothelial cells (ECs) was investigated.

Methods and Findings.—Bovine coronary venular ECs were stably transfected with a *lacZ* gene (lacZ-EC), rat arginase I cDNA (AI-EC), or mouse arginase II cDNA (AII-EC). Cell-proliferation assays demonstrated that EC proliferation was greatly elevated in the AI-EC and AII-EC conditions compared with lacZ-EC. In addition, proliferating cell nuclear antigen expression was enhanced in the AI-EC and AII-EC groups.

An irreversible inhibitor of ornithine decarboxylase, DL-α-difluoromethylornithine (DFMO), established the fact that increased polyamine synthesis was involved in mediating enhanced AI-EC and AII-EC growth. Adding 5 mmol of DFMO to the culture medium totally eliminated the differences in cellular putrescine levels and decreased the differences in spermidine levels in all conditions. In addition, DFMO prevented an increase in AI-EC and AII-EC proliferation compared with lacZ-EC. Adding 10 and 50 μmol putrescine increased AI-EC, AII-EC, and lacZ-EC growth to the same degree, in a dose-dependent fashion.

Conclusion.—Arginase normally limits endothelial cell proliferation. Thus, increased expression of either arginase isoform results in increased EC proliferation through an increase in polyamine synthesis from L-arginine.

▶ This interesting article provides data to suggest that polyamines modulate bovine coronary vascular endothelial cell proliferation. Polyamines are polycationic proteins essential for cell growth. They are known to interact with nucleic acids, proteins, and other negatively charged molecules. In this study, the experimental design used straightforward transfection protocols. The authors suggest their findings are relevant for cardiovascular disease because endothelial cells in the spontaneously diabetic BB rat (an animal model for human type 1 diabetes) are severely deficient in arginase activity. However, the authors also point out that proliferative dependence on arginase activity is shared by Chinese hamster ovary cells, caco-2 human colon cancer cells, and some human breast cancer cell lines. Thus, the true relevance of polyamines to cardiovascular disease must be questioned.

M. T. Watkins, MD

Alcohol Consumption and Risk of Peripheral Arterial Disease: The Rotterdam Study
Vliegenthart R, Geleijnse JM, Hofman A, et al (Erasmus Univ, Rotterdam, The Netherlands; State Univ Groningen, The Netherlands; Agricultural Univ, Wageningen, The Netherlands; et al)
Am J Epidemiol 155:332-338, 2002   1–18

Background.—Moderate alcohol intake is known to be associated with a decreased risk of cardiovascular disease, but little is known about the relationship of alcohol intake and atherosclerosis. The association between alcohol consumption and the risk of peripheral arterial disease was investigated in a cross-sectional study.

Methods.—Data were obtained on 3975 participants in the population-based Rotterdam Study of men and women aged 55 years and older. The participants were free of symptomatic cardiovascular disease. Information on alcohol intake and peripheral arterial disease, as measured by the ankle/brachial blood pressure index, was available for each participant.

Findings.—Male drinkers reported drinking beer, wine, and liquor, and female drinkers reported drinking mostly wine and fortified wine types. Women, but not men, had an inverse relationship between moderate alcohol intake and peripheral arterial disease. Among nonsmoking men, the odds ratio for a daily alcohol intake of 10 g or less was 0.86 compared with non-drinking; for 11 to 20 g, it was 0.75; and for more than 20 g, it was 0.68. Among nonsmoking women, these odds ratios were 0.65, 0.66, and 0.41, respectively.

Conclusion.—In this large population-based study, moderate alcohol intake was associated inversely with peripheral arterial disease in women but not men. When only nonsmokers were included in the analysis, an inverse association was observed in both men and women.

▶ It appears my residents will live forever and I will die young. What is the virtue in that?

G. L. Moneta, MD

Antioxidant Vitamins and the Risk of Carotid Atherosclerosis: The Perth Carotid Ultrasound Disease Assessment Study (CUDAS)

McQuillan BM, Hung J, Beilby JP, et al (Gairdner Campus of the Heart Research Inst of Western Australia, Perth; Univ of Western Australia, Perth; QEII Med Ctr, Nedlands, Perth)
J Am Coll Cardiol 38:1788-1794, 2001   1–19

Background.—Animal studies have shown that antioxidants inhibit lipid oxidation and limit the development of atherosclerosis, yet epidemiologic studies and randomized clinical trials have yielded conflicting results regarding the beneficial effect of antioxidant intake. The role of antioxidant vitamins in reducing the risk of carotid atherosclerosis was investigated in a large, randomly selected, cross-sectional Australian population.

Methods.—The study included 558 men and 553 women (age, 27-77 years; mean age, 53 years) who were enrolled in the Perth Carotid Ultrasound Disease Assessment Study. Each age decade contained a similar number of men and women. Fasting venous blood samples were obtained to determine plasma levels of antioxidant vitamins (vitamins A, C and E, alpha- and beta-carotene and lycopene) and homocysteine. Data on history of hypertension, hyperlipidemia, diabetes, angina pectoris, myocardial infarction, and stroke were collected by a self-administered questionnaire. Participants also underwent bilateral carotid artery B-mode US imaging.

Results.—Women were more likely than men to consume antioxidant-containing vitamin supplements. Supplement use did not differ, however, across age deciles or in subgroups defined by history of smoking, diabetes, hypertension, or hyperlipidemia. With increasing quartiles of dietary vitamin E intake in men and after adjustment for age and risk factors of interest, a progressive decrease in mean carotid artery intima-media (wall) thickness (IMT) was noted, an indication of carotid artery plaque; among women, a trend for this association was nonsignificant. For plasma antioxidant vitamins, only women showed an inverse association between carotid artery mean IMT and plasma lycopene. No independent association was seen between any dietary or plasma antioxidant vitamins and focal plaque.

Conclusion.—Supplemental antioxidant vitamin use was not associated with mean IMT or carotid artery plaque in this large population of men and women. The findings offer only limited support for the hypothesis that the risk of atherosclerosis may be lowered by an increase in dietary intake of vitamin E and plasma lycopene.

▶ I am sure this study, which shows no effect of supplemental antioxidants on the development of atherosclerosis, will not have a whit of effect on the antioxidant fanatics. Where there is money to be made, objectivity can be in short supply.

G. L. Moneta, MD

Blood Thrombogenicity in Type 2 Diabetes Mellitus Patients Is Associated With Glycemic Control

Osende JI, Badimon JJ, Fuster V, et al (Zena and Michael A. Wiener Cardiovascular Inst, New York; Mount Sinai School of Medicine, New York)
J Am Coll Cardiol 38:1307-1312, 2001   1–20

Background.—Type 2 diabetes mellitus (T2DM) is a major independent risk factor for coronary artery disease. Patients with T2DM display not only accelerated atherosclerosis but also increased morbidity and mortality rates after percutaneous coronary interventions because of thrombotic complications of atherosclerosis. This increased risk is only partially explained by the association of T2DM with other classic risk factors; other factors, such as a hypercoagulable state, are also possible and may contribute to the increased risk in patients with T2DM. The procoagulant state associated with T2DM is manifested clinically by a high rate of acute arterial thrombotic episodes. It was hypothesized that the observed increase in blood thrombogenicity is partially mediated by chronic glycemic control. This hypothesis was tested by comparing the effects of a conservative versus an intensive approach to the management of diabetes.

Methods.—The study group comprised 40 patients with T2DM with glycosylated hemoglobin (HbA1c) equal to 7.5% or more. Patients maintained their current hypoglycemic therapies and were randomized to a conservative diet (diet modification plus placebo) or to a diet with an intensive hypoglycemic regimen (diet modification plus troglitazone). Patients maintained the diet for 3 months. Thrombogenicity was measured at baseline and after 3 months with the Badimon ex vivo perfusion chamber and assessed as platelet-thrombus formation. Repeated measurements enabled patients to be their own control subjects.

Results.—Glucose control was improved in 48% of patients in the conservative diet group and 74% of patients in the intensive diet group, with an overall HbA1c reduction of 0.5% or more, demonstrating a significant reduction increase in blood thrombogenicity. A significant positive correlation was noted between the reduction in thrombus formation and the reduction of HbA1c, and the reduction in HbA1c was comparable for both groups. Patients who did not have glycemic improvement also did not have a change in blood thrombogenicity. The only significant predictor of a decrease in blood thrombogenicity was improved glycemic control.

Conclusions.—An association was observed between improved glycemic control and blood thrombogenicity reduction in patients with T2DM. Further studies of the relationship between glycemic control and thrombotic complications are warranted.

▶ Another bit of evidence good blood sugar control is important in potentially reducing acute as well as long-term complications in diabetes. Decreased thrombogenicity associated with decreased HbA1c levels suggests perioperative thrombotic complications of diabetes may be reduced by a period of tight glycemic control prior to operation. (See also Abstract 5–18.)

G. L. Moneta, MD

Body Fatness and Fat Distribution as Predictors of Metabolic Abnormalities and Early Carotid Atherosclerosis
Takami R, Takami K, Takeda N, et al (Matsunami Gen Hosp, Kasamatsu, Japan; Gifu Univ, Japan)
Diabetes Care 24:1248-1252, 2001   1–21

Background.—Obesity is an increasingly prevalent disorder in many countries, and the potential links between obesity and cardiovascular disease are receiving increased attention. Beginning in the 1980s, reports based on anthropometric measurements indicated that abdominal distribution of fat is a significant risk factor for the development of diabetes, dyslipidemia, and cardiovascular disease. As a result of the use of CT and MRI, which allowed the direct measurements of abdominal fat distribution and a precise analysis of the relationship between fat topography and metabolic abnormalities, intra-abdominal fat has been proposed as the most important determinant of obesity-related metabolic abnormalities. The hypothesis that intra-abdominal fat is more strongly associated with metabolic abnormalities and atherosclerosis than general adiposity was tested in a cross-sectional study of carotid artery atherosclerosis.

Methods.—The study included 849 Japanese men (mean age, 50.3 years) with a mean body mass index (BMI) of 23.5 kg/m². US was used to measure intimal-medial thickness (IMT) of the carotid artery. General adiposity was assessed by BMI. Abdominal fat was determined by measurement of waist circumference and waist-to-hip ratio. CT was used to determine abdominal subcutaneous fat area and intra-abdominal fat area. Correlations between these measurements and carotid IMT were then analyzed. The interaction of generalized adiposity (BMI) and intra-abdominal fat area in relation to metabolic variables, such as glucose tolerance, insulin resistance, and serum lipids, was also evaluated.

Results.—Correlations were observed between carotid IMT and BMI, waist circumference, waist-to-hip ratio, abdominal subcutaneous fat area, and intra-abdominal fat area. Adjustment for BMI eliminated the associations between IMT and waist circumference, abdominal subcutaneous fat area, and intra-abdominal fat area, but the correlation between IMT and waist-to-hip ratio remained significant. BMI and intra-abdominal fat area were independently associated with insulin resistance, glucose tolerance, HDL cholesterol, and blood pressure. Intra-abdominal fat area was independently correlated with serum triglyceride levels, but BMI was not.

Conclusions.—The hypothesis that intra-abdominal fat is more strongly associated with metabolic abnormalities and atherosclerosis than general adiposity for carotid atherosclerosis was not confirmed. Caution should be observed when relying on waist-to-hip ratio as a measure of abdominal fat. The role of intra-abdominal fat area in metabolic abnormalities may not be as extensive as is conventionally believed. These findings indicate that BMI and waist-to-hip ratio are simple and better clinical predictors than intra-abdominal fat area for carotid atherosclerosis.

▶ This study is unconvincing that the distribution of body fat predicts metabolic abnormalities or atherosclerosis development. Fat appears to be fat. How it is distributed more likely is related to genetics and gender. No matter where it is, it is not good for you. There is no good fat, and probably no distribution pattern that suggests lower risks of obesity-related complications.

G. L. Moneta, MD

Decreased Rate of Coronary Restenosis After Lowering of Plasma Homocysteine Levels

Schnyder G, Roffi M, Pin R, et al (Univ Hosp, Bern, Switzerland; Kardiologische Praxis, Bremen, Germany; Univ of California, San Diego)
N Engl J Med 345:1593-1600, 2001   1–22

Background.—Restenosis is an important limitation of percutaneous coronary angioplasty, and effective pharmacotherapy has been elusive. The total plasma homocysteine level is an important predictor of cardiovascular risk and correlates with the severity of coronary artery disease. This has spurred interest in its possible role in restenosis. In a previous study, an association was shown between elevated total plasma homocysteine levels and restenosis after percutaneous coronary angioplasty. The effects of lowering plasma homocysteine levels on restenosis after coronary angioplasty were evaluated.

Methods.—A group of 205 patients (mean age, 61 years) underwent folate treatment or placebo treatment for 6 months after successful coronary angioplasty in this prospective, double-blind, randomized trial. Folate treatment consisted of a combination of folic acid, vitamin B12, and pyridoxine. The study's primary end point was restenosis within 6 months, as determined by quantitative coronary angiography. The secondary end point was a composite of major adverse cardiac events.

Results.—The 2 groups had similar baseline characteristics and initial angiographic results after coronary angioplasty. The folate treatment group experienced significantly lowered plasma homocysteine levels (from 11.1 ± 4.3 to 7.2 ± 2.4 µmol/L). At follow-up evaluation, the folate treatment group had a significantly larger minimal luminal diameter and a less severe degree of stenosis (39.9% ± 20.3%) compared with the placebo group (48.2% ± 28.3%). The patients who received folate treatment also had a significantly lower rate of restenosis (19.6%) than those who received placebo (37.6%) and less need for revascularization of the target lesion (10.8% vs 22.3%) (Fig 3).

Conclusion.—A combination treatment with folic acid, vitamin B12, and pyridoxine significantly reduces homocysteine levels and decreases the rate of restenosis after coronary angioplasty. The need for revascularization of the target lesion was also reduced with this therapy. Folate therapy is inex-

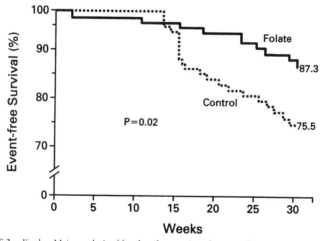

FIGURE 3.—Kaplan-Meier analysis of freedom from major adverse cardiac events in 196 patients. The rate of event-free survival was significantly higher among patients assigned to folate treatment than among control patients. The relative risk of a major cardiac event with folate treatment was 0.52 (95% confidence interval, 0.28-0.98). Revascularization of the target lesion (relative risk, 0.48; 95% confidence interval, 0.25-0.94) accounted for most of the observed events. (Reprinted by permission of *The New England Journal of Medicine* from Schnyder G, Roffi M, Pin R, et al: Decreased rate of coronary restenosis after lowering of plasma homocysteine levels. *N Engl J Med* 345:1593-1600, 2001. Copyright 2001, Massachusetts Medical Society. All rights reserved.)

pensive and has minimal side effects. It should be considered as adjunctive therapy for patients who are undergoing coronary angioplasty.

▶ A large number of studies have demonstrated that elevated plasma homocysteine is an independent risk factor for atherosclerotic disease, and a nearly equally large number of studies have shown that plasma homocysteine levels can be lowered with folate therapy. To my knowledge, this is the first clinical trial that has demonstrated clinical benefit as a result of homocysteine lowering therapy. A number of caveats are in order. The study was small, and the primary end point, postangioplasty coronary restenosis, was studied at only a single time point (6 months postangioplasty). If the restenosis rates converge at 12 months, different conclusions may be in order. No matter, this is a significant study. At least 9 much larger randomized trials of similar therapy with multiple end points are currently under way. I don't think this study is enough evidence that those trials should be stopped, but it does rightfully claim the distinction of being the first to show benefit. I hope it is not the only.

L. M. Taylor, Jr, MD

Effect of Controlled Release/Extended Release Metoprolol on Carotid Intima-Media Thickness in Patients With Hypercholesterolemia: A 3-Year Randomized Study
Wiklund O, Hulthe J, Wikstrand J, et al (Sahlgrenska Univ, Sweden; Göteborg Univ, Gothenburg, Sweden; AstraZeneca, Mölndal, Sweden)
Stroke 33:572-577, 2002   1–23

Background.—The ability of β-adrenergic blockers to improve survival in patients who suffer myocardial infarction has been attributed to the mediation of better myocardial function, antihypertensive or antiarrhythmic effects, or reduced myocardial oxygen consumption, but evidence now indicates that these agents exert an additional antiatherosclerotic effect. In addition, β-blocker treatment has been shown to inhibit development of atherosclerosis and endothelial injury caused by psychosocial stress in cynomolgus monkeys. The binding of low-density lipoproteins to arterial proteoglycans can be reduced by therapy with a β-blocker (controlled release/extended release [CR/XL] metoprolol succinate). It was hypothesized that CR/XL metoprolol would provide an antiatherosclerotic effect for patients with hypercholesterolemia taking lipid-lowering therapy (statins) concomitantly and that this effect could be quantified using carotid intima-media thickness (IMT) determinations. The validity of this hypothesis was investigated.

Methods.—The study included 40 patients who were given CR/XL metoprolol and 40 patients who were given placebo. The metoprolol was given in 100 mg once daily doses to patients with hypercholesterolemia and signs of early atherosclerosis of the carotid artery. Thirty-eight of the placebo patients and 48 of the metoprolol patients were available for 2-year follow-up evaluation, and 35 placebo and 44 metoprolol patients for the 3-year follow-up assessment.

Results.—At baseline, among the placebo patients, total cholesterol levels were 8.6 mmol/L; in the metoprolol group, they were 9.4 mmol/L. At 1-year follow-up, the IMT of the carotid bulb declined significantly in the group receiving CR/XL metoprolol when compared with those receiving placebo. However, no significant difference in change of common carotid IMT was found between the 2 groups at that time. After 1 year, the progression rate of the composite variable carotid bulb IMT plus common carotid IMT showed a highly significant difference between the placebo and CR/XL metoprolol groups. This effect persisted to the 3-year assessment. After 3 years, the 2 groups showed a significant difference in progression rate of the common carotid IMT, but not in the carotid bulb IMT. Both groups had total cholesterol reductions to 6.4 mmol/L by the end of follow-up, and LDL cholesterol levels decreased to a similar degree.

Conclusions.—Patients taking statins for hypercholesterolemia who are also given β-blockers show an antiatherosclerotic effect of the β-blockade detectable on IMT measurement. Thus, both statins and β-blockers appear to influence disparate mechanisms in the process of atherosclerosis, and an additive benefit can be achieved.

▶ β-Blocker therapy has been shown to be associated with improved survival after vascular surgical operations. While beneficial cardiac effects of β-blockers can be evoked to account for the perioperative benefit of β-blockers, it has always been a bit of a mystery why *perioperative* β-blockers would improve long-term survival. In this study, β-blockers administered daily during the 36 months of the study resulted in decreased IMT, a marker of atherosclerotic activity, in the treated patients. Given the long-term mortality benefits of *perioperative* β-blockers, perhaps a short course of β-blockers is all that is needed to achieve an anti-atherogenic effect and a reduction of IMT.

G. L. Moneta, MD

Homocysteine Decreases Endothelium-Dependent Vasorelaxation in Porcine Arteries

Chen C, Conklin BS, Ren Z, et al (Veterans Affairs Med Ctr, Decatur, Ga; Emory Univ, Atlanta, Ga)
J Surg Res 102:22-30, 2002   1–24

Background.—Hyperhomocysteinemia is defined as plasma homocysteine levels exceeding 15 µmol/L and is a recognized independent risk factor for vascular disease. The cellular and molecular mechanisms involved in the pathogenesis of homocysteine are generally unknown. The effect of homocysteine on endothelium-dependent vasorelaxation in porcine coronary and common carotid arteries was assessed, along with the immunoreactivity of endothelial nitric oxide synthase (eNOS) of treated vessels.

Methods.—Various concentrations of homocysteine were used to incubate pig coronary artery rings for 24 hours, then myographic analysis was done with thromboxane A_2 analogue U46619 (causing contraction) and bradykinin or sodium nitroprusside (causing relaxation). Three treatment groups (control, 50 μmol/L homocysteine, and 100 μmol/L homocysteine) were compared with respect to changes in the diameter of the porcine carotid arteries in response to norepinephrine and acetylcholine. Histologic tests were used to measure endothelial morphologic changes and eNOS levels.

Results.—No significant differences were found between control and homocysteine-treated rings in maximum vessel tension after challenge with thromboxane A_2 analogue U46619, but a significant decrease in endothelium-dependent vasorelaxation was noted after homocysteine treatment in response to bradykinin challenge (Fig 1). A single high dose of sodium nitroprusside inhibited the effect on maximal relaxation after homocysteine treatment. Homocysteine showed specific impairment of endothelium-dependent vasorelaxation but did not affect smooth muscle cell function in pig coronary artery ring assessments. The function of endothelium-dependent vasorelaxation was significantly decreased in vessels treated with homocysteine compared with control rings (Fig 2); no effect was seen in smooth muscle contractility after homocysteine treatment. Homocysteine was also able to produce endothelial cell injury and inhibit the expression of eNOS. Significant decreases in immunoreactivity of eNOS were found in the 50 μmol/L– and 100 μmol/L–homocysteine-treated vessels (coronary and carotid arteries).

Conclusions.—Homocysteine impaired the endothelium-dependent vasorelaxation of coronary arteries in these tests. Among the significant

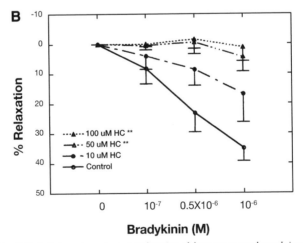

FIGURE 1.—B, Endothelium-dependent vasorelaxation of the precontracted vessel rings in response to bradykinin (0.1 μmol/L, 0.5 μmol/L, and 1 μmol/L), showing significant reductions in homocysteine-treated groups compared to the control group. **$P < .01$, $n = 5$). *Abbreviation: HC,* Homocysteine. (Courtesy of Chen C, Conklin BS, Ren Z, et al: Homocysteine decreases endothelium-dependent vasorelaxation in porcine arteries. *J Surg Res* 102:22-30, 2002.)

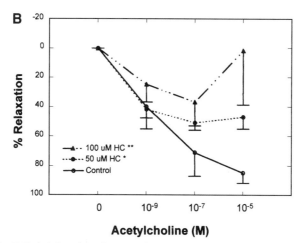

Acetylcholine (M)

FIGURE 2.—B, Endothelium-dependent vasorelaxation of the carotid arteries in response to acetylcholine (0.001 μmol/L, 0.1 μmol/L, and 10 μmol/L), showing significant reductions in homocysteine-treated groups compared to the control group (**$P < .01$, *$P < .05$, $n = 4$). *Abbreviation: HC*, Homocysteine. (Courtesy of Chen C, Conklin BS, Ren Z, et al: Homocysteine decreases endothelium-dependent vasorelaxation in porcine arteries. *J Surg Res* 102:22-30, 2002.)

mechanisms of homocysteine-induced formation of vascular lesions are eNOS downregulation and endothelial injury.

▶ Since elevated plasma homocysteine was established as an independent risk factor for atherosclerotic disease in the 1980s, multiple laboratories have looked for a mechanistic explanation. Many have been found, in nearly all aspects of coagulation, cellular proliferation, plaque formation, and, as exemplified by this article, in vascular wall physiology. Whether all, any, or none of the myriad of demonstrated laboratory effects of homocysteine is important in humans is unknown.

L. M. Taylor, Jr, MD

Perianeurysmal Fibrosis: A Relative Contra-indication to Endovascular Repair
Vallabhaneni SR, McWilliams RG, Anbarasu A, et al (Royal Liverpool Univ, England)
Eur J Vasc Endovasc Surg 22:535-541, 2001   1–25

Background.—Open surgical repair of inflammatory abdominal aortic aneurysm (IAAA) in patients with perianeurysmal fibrosis (PAF) is associated with higher morbidity and mortality than open repair of noninflammatory aneurysms. Therefore, endovascular repair (EVAR) is an attractive approach to patients with IAAA and PAF. However, animal studies have shown that EVAR can cause an immediate local inflammatory response around the stent-graft. This retrospective human study was undertaken to examine whether EVAR can induce or worsen PAF in patients with IAAA.

Methods.—The subjects were 61 patients with IAAA who underwent EVAR and who had 6 months or more of follow-up (median, 18 months). Three radiologists independently graded preoperative and postoperative CT images on a 6-point scale to assess PAF. The influence of preoperative PAF on outcomes and the prevalence of de novo PAF after EVAR were evaluated.

Results.—Most patients (45, or 74%) had no evidence of PAF either before or after EVAR. Six (10%) had PAF present before EVAR. PAF persisted at 6 to 36 months of follow-up in 5 of these 6 patients and in 1 patient, PAF actually progressed to the point at which ureteric stenting was required for hydronephrosis and ureteric obstruction (Fig 3). The remaining 10 patients (16%) had no evidence of PAF on preoperative CT scans but developed CT evidence of PAF as early as 3 months after EVAR. Most cases of de novo PAF were low grade, but in one 76-year-old patient, PAF more than 8 mm thick had developed by 6 months after EVAR; the patient died of sepsis 24 months after the procedure.

Conclusion.—In patients with IAAA who have PAF before EVAR, surgery does not appear to reduce PAF, and it may exacerbate it. EVAR also appears

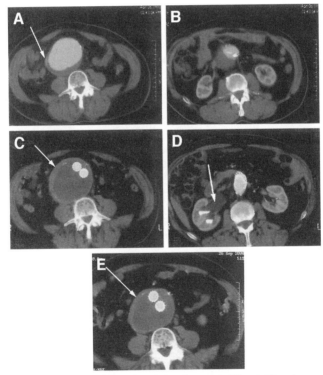

FIGURE 3.—CT scans showing localized grade 1 perianeurysmal fibrosis (**A**) and normal kidneys (**B**) before operation. Perianeurysmal fibrosis had worsened significantly by 9 months after operation (**C**), and this was associated with development of right hydronephrosis (**D**). Perianeurysmal fibrosis had not reduced more than 2 years after operation (**E**). (Reprinted from Vallabhaneni SR, McWilliams RG, Anbarasu A, et al: Perianeurysmal fibrosis: A relative contra-indication to endovascular repair. *Eur J Vasc Endovasc Surg* 22:535-541, 2001. Copyright 2001, by permission of the publisher.)

to induce de novo PAF (16% in this study) of patients with no preoperative CT evidence of PAF. Thus, clinicians should consider the risks associated with PAF when planning EVAR for patients with IAAA—even those without PAF preoperatively.

▶ Data are always so much more difficult to deal with than logic, especially when data conflict with logic. It seems so logical to treat inflammatory aneurysm with EVAR. However, the limited data presented in this article suggest PAF may worsen rather than improve as the result of EVAR. Obviously, this is a small study; however, perhaps the presence of an inflammatory aneurysm may actually be a contraindication to EVAR.

G. L. Moneta, MD

Ubiquitin-Proteasome Pathway as a New Target for the Prevention of Restenosis
Meiners S, Laule M, Rother W, et al (Humboldt-Universität zu Berlin; Schering AG, Berlin)
Circulation 105:483-489, 2002

1–26

Introduction.—The ubiquitin-proteasome system is the primary intracellular protein degradation pathway in eukaryotic cells. It is responsible for regulation of central mediators of proliferation, inflammation, and apoptosis that are fundamental pathomechanisms in the development of vascular restenosis. The influence of proteasome inhibition on neointimal formation was evaluated in a balloon injury model with use of a rat carotid artery.

Methods and Findings.—The local application of the proteasome inhibitor MG132 (1 mmol/L) resulted in marked inhibition of intimal hyperplasia (by 74%; $P = .008$). This effect was accompanied by reduced proliferation, diminished infiltration of macrophages, and prolonged apoptosis, determined via immunohistochemical and terminal deoxynucleotidyl transferase–mediated dUTP nick end labeling (TUNEL) analyses. The functional effects of proteasome inhibition on proliferation, activation of nuclear factor kappa B, and apoptosis were further identified in rat primary vascular smooth muscle cells. The presence of MG132 inhibited vascular smooth muscle proliferation in a dose-dependent fashion; 50% inhibition occurred at 10 µmol/L. Tumor necrosis factor-α-induced degradation of IκBα and β was blocked. The activation of nuclear factor kappa B was inhibited in a concentration-dependent fashion in bandshift assays. The proteasome inhibition (1-50 µmol/L MG132) induced apoptotic cell death up to 80%, as verified by DNA/histone enzyme-linked immunosorbent assay and TUNEL-fluorescence activated cell sorter (FACS) analysis. The specificity of proteasome inhibition was identified by accumulation of multiubiquitinylated proteins and accumulation of specific proteasomal substrates.

Conclusion.—Inhibition of the ubiquitin-proteasome system effectively decreases neointimal formation in vivo. This corresponds to strong antiproliferative, anti-inflammatory, and proapoptotic influences in vitro and in vivo. The ubiquitin-proteasome system may be a new target in the prevention of vascular restenosis.

▶ This rat model demonstrates another potential target to reduce intimal hyperplasia after arterial injury. Of course, it is a long way from the rat to the human, at least to most humans. Perhaps preventing restenosis by targeting the ubiquitin-proteasome pathway is interesting. This may be a potentially new mechanism to target restenosis. However, based on previous "major breakthroughs" in restenosis, the likely result is more grants, but no clinical efficacy.

G. L. Moneta, MD

Understanding the Treatment Preferences of Seriously Ill Patients
Fried TR, Bradley EH, Towle VR, et al (West Haven Veterans Affairs Connecticut Healthcare System, Conn; Yale Univ, New Haven, Conn)
N Engl J Med 346:1061-1066, 2002   1–27

Introduction.—Honoring the treatment preferences of patients who are terminally ill is important in the provision of high-quality care at the end of life. The effects of the burden of treatment and a variety of possible outcomes on the preferences for care expressed by older patients with serious illnesses were examined.

Methods.—A questionnaire concerning treatment preferences was administered to 226 individuals who were 60 years or older and who had a limited life expectancy due to cancer, congestive heart failure, or chronic obstructive pulmonary disease. Participants were asked whether they would want to receive a particular treatment, first when the outcome was known with certainty and then with various likelihoods of an adverse outcome. The outcome without treatment was stipulated as death from the underlying disease. The burden of treatment included the length of the hospital stay, the extent of testing, and the invasiveness of interventions.

Results.—The burden of treatment, outcome, and likelihood of the outcome all affected treatment preferences. For a low-burden treatment with the restoration of current health, 98.7% of patients indicated they would choose to receive treatment versus not receive it and die; 11.2% responded that they would not choose the treatment if it had a high burden. If the outcome was survival in the presence of severe functional impairment or cognitive impairment, 74.4% and 88.8%, respectively, indicated that they would not choose the treatment. The number of participants who indicated that they would choose treatment diminished as the likelihood of an adverse outcome rose; fewer participants chose treatment when the possible outcome was functional or cognitive impairment than when it was death. Preferences did not vary by primary diagnosis.

Conclusion.—Patients' attitudes concerning the burden of treatment, possible outcomes, and the likelihood of these outcomes need to be considered in advance care planning. The likelihood of adverse functional and cognitive treatment outcomes needs explicit consideration.

▶ All physicians who take care of seriously ill patients know most patients would rather be dead than seriously impaired. This type of research makes great press, but it doesn't tell doctors who actually take care of sick patients anything useful.

G. L. Moneta, MD

A Decade of Decline: An Analysis of Medicare Reimbursement for Vascular Surgical Procedures
York JW, Lepore MR, Opelka FG, et al (Alton Ochsner Med Found, New Orleans, La)
Ann Vasc Surg 16:115-120, 2002   1–28

Introduction.—Standard Medicare reimbursements for vascular surgical procedures have progressively declined. Changes in Medicare fee schedules particularly affect vascular surgeons because up to 70% of all patients requiring vascular surgery are funded by Medicare. The reduction in vascular surgical procedure reimbursements during the past decade was analyzed quantitatively and objectively.

Methods.—Data for analysis of specific vascular surgical procedures were gathered from the National Center for Health Statistics-National Hospital Discharge Survey (NCHS-NHDS) for all vascular procedures as reported by ICD-9-CM codes. The average Medicare reimbursements for all of the specified procedures for 1990 were compared with those of 2001. The percentage change in the average reimbursement during this time was determined. Comparisons between 1990 and 2001 dollar amounts were made after correcting for inflation. The consumer price index was used as a guide. This correction factor permits the calculation of the actual percentage decrease in "real dollars" that is reflected in buying power.

Results.—Significant reductions were observed for Medicare reimbursement for every vascular procedure included in the analysis (Fig 1). An average reduction in buying power of 41% per case was demonstrated for vascular surgical procedures during the past decade.

Conclusion.—Medicare reimbursements for vascular surgical procedures have decreased markedly during the past decade. As the demand for health care in the United States increases and as the age of the US population increases, the value of services provided by vascular surgeons also should increase.

▶ One might ask why such an article is included in the "Basic Considerations" section of the YEAR BOOK OF VASCULAR SURGERY. Basically, I include it because if these patterns of reimbursement continue, the continuing existence of vascular surgery as an economically viable independent specialty is doubtful.

G. L. Moneta, MD

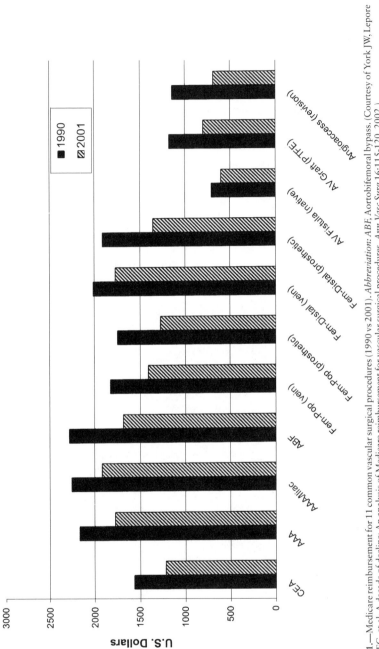

FIGURE 1.—Medicare reimbursement for 11 common vascular surgical procedures (1990 vs 2001). *Abbreviation: ABF,* Aortobifemoral bypass. (Courtesy of York JW, Lepore MR, Opelka FG, et al: A decade of decline: An analysis of Medicare reimbursement for vascular surgical procedures. *Ann Vasc Surg* 16:115-120, 2002.)

2 Endovascular

A Randomized Comparison of a Sirolimus-Eluting Stent With a Standard Stent for Coronary Revascularization
Morice M-C, for the RAVEL Study Group (Institut Cardiovasculaire Paris Sud, Massy, France; et al)
N Engl J Med 346:1773-1780, 2002   2–1

Background.—The increasingly common use of stents has improved outcomes in percutaneous coronary revascularization. However, the long-term success of this approach continues to be limited by in-stent restenosis. Sirolimus (rapamycin) is a macrocyclic lactone that inhibits cytokine-mediated and growth-factor-mediated proliferation of lymphocytes and smooth-muscle cells. This study compared the performance of a coronary stent that slowly releases sirolimus over 30 days with the performance of a standard uncoated stent in patients with ischemic heart disease.

Methods.—A randomized double-blind trial compared sirolimus-releasing and uncoated stents for revascularization of single, primary lesions in native coronary arteries. The study group comprised 238 patients treated at 19 medical centers. The primary outcome was in-stent late luminal loss (the difference between the minimal luminal diameter immediately after the procedure and the diameter of 6 months). Secondary outcomes included the percentage of in-stent stenosis of the luminal diameter and the rate of restenosis (luminal narrowing of 50% or more). The study also analyzed a composite clinical end point comprising death, myocardial infarction, and percutaneous or surgical revascularization at 1, 6, and 12 months.

Results.—The degree of neointimal proliferation was significantly lower in the sirolimus stent group compared with the standard stent group. None of the patients in the sirolimus stent group had restenosis of 50% or more of the luminal diameter, while restenosis of 50% or more occurred in 26.6% of patients in the standard stent group. There were no episodes of stent thrombosis in either group. In 1 year of follow up, the overall rate of major cardiac events was 5.8% in the sirolimus stent group and 28.8% in the standard stent group. This difference was attributable solely to a higher rate of revascularization of the target vessel in the standard stent group.

Conclusions.—A sirolimus-eluting stent showed significant potential for preventing neointimal proliferation, restenosis, and associated clinical events compared with a standard coronary stent.

▶ Drug-eluting stents are big news and potentially big business. Sirolimus (rapamycin) in animal studies inhibits cytokine and growth factor-mediated neointimal proliferation. It can be applied to stents as a mixture of drug and a nonerodable polymer. It is then eluted by the stent for about 30 days. The short-term results of this study are very impressive. The drug coated stents appear to virtually eliminate neointimal in-stent restenosis at 6 months. Although this follow-up is short-term, we know the primary time for development of neointimal lesions is within the first 6 months of stent implantation. Furthermore, most of this starts within 30 days of stent implantation, which is the period of time the stent elutes the drug. There appears to be real potential with this type of therapy.

G. L. Moneta, MD

Ten-Year Experience With Endovascular Therapy in Aortic Aneurysms

Parodi JC, Ferreira LM (Instituto Cardiovascular de Buenos Aires, Argentina)
J Am Coll Surg 194:S58-S66, 2002   2–2

Background.—Endoluminal treatment of abdominal aortic aneurysms (AAAs) has emerged as a potential therapeutic alternative to open surgery. Initial and midterm results of endoluminal aneurysm exclusion are encouraging, but late adverse events may represent a significant limitation to the technique.

Methods.—Available data for a consecutive group of patients were retrospectively reviewed to obtain information about the long-term results of endoluminal treatment of abdominal aortic aneurysms (AAA) with the homemade Parodi endograft, using both an aorto-aortic and aorto-uni-iliac design. In addition, data on a group of 136 consecutive patients treated with the Vanguard endograft were analyzed. Patients were followed up every 6 months with clinical examination, plain x-ray films of the abdomen, color duplex, and contrast-enhanced CT.

Results.—Results for the Parodi aorto-aortic design were presented for patients in whom follow-up was available for 5 years after implantation. The aorto-aortic endograft design for the Parodi endograft failed in 12 of 15 patients, for a failure rate of 80%. In all cases the failures were due to the development of a distal endoleak. The aneurysm increased in size in 8 patients. The aorto-uni-iliac design for the Parodi endograft provided successful long-term results in 10 of 15 patients. In these 10 patients the aneurysm decreased in size, and there were no endoleaks. There were 5 late (types I and II) endoleaks among these 15 patients. All these patients with late endoleaks had their aneurysms enlarge. The totally supported Vanguard device had a high rate of midterm failure. A secondary procedure was needed in 22% of the patients after a mean follow-up of 28 months. Of the 5 causes of failure in the Vanguard device, 4 were device-related. These aneurysms ruptured due to acute development of a type III endoleak.

Conclusions.—Dilatation of the distal neck is responsible for the high failure rate of aorto-aortic endografts. The aorto-uni-iliac configuration of the Parodi endograft provided acceptable long-term results. Late endoleak leads to aneurysm enlargement. Further experience with endografts is required before widespread use can be recommended.

▶ Parodi and Ferreira have updated their long experience with endovascular repair, including 30 patients with the original tubular or tapered endograft that had over 5-year follow-up and 136 patients with serial versions of a commercial modular endograft. They found there was no significant dilation of the proximal neck with balloon-expandable proximal stents. This is in sharp contrast to aorto-aortic tube grafts where the distal attachment is unstable due to neck dilation, resulting in abandonment of this configuration for primary treatment of AAAs. This article also reviews late device-related failures, including dislocation of modular components, occlusion of limbs, wearing of graft fabric, migration, and metal fractures. Some of these complications are related to initial exclusion with aneurysm shrinkage and subsequent device deformation leading to aneurysm rupture. Based on direct postmortem observation of an atrophic sac wall, it was hypothesized that late onset endoleaks in a sac free of endoleak may be more likely to lead to rupture. The authors conclude that endovascular repair should be limited to experienced centers and offered to high-risk patients harboring large or symptomatic aneurysms.

J. S. Matsumura, MD

Impact of Exclusion Criteria on Patient Selection for Endovascular Abdominal Aortic Aneurysm Repair
Carpenter JP, Baum RA, Barker CF, et al (Univ of Pennsylvania, Philadelphia)
J Vasc Surg 34:1050-1054, 2001   2–3

Introduction.—Wide-ranging predictions have been made regarding the usefulness of endovascular repair for patients with abdominal aortic aneurysms (AAAs). The availability of US Food and Drug Administration approved devices has eliminated many restrictions concerning patient selection, which had been controlled by device trials. The applicability of endovascular repair of abdominal aortic aneurysms (EVAR) in current practice was examined, along with identification of the anatomic barriers to successful endovascular AAA repair that should guide future device development.

Methods.—All patients seen between April 1998 and June 2000 for infrarenal AAA repair were offered evaluation for endovascular repair. Patients underwent thin-cut spiral CT scans and arteriograms. Anatomic features were prospectively entered into a database. The use of a wide selection of available devices allowed the treatment of diverse AAA anatomic characteristics.

Results.—Of 307 patients evaluated, 264 were men and 43 were women. Of these, 204 (66%) underwent endovascular repair; 103 (34%) were rejected. The reasons for exclusion were short aneurysm neck (56; 54%), insufficient access because of small iliac arteries (48; 47%), wide aneurysm neck (41; 40%), presence of bilateral common iliac aneurysms that extend to the hypogastric artery (22, 21%), excessive neck angulation (14, 14%), extensive mural thrombus in the aneurysm neck (10, 10%), extreme tortuosity of the iliac arteries (10, 10%), accessory renal arteries originating from the AAA (6; 6%), malignancy detected during the evaluation (5; 5%), and death during the examination interval (2; 2%). Patients who were rejected had an average of 1.9 exclusion criteria (range, 1-4). A disproportionate number of women were excluded because of anatomic findings (P = .0009). Eighty percent of patients at low risk for surgery qualified for endovascular repair; only 49% of patients at high risk for surgery were acceptable candidates (P < .001). Of the 103 patients who were excluded, 34 (33%) underwent open surgical repair, and 69 (67%) were considered unfit for open surgery. Endograft placement failed in 3 patients (1.4%) because of inadequate vascular access.

Conclusion.—Most infrarenal AAAs (66%) are able to be treated with endovascular devices available commercially or through clinical trials approved by the US Food and Drug Administration. Patients at high risk for surgery who could benefit most from EVAR are less likely to qualify for the procedure (49%). Men are more likely than women to meet anatomic criteria for EVAR. Problems with vascular access and attachment site geometry are major reasons for exclusion. Smaller profile devices that can negotiate small and tortuous iliac arteries are needed. Proximal and distal attachment site problems need devices that can accommodate wide and angulated aortic necks and achieve short seal zones.

▶ Carpenter et al have reviewed their series of patients considered for endovascular repair with a number of approved and investigational devices and enumerated the reasons for exclusion. They found short infrarenal necks (54%), inadequate iliac access (47%), and wide aneurysm necks (40%) to be the predominant reasons for rejection. Excessive neck angulation (10%), extensive mural thrombus in the neck (10%), iliac tortuosity (10%), and accessory renal arteries (6%) were less frequent reasons for exclusion. They found 56% of women, compared with 30% of men, were unacceptable anatomic candidates for endovascular repair. These frequencies of exclusion are likely to vary with availability of novel devices and physician willingness and ability to treat patients with borderline anatomy.

J. S. Matsumura, MD

Endoluminal Graft Repair for Abdominal Aortic Aneurysms in High-Risk Patients and Octogenarians: Is It Better Than Open Repair?

Sicard GA, Rubin BG, Sanchez LA, et al (Washington Univ, St Louis)
Ann Surg 234:427-437, 2001

2–4

Background.—An experience with endoluminal repair of AAAs is reported, focusing on the results for octogenarians.

Methods.—The analysis included 470 consecutive patients who underwent elective AAA repair from 1997 to 2000. Two hundred ten patients had conventional open surgery, and 260 underwent endoluminal graft repair. Ninety patients were aged 80 years or older: of these, 52 underwent endoluminal repair and 38 open surgery. The mean follow-up in the series overall was 26 months for patients undergoing open surgery and 17 months for those undergoing endoluminal repair.

Results.—Patients undergoing the 2 procedures had similar characteristics and risk factors, including those aged 80 years and older. Postoperative complication rates were significantly lower with endoluminal repair. For patients of all ages, the complication rate was 30% for open surgery versus 8.5% for endoluminal repair. Values in the 80-and-over group were 37% and 11.5%, respectively. For the older patients, postoperative mortality rates were not significantly lower with endoluminal repair (Fig 2).

Conclusions.—At short- to-midterm follow-up, the results of open versus endoluminal repair of AAA are comparable, including low mortality rates with both techniques. For patients aged 80 years and older, endoluminal AAA repair offers lower rates of morbidity, including a lower rate of serious complications. Long-term follow-up studies of endoluminal graft repair are

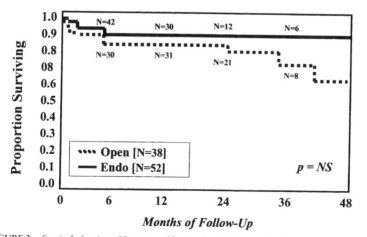

FIGURE 2.—Survival of patients 80 years or older. Kaplan-Meier analysis. (Courtesy of Sicard GA, Rubin BG, Sanchez LA, et al: Endoluminal graft repair for abdominal aortic aneurysms in high-risk patients and octogenarians: Is it better than open repair? *Ann Surg* 234:427-437, 2001.)

needed, with special attention to the results in very elderly and high-risk patients.

▶ The results of this study are pretty much what you would expect. Properly selected 80-year-olds basically do the same as younger patients with either open or endoluminal repair. More and more it is clear that it is physiologic rather than chronologic risk factors that make the difference in getting people through an operation. The cost-effectiveness of operating on the elderly in terms of remaining years of life is, however, another question.

G. L. Moneta, MD

Efficacy of a Bifurcated Endograft Versus Open Repair of Abdominal Aortic Aneurysms: A Reappraisal
Makaroun MS, Chaikof E, Naslund T, et al (Univ of Pittsburgh, Pa; Emory Univ, Atlanta, Ga; Vanderbilt Univ, Nashville Tenn; et al)
J Vasc Surg 35:203-210, 2002   2–5

Introduction.—Late complications and graft failures of endovascular repair of abdominal aortic aneurysms (AAAs) have necessitated further evaluation of this alternative approach to open procedures. The outcomes of a multicenter trial comparing a bifurcated endograft (AB) with standard open repair (OR) were examined to determine the late findings of both methods of AAA treatment.

Methods.—Two hundred forty-two patients with AAA who were successfully treated with an AB and 111 control patients consecutively treated concurrently with OR between December 1995 and February 2000 were followed up at least yearly. Twenty-five immediate conversions were not included in late follow-up. All imaging modalities taken during follow-up were examined by a core laboratory for AAA size, endoleaks, migration, and device integrity. Clinical findings from yearly visits were compared. Death reports were read to determine the cause of death.

Results.—The average follow-up for the AB group was 36 months; data were available for 194 patients at 3 years and for 55 patients at 4 years. The cumulative mortality rate was 15.7% for the AB group and 12.6% for the OR group ($P = .59$). The significant early benefit to the AB group in cardiopulmonary complications was no longer obvious at 3-year follow-up. The AB advantage in total and bowel complications persisted, but so did the higher renal complication rates in the AB group. At 3-year follow-up, 73.7% of patients had a significant decrease in size of their AAA; 25.7% still had an endoleak. One migration and 2 single hook fractures occurred. Fifty patients (20%) underwent graft-associated reinterventions (Fig 2); there were no deaths. Twenty-eight (11.6%) patients underwent interventions for limb flow compromise; 25 were treated for endoleak. Late conversion to OR was needed in 5 patients (2%). No AAA ruptures occurred in either group.

Conclusion.—The rupture-free survival rate after AAA treatment with the bifurcated AB was similar to that of OR. The proximal attachment sys-

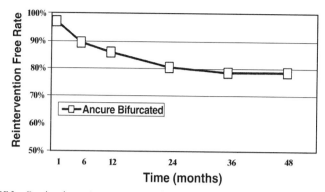

FIGURE 2.—Freedom from reintervention curve for AB group over 4 years. (Courtesy of Makaroun MS, Chaikof E, Naslund T, et al: Efficacy of a bifurcated endograft versus open repair of abdominal aortic aneurysms: A reappraisal. *J Vasc Surg* 35:203-210, 2002.)

tem was relatively stable, and the AAA shrunk in 75% of patients treated. Most late procedures were percutaneous. Patients need to be aware that there may be a need for future interventions.

▶ This study represents late follow-up of the EVT Trial. Basically, the patients treated with endografting versus open repair did the same over time in terms of survival, and no ruptures were reported. The endograft patients, however, required many more additional procedures. I am not sure this is all that bad, as long as the reintervention rate does not continue to climb over time. In fact, in this article, most of the reinterventions were within the first year of stent-graft implantation. We certainly accept the 20% reintervention rate with vein grafts for lower extremity bypass. However, if the reintervention rate gets much higher for stent-grafts, especially if it rises at a steady rate, the whole concept of endografting will have to be rethought. Endografts may be able to deal with the aneurysm, but not with the biology of the disease.

G. L. Moneta, MD

Serious Complications That Require Surgical Interventions After Endoluminal Stent-Graft Placement for the Treatment of Infrarenal Aortic Aneurysms

Schlensak C, Doenst T, Hauer M, et al (Univ of Freiburg, Germany)
J Vasc Surg 34:198-203, 2001   2–6

Introduction.—The long-term morbidity of endoluminal stent-graft placement, specifically complications requiring surgical treatment, was examined in 150 patients with abdominal aortic aneurysms (AAAs).

Methods.—The mean age of 142 men and 8 women with AAAs treated between September 1994 and December 1998 was 69.6 years. All underwent placement of an intravascular nitinol stent-graft (Stentor [55] and Vanguard-System [95]); 8 tubular and 142 bifurcated grafts were used. Of these, 144 were placed successfully. The mean follow-up was 49 months.

The following complications were observed in 13.3% of stent-graft placements: 4 cases of migration or dislocation of the prosthesis (30.5 months after placement); 2 ruptures of the aorta (26.7 and 15.0 months after placement); 3 endoleaks (27.5 months after placement); and 5 infections of the prosthesis (26.6 months after placement). There was no relationship between complications and the type of stent used. All patients with complications underwent surgical replacement of the prosthesis with a Dacron graft.

Conclusion.—Most complications are the result of a continuation of the disease process, leading to loosening of the prosthesis. Explantation of the prosthesis and surgical repair is possible. Because it is not possible to predict the onset of reperfusion of the excluded aneurysms, all patients with infrarenal aortic stent-grafts need frequent tomographic follow-up. Improvements in stent-graft design are needed.

▶ Some endograft complications are serious and technically or biologically not amenable to percutaneous techniques. The rate of complications requiring open surgical intervention is much higher in this series than others (13.3% in this article vs less than 3% in the previous article) and may be due primarily to the type of prosthesis utilized in this study. Whatever the reasons, the breadth and seriousness of the late complications in this series are unacceptable. Hopefully, it reflects stent-graft design and not a problem with the whole concept of endografting. I like to point out endografts are not like laparoscopic cholecystectomies where the same operation is done differently. Endografting is a whole different operation than open repair. It basically ignores the biology of the underlying disease. How long Mother Nature can be fooled is the $64 question.

G. L. Moneta, MD

Endovascular Repair of Ruptured Abdominal Aortic Aneurysm: A Challenge to Open Repair? Results of a Single Centre Experience in 20 Patients
Hinchliffe RJ, Yusuf SW, Macierewicz JA, et al (Univ Hosp, Nottingham, England)
Eur J Vasc Endovasc Surg 22:528-534, 2001   2–7

Background.—There is significant morbidity and mortality attendant to the repair of ruptured abdominal aortic aneurysms (rAAAs). There has been little change in the surgical technique for management of this condition during the past few decades, and the perioperative mortality remains near 50% and major morbidity near 70%. The technique of endovascular repair of aneurysms has evolved significantly during the past decade, but the experience has been largely confined to elective repair. Endovascular repair of AAAs has been shown to be associated with reduced physiologic stress during elective repair. It was hypothesized that reduced physiologic stress associated with endovascular repair may improve the outcome in patients with rAAAs.

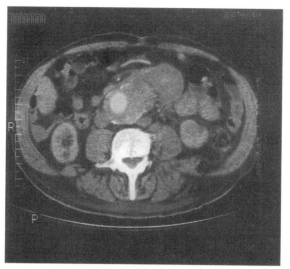

FIGURE 2.—Preoperative ruptured AAA. (Courtesy of Hinchliffe RG, Yusuf SW, Macierewicz JA, et al: Endovascular repair of ruptured abdominal aortic aneurysm: A challenge to open repair? Results of a single centre experience in 20 patients. *Eur J Vasc Endovasc Surg* 22:528-534, 2001. Reprinted by permission of Harcourt Publishers Ltd.)

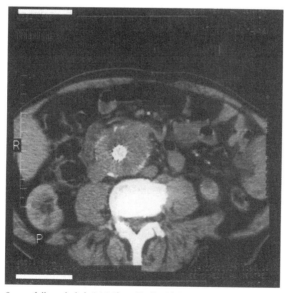

FIGURE 3.—Successfully excluded rAAA (from Fig 2) with EVG. (Courtesy of Hinchliffe RG, Yusuf SW, Macierewicz JA, et al: Endovascular repair of ruptured abdominal aortic aneurysm: A challenge to open repair? Results of a single centre experience in 20 patients. *Eur J Vasc Endovasc Surg* 22:528-534, 2001. Reprinted by permission of Harcourt Publishers Ltd.)

Methods.—A feasibility study of endovascular repair of rAAAs was conducted in the United Kingdom from 1994 to 2000. Patients admitted with rAAAs were assessed by an experienced surgical team, and most underwent spiral CT angiography. The patients were then transferred to the operating room for endovascular repair of the ruptured aneurysm.

Results.—A total of 20 patients underwent repair (Fig 2). Of these patients, 7 were referred from another hospital. Eight patients were considered unfit for open repair. The median duration of the procedure was 180 minutes, and the median blood loss was 1200 mL. The overall perioperative mortality rate was 45%. Several intraoperative and perioperative procedures were needed to ensure exclusion of the aneurysm and to address the complications of endovascular surgery (Fig 3).

Conclusions.—The treatment of rAAAs continues to challenge surgeons. There are a number of advantages to endovascular repair for the treatment of AAAs, and these findings indicate that endovascular repair is a promising technique. Yet more experience is need to determine the efficacy of this approach in comparison with open repair.

▶ Hinchliffe et al have reported a feasibility study of endovascular repair of rAAAs. The experience with 20 patients spanned 7 years and included the evolution of techniques. They had a 45% perioperative mortality, and many perioperative procedures were necessary to accommodate difficult anatomy. Although some patients were referred from other hospitals, the series included patients with hemodynamic instability, including preprocedure cardiac arrest. Enrollment was limited by the need for an endovascular call team. A critical comparison of this article with other series of open and endovascular repair is difficult because of potential selection bias inherent to institutional peculiarities of management of this disease.

J. S. Matsumura, MD

Clinical Implications of Internal Iliac Artery Embolization in Endovascular Repair of Aortoiliac Aneurysms

Lyden SP, Sternbach Y, Waldman DL, et al (Strong Mem Hosp, Rochester, NY; Univ of Rochester, NY)

Ann Vasc Surg 15:539-543, 2001   2–8

Introduction.—To overcome constraints imposed by iliac artery anatomy, the anatomic inclusion for endovascular aortic aneurysm repair can be broadened by the use of intentional coil occlusion of 1 or both internal iliac arteries (IIAs) and extension of the distal limb of the graft into an external iliac artery. The results and clinical outcome of patients requiring IIA embolization to facilitate endoluminal repair of aortoiliac aneurysms were reviewed to ascertain the safety and efficacy of this approach.

Methods.—During a 30-month period, 84 patients with aortic and aortoiliac aneurysms underwent endovascular abdominal aortic aneurysm repair with a variety of endovascular stent grafts. Of these, 23 underwent intentional unilateral (n = 22) or bilateral (n = 1) internal iliac occlusion. Morbidity, mortality, and long-term clinical outcomes were assessed in these 23 patients. Patients were interviewed by telephone regarding preprocedure and postprocedure symptoms of pain or pressure in the buttocks or thighs at rest or at their usual level of daily activity, change in buttock or thigh pain or pressure, sexual dysfunction, pelvic or lower extremity pain, parasthesias or weakness, or onset of bowel or bladder incontinence.

Results.—Successful stent-graft deployment was achieved in all 84 patients. In patients requiring IIA embolization, there were 22 men and 1 woman. The mean length of hospital stay was similar for the embolized and nonembolized groups ($P < .9$). Five of the 23 patients (22%) in the embolized group died during the 30-day perioperative period compared with 4 (4.7%) in the nonembolized group. There were 3 late deaths (13%). Morbidity directly attributable to IIA occlusion was observed in 9 patients (39%). Seven (30%) patients had postoperative pelvic or hip claudication or ischemia. The 6 surviving ambulatory patients described their symptoms as mild and not interfering with their lifestyle. Three patients (13%) had neurologic deficits develop in the lower extremities postoperatively. Six male patients had impotence; 4 had impotence before IIA embolization.

Conclusion.—Intentional internal iliac artery embolization to permit endovascular repair of abdominal aortic aneurysms is accompanied by significant morbidity and needs to be used with caution.

▶ Preoperative embolization of hypogastric arteries has become a common adjunctive procedure for treating more complex aortoiliac aneurysms by open and endovascular approaches. Lyden et al have reviewed their results with 23 patients having this procedure (22 unilateral and 1 bilateral). Nine patients (39%) had morbidity directly related to the embolization procedure, including seven with pelvic or hip claudication. More importantly, 3 patients had neurologic deficits develop; 2 of these had operative complications of aorto-monoiliac grafts that resulted in the contralateral IIA becoming occluded and both patients died with complications related to pelvic ischemia. The authors were unable to demonstrate any association with staging of embolization or location of coil placement, although bilateral internal iliac occlusion should be avoided.

J. S. Matsumura, MD

Iliac Arterial Injuries After Endovascular Repair of Abdominal Aortic Aneurysms: Correlation With Iliac Curvature and Diameter
Tillich M, Bell RE, Paik DS, et al (Stanford Univ, Calif)
Radiology 219:129-136, 2001   2–9

Background.—Abdominal aortic aneurysms (AAAs) may be associated with narrow, tortuous iliac arteries and is an important consideration in the endovascular repair of these AAAs. The diameter and curvature of the iliac arteries, along with the vessel wall's morphologic characteristics, must be accurately portrayed before stent-graft deployment. It was hypothesized that greater degrees of iliac arterial curvature increases the risk of injury or rupture of the intima during deployment of the stent-graft, and that injuries to the intima of the iliac arteries are often associated with small-diameter iliac arteries.

Methods.—Forty-two patients who were having transfemoral delivery of aortic stent-grafts underwent helical CT scanning. From these data, the iliac artery curvature values and orthogonal cross-sectional areas were quantified at every millimeter along the median centerline of the iliac artery. The iliac tortuosity index was determined as the sum of the curvature values for all points with a curvature of at least 0.3 cm^{-1}; this index indicated global iliac tortuosity. The mean cross-sectional diameter was determined from the cross-sectional area indexed for all points. After the stent-graft was deployed, helical CT data analysis was carried out to determine whether iliac artery dissections were present.

Results.—Sixteen patients had 18 acute iliac arterial dissections (prevalence of 0.21); in 11 patients, the dissections were at the primary site where the stent-graft was deployed; in 3, it was at the secondary site; and in 2, it was bilateral. The dissected iliac segment was 10 to 215 mm long (mean, 85 mm). The iliac tortuosity index was greater in iliac arteries that had dissections than in those without dissections, even in the same patient; this difference reached statistical significance. In 10 of the 11 iliac dissections, the tortuosity index was greater ipsilateral to the primary component delivery when the dissection developed along the route to the primary component delivery site. When the dissection occurred in the secondary site, the tortuosity index was greater than in the nondissected primary site.

Conclusion.—The method developed to quantify iliac tortuosity is founded on a 3-dimensional evaluation of the arterial lumen. The magnitude of the tortuosity index correlated significantly with the likelihood of intimal injury occurring after stent-graft deployment. This tortuosity index may reliably predict risk for intimal injury to the access route after stent-graft delivery.

▶ I don't like articles like this one. They are an attempt to quantify judgement, and never really provide absolute guidelines. In addition, the end point in this article was dissection of the iliac artery, a problem frequently fixed with deployment of the graft. I would have been interested in knowing how frequently these dissections actually adversely impacted the outcome of the stent-graft procedure.

G. L. Moneta, MD

Endovascular Repair of Abdominal Aortic Aneurysms: Stent-Graft Fixation Across the Visceral Arteries

Burks JA Jr, Faries PL, Gravereaux EC, et al (Mount Sinai School of Medicine, New York)
J Vasc Surg 35:109-113, 2002
2–10

Background.—Endovascular grafting is an alternative method for the repair of appropriately selected abdominal aortic aneurysms (AAAs). However, not all AAAs can be repaired with an endovascular approach. Recently, transrenal artery fixation of endovascular stent-grafts has been recommended as a safe and effective means of reducing the risk of type I endoleaks, particularly in the setting of short infrarenal necks. In this approach, the close proximity of the superior mesenteric and celiac arteries to the renal arteries commonly results in the placement of the stent struts across all the vessels of the visceral segment of the aorta. The incidence and impact of transvisceral artery fixation during aortic stent-graft deployment for the treatment of AAAs were determined.

Methods.—Between January 1997 and June 1999, 192 patients (mean age, 82 years) who had AAAs were treated with an endovascular graft secured proximally to the aorta with a long (15 mm) uncovered stent segment. Preoperative and postoperative abdominal aortograms and intravenous contrast–enhanced spiral CT scans were performed, and follow-up CT scans were obtained at 3, 6, and 12 months and then annually to determine stent position and patency of the visceral arteries.

Results.—The uncovered stent was at or above the level of the superior mesenteric artery in 95 patients (49%). In 23 patients (12%), the stent extended to the level of the celiac axis (Fig 3). Serum creatinine levels remained stable during a mean follow-up period of 25 months, and no stenoses or occlusions occurred in the celiac, superior mesenteric, or renal arteries. No evi-

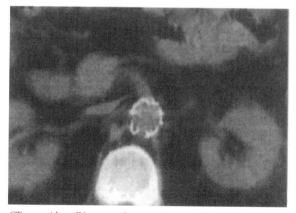

FIGURE 3.—CT scan without IV contrast demonstrating stent struts projecting across the origin of the superior mesenteric artery (SMA). (Courtesy of Burks JA Jr, Faries PL, Gravereaux EC, et al: Endovascular repair of abdominal aortic aneurysms: Stent-graft fixation across the visceral arteries. *J Vasc Surg* 35:109-113, 2002.)

dence of renal, hepatic, splenic, or intestinal infarction was observed on contrast-enhanced spiral CT scans, and there were no type I endoleaks.

Conclusions.—Transvisceral fixation of the uncovered proximal aortic stent occurs frequently during the deployment of devices for use in transrenal fixation. There is no early morbidity associated with transvisceral fixation; however, long-term follow-up is necessary to ensure that transvisceral fixation is not associated with late sequelae.

▶ Burks et al have reviewed their extensive endovascular experience and culled 192 patients with uncovered suprarenal stents. They found that 95 of these patients, or about half (49%), had extension of the stent across the superior mesenteric artery and 23 patients had extension to the celiac artery. These 95 patients with transvisceral fixation were followed up for a mean of 25 months (range, 6-44 months) with periodic physical examination, serum creatinine, and spiral CT scan (3, 6, 12 months, and annual). No data are given on compliance with follow up testing. There were 2 patients with inadvertent coverage of a renal artery with graft material who had increased serum creatinine and unilateral renal infarction. These investigators were unable to identify any patients with visceral artery stenosis, occlusion, or radiologic/clinical bowel ischemia. They found no other evidence of renal, hepatic, or splenic infarction. They conclude that the technique is safe, although they acknowledge the downside of increased complexity of conversion to open repair. These results are unusually impressive compared to other reports of infrequent renal mass loss, segmental renal infarcts, and elevated serum creatinine after infrarenal open and endovascular repairs without transrenal fixation. Further, it is unclear how sensitive CT is compared with arteriography in identifying stenosis in areas with metallic stents. Lastly, when stents "jail" coronary branches, the amount of stent area has been correlated with frequency of occlusion, and it is unclear if results can be extrapolated to other transvisceral devices.

J. S. Matsumura, MD

Histopathologic Analysis of Endovascular Stent Grafts From Patients With Aortic Aneurysms: Does Healing Occur?
McArthur C, Teodorescu V, Eisen L, et al (Mount Sinai School of Medicine, New York)
J Vasc Surg 33:733-738, 2001   2–11

Background.—Optimal long-term success with endovascular graft therapy of aortic aneurysms requires the tissues heal in a way that promotes stent-artery incorporation. The clinical use of prosthetic vascular grafts placed endoluminally is relatively new and data are limited to those gathered from explanted human grafts. Specimens recovered from patients who had endoluminal repair of aortic aneurysms were analyzed. The analyses covered a period of 7 years.

Methods.—Endovascular grafts were used for 313 patients placed to exclude arterial aneurysms of the thoracic or abdominal aorta. Eleven grafts

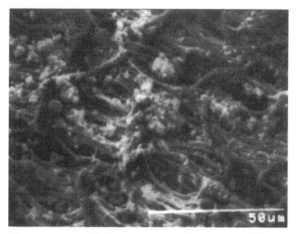

FIGURE 3.—Electron microscopy performed on aortic endograft explanted 2 months after aortic endografting. Nodal pattern of polytetrafluoroethylene graft material is seen with adherent platelets and fibrin but no organized cellular layer. (Courtesy of McArthur C, Teodorescu V, Eisen L, et al: Histopathologic analysis of endovascular stent grafts from patients with aortic aneurysms: Does healing occur? *J Vasc Surg* 33:733-738, 2001.)

were recovered for analysis, 5 of which were removed during open aortic surgery and 6 at autopsy after the patient died from nonendovascular graft–related causes. Specimens were analyzed for adherence of the graft to the vessel wall and appropriately categorized.

Results.—Eight of the grafts were deemed firmly adherent to the arterial wall at the sites of the stent attachments. Loose adherence to the thrombus in the aneurysmal sac was noted for all grafts. A translucent film of fragile thrombotic material spanned the artery-graft interface in each of the endografts. In 3 patients, the grafts were readily separated from the luminal surface at the stent anastomotic site; 2 of these had endoleaks (1 proximal and 1 distal) that were clinically detectable. These leaks increased the ability to separate the endograft from the aorta. On microscopic analysis of the interface between the stent and the graft, compacted fibrin was found in 1 patient and a small amount of cellular or fibrous tissue in the other. One patient with recurrent infection had an area of communication between the aneurysm sac that had been excluded and the duodenum, requiring graft excision and aortic ligation. No significant stent graft incorporation was found at the anastomotic sites in the specimens evaluated. Myointimal cells were absent, with only compacted fibrin and thrombus (Fig 3).

Conclusion.—The 11 explanted grafts assessed had minimal tissue incorporation of the grafts, even though there was an apparently tight adherence between the graft and arterial wall. Thus, the attachment system of an endovascular graft device is crucial to fixation of the graft. Long-term fixation is not guaranteed.

▶ Possible healing of endografts has been suggested by animal studies. It seems, however, healing of stent-grafts is likely to be wishful thinking. While graft healing is desirable, healing in a bed of thrombus in aortic sacs does not appear to happen. If healing is to occur, it would seem most likely to occur at the attachment sites. This study, however, failed to show endothelialization of even attachment sites, once again proving people are different than dogs and pigs.

G. L. Moneta, MD

External Transabdominal Manipulation of Vessels: A Useful Adjunct With Endovascular Abdominal Aortic Aneurysm Repair

Sternbergh WC III, Money SR, Yoselevitz M (Ochsner Clinic and Found, New Orleans, La)
J Vasc Surg 33:886-887, 2001   2–12

Background.—Relatively large, stiff delivery systems are used for endografts in the endovascular treatment of abdominal aortic aneurysms (AAAs). These can produce difficulties in patients who have major aortic neck angulation or tortuous iliac arteries. An adjunct was developed to facilitate the delivery of these devices when the patient presents difficult anatomical situations.

Technique.—The patient is prepped and draped, including the entire abdomen. An assistant applies abdominal pressure from lateral to the midline if passage of a large sheath or device meets significant resistance. This pressure can straighten the tortuous segment (Figs 1 and 2). As the assistant maintains pressure—which must be deep to change the vessel's position—the device is advanced. If needed, force can be applied cephalad-central or caudal-central. When this maneu-

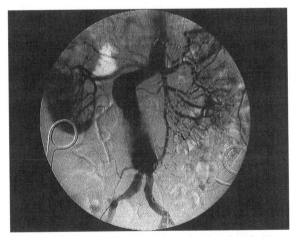

FIGURE 1.—Abdominal aortic aneurysm with highly angulated aortic neck. (Courtesy of Sternbergh WC III, Money SR, Yoselevitz M: External transabdominal manipulation of vessels: A useful adjunct with endovascular abdominal aortic aneurysm repair. *J Vasc Surg* 33:886-887, 2001.)

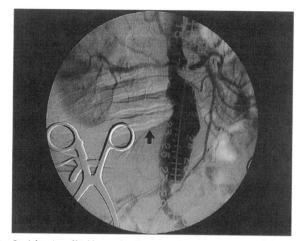

FIGURE 2.—Straightening of highly angulated aortic neck with external abdominal manipulation. Note digital pressure from patient's right side toward midline (*arrow*). (Courtesy of Sternbergh WC III, Money SR, Yoselevitz M: External transabdominal manipulation of vessels: A useful adjunct with endovascular abdominal aortic aneurysm repair. *J Vasc Surg* 33:886-887, 2001.)

ver is needed, the position of the lowest renal artery must be reconfirmed after the device is placed and before deployment. After the angulated segment of vessel is passed, transabdominal pressure is released, and the endograft can be deployed.

Results.—The technique described was used in 20% to 30% of 141 endovascular AAA repairs and proved most useful with highly angulated aortic necks. If the aortic angulation is severe, suboptimal apposition of the endograft to the aortic neck may occur, there may be an increased risk for early or delayed migration of the endograft, or a proximal type I endoleak may occur. The risk of kinking of the iliac vessel and subsequent occlusion of the limb is increased with severe tortuosity. Tortuous iliac arteries in patients who are fairly thin may also benefit from the technique. Thus, patients must be selected with attention to these difficulties. A successful endovascular repair of AAA is not guaranteed, even if the difficult anatomy is traversed.

Conclusion.—The simple adjunct described can significantly facilitate the delivery of endografts for use in AAA repair in patients with challenging anatomy. It should be noted that the hand applying pressure will be placed close to the source of radiation and may be protected by a lead glove, along with a ring radiation badge, to quantify the amount of radiation exposure.

▶ This is "pushing" things a bit too far for my taste.

G. L. Moneta, MD

Exclusion of Accessory Renal Arteries During Endovascular Repair of Abdominal Aortic Aneurysms
Aquino RV, Rhee RY, Muluk SC, et al (Univ of Pittsburgh, Pa)
J Vasc Surg 34:878-884, 2001   2–13

Introduction.—Adequate proximal neck length is critical for proper endovascular treatment of abdominal aortic aneurysms (AAAs). Placement of endografts in AAAs with relatively short proximal necks may necessitate covering the origin of accessory renal arteries. Regional renal ischemia with loss of parenchyma or worsening hypertension may occur with exclusion of these arteries. An experience with accessory renal exclusions during endovascular AAA repair was reviewed to determine the incidence and severity of complications.

Methods.—Complete records were available for 311 of 325 consecutive patients who underwent endovascular grafts for AAAs from February 6, 1996, to March 15, 2001. The presence of accessory renal arteries was de-

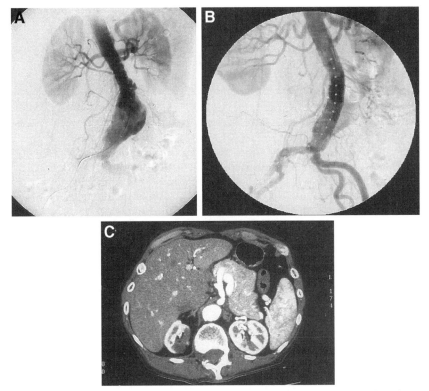

FIGURE 2.—**A,** Preoperative angiogram demonstrating small right accessory renal artery above the aneurysm. **B,** Intraoperative angiogram showing the exclusion of the right accessory renal artery. **C,** Follow-up CT scan depicting a right segmental infarction. (Courtesy of Aquino RV, Rhee RY, Muluk SC, et al: Exclusion of accessory renal arteries during endovascular repair of abdominal aortic aneurysm. *J Vasc Surg* 34:878-884, 2001.)

termined from preoperative/intraoperative aortography or from CT scanning (Fig 2). Size of the accessory renal arteries was determined by using the main renal arteries as a reference. Consideration for excluding the accessory renal arteries was based on the likelihood of successful proximal attachment to healthy aorta, an accessory vessel whose size was not greater than the diameter of the main renal artery, and the absence of renal disease.

Results.—The mean follow-up was 11.5 months. Fifty-two accessory renal arteries were observed in 37 patients (12%) (range, 1-3 or more per patient). Twenty-six accessory renal arteries were covered in 24 patients (20 men, 4 women; mean age, 74.1 years; range, 57-85 years). For 23 patients, the Ancure device was used; the Excluder device was used in 1 patient. Twenty-two of the 26 excluded accessory renal arteries originated above the aneurysm, and 4 originated directly from the aneurysm. No perioperative mortalities were recorded. One patient died 5 months after endovascular repair of an unrelated condition. There was one type I (distal) endoleak. No type II endoleaks occurred. Five patients (21%) had segmental renal infarction related to the side of accessory renal artery exclusion. One patient with segmental infarction had significant postoperative hypertension for which blood pressure medication was changed. The blood pressure returned to normal 3 months later. One patient with a stenotic left main renal artery needed exclusion of the accessory renal artery for successful proximal attachment. Serum creatinine levels continued to be unchanged throughout follow-up in all except one patient, for whom progressive postoperative renal failure developed in spite of a normal renal flow scan.

Conclusion.—Exclusion of accessory renal arteries to facilitate endovascular AAA repair seems to be well tolerated. Complications were rare and mild. Endovascular therapy in patients with relatively short proximal necks may necessitate the sacrifice of accessory renal vessels, particularly in high-risk patients who may benefit from this form of AAA treatment.

▶ A frequent finding during preoperative imaging evaluation for endovascular repair are accessory renal arteries. Aquino et al reviewed their institutional series and identified 37 patients with 52 accessory renal arteries, and considerations for optimal proximal sealing resulted in coverage of 26 of these arteries. Of these, 5 patients had segmental renal infarction and 1 patient had transient worsening of hypertension. This report provides helpful data on the sequelae of accessory renal artery coverage when deemed necessary.

J. S. Matsumura, MD

Causes and Outcomes of Open Conversion and Aneurysm Rupture After Endovascular Abdominal Aortic Aneurysm Repair: Can Type II Endoleaks Be Dangerous?

Buth J, Harris PL, van Marrewijk C (Catharina Hosp, Eindhoven, The Netherlands; Royal and Univ Hosp, Liverpool, England)
J Am Coll Surg 194:S98-S102, 2002   2–14

Background.—Late complications have plagued the stent-graft approach to treatment of abdominal aortic aneurysms (AAAs), with rupture of the aneurysm being the most dramatic evidence of treatment failure. Late conversion to open surgery is performed either for manifest rupture of the aneurysm or for impending rupture. There is uncertainty as to which signs and findings obtained by regular imaging are an accurate indicator of an increased risk of conversion to open surgery or aneurysm rupture. The role of endoleaks, particularly type II or side branch perfusion endoleaks, is controversial. These and other aspects of EVAR were evaluated in this overview of the EUROSTAR series. The EUROSTAR database was established in 1996 for the purpose of collation and analysis of data from patients who undergo endovascular treatment for AAA.

Methods.—Data for 3539 patients who underwent treatment between January 1994 and July 2001 were collected and entered in the database. In addition, 454 patients were enrolled as a separate retrospective cohort. Preoperative medical risk factors and morphologic variables were prospectively

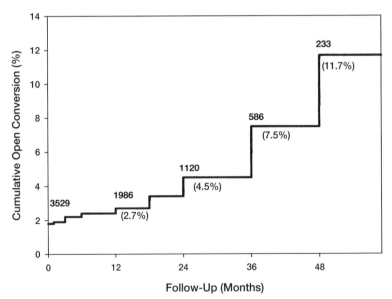

FIGURE 2.—Freedom from conversion in 3529 patients. *Significantly different from simvastatin, *P* < .0001. (Courtesy of Buth J, Harris PL, van Marrewijk CL: Causes and outcomes of open conversion and aneurysm rupture after endovascular abdominal aortic aneurysm repair: Can type II endoleaks be dangerous? *J Am Coll Surg* 194:S98-S102, 2002. By permission of the American College of Surgeons.)

recorded, along with the details of the endovascular procedure, the completion angiogram, and the postoperative course. Imaging surveillance was included in the follow-up visits, which occurred on a fixed schedule.

Results.—In the current series, 149 patients (4.2%) required an open conversion, with 67 needing conversion during the initial procedure or later in the postoperative month and 82 patients needing conversion during follow-up. The most common reasons for primary conversion were access problems and device migration. Secondary conversions were performed for rupture in 16 patients, and elective conversion was associated with persistent endoleak with or without aneurysmal growth in 35 patients. Overall, the cumulative rate of conversion was 11.7% at 4 years (Fig 2).

Conclusions.—Late conversion and aneurysm rupture are associated with each other, and these 2 events have several common patient and morphologic risk factors. Type I endoleaks usually are caused by errors in physician judgment. Type III endoleaks need to be resolved by improved design of endografts. Type II endoleaks are usually innocuous, but if the aneurysm is enlarged considerably a more aggressive intervention may be necessary.

▶ The EUROSTAR collaborators have updated their voluntary registry of over 3500 patients to ascertain the clinical dangers of type II endoleaks; 7.8% of patients had an isolated type II endoleak, and a correlation was found with secondary interventions (22% vs 6% without type II endoleak) and multivarate regression analysis confirmed a relationship with secondary conversions. However, there was no significant relationship of type II endoleaks with aneurysm enlargement at 3 years (10% vs 5.4%), any conversion to open surgery at 2 years (2.6% vs 1.0%), aneurysm rupture at 2 years (1.8% vs 0.7%), or survival at 3 years (81% vs 83%). While type II endoleaks do not appear dangerous at a statistically significant level and survival is comparable, these trends are concerning. Further, the Kaplan-Meier curves for conversion and aneurysm rupture have no evidence of plateau effect in the first 5 years. Although many groups have an initially conservative approach to branch endoleaks, these data support long-term surveillance and reintervention for type II endoleak associated with aneurysm enlargement.

J. S. Matsumura, MD

Rupture of an Abdominal Aortic Aneurysm Secondary to Type II Endoleak
Hinchliffe RJ, Singh-Ranger R, Davidson IR, et al (Univ Hosp, Nottingham, England)
Eur J Vasc Endovasc Surg 22:563-565, 2001   2–15

Introduction.—Most aneurysm sac ruptures after endovascular aneurysm repair (EVAR) are due to graft migration and a resulting type I endoleak. Attachment-site endoleaks cause persistent or continued pressurization of the aneurysm sac and eventual rupture. However, the significance of the much more frequent type II, or retrograde endoleak, is not known. A case of fatal aneurysm sac rupture secondary to a known type II endoleak of the inferior mesenteric artery is discussed.

> *Case Report.*—Man, 80, underwent EVAR of an 8.9-cm (maximal anteroposterior diameter) AAA. He had a bifurcated endovascular stent-graft placement with no intraoperative complications or evidence of an endoleak. Spiral computerized tomographic angiography (SCTA) at 1 week was satisfactory. The maximal anteroposterior aneurysm diameter was 9.1 cm at this time. Follow-up SCTA at 8 months revealed a satisfactory position and alignment of the endograft with no notable angulation or distortion. The aneurysm sac diameter was 10.2 cm, and no evidence of an endoleak was found. At 12 months, the patient was admitted complaining of abdominal pain. Radiographic contrast was seen in the 11-cm aneurysm sac (endoleak). Digital subtraction angiography with selective catheterization of the superior mesenteric artery revealed a patent inferior mesenteric artery (IMA). Contrast was not clearly seen to enter the aneurysm sac, and embolization was not performed. The patient was discharged. He was seen shortly afterwards with a 1-hour history of sudden onset, generalized abdominal pain. During SCTA, he became hemodynamically unstable, deteriorated rapidly, and died of hypovolemic shock. The SCTA verified aneurysm rupture. No graft migration was observed, and the graft was patent. Postmortem examination showed a left-sided anterolateral aneurysm sac rupture. The stent-graft was well positioned into the aortic wall proximally and in the common iliac arteries distally. The stent-graft body was intact, along with the joint between the main body and iliac limbs. A fresh thrombus was seen within the aneurysm sac. The IMA was not seen because of the distortion created from the large hematoma. No other intra-abdominal pathologic disorders were found.

Conclusion.—These findings confirm the danger of not treating a type II endoleak associated with aneurysm sac enlargement. Such endoleaks should be treated to prevent aneurysm rupture.

▶ In this case, aneurysm rupture after endograft repair was associated with a type II endoleak involving the inferior mesenteric artery. A previous case report[1] reported rupture associated with an endoleak involving an accessory renal artery. Obviously, not all type II endoleaks are equal and not all are benign. I wonder if endoleaks involving the IMA or accessory renals have the same prognosis as those just involving lumbar vessels? (See also Abstracts 2–14 and 2–16.)

G. L. Moneta, MD

Reference

1. White RA, Donayre C, Walot I, et al: Abdominal aortic aneurysm rupture following endoluminal graft deployment: Report of a predictable event. *J Endovasc Ther* 7:257-262, 2000.

Endovascular Stent-Graft in Abdominal Aortic Aneurysms: The Relationship Between Patent Vessels That Arise From the Aneurysmal Sac and Early Endoleak

Fan C-M, Rafferty EA, Geller SC, et al (Massachusetts Gen Hosp, Boston)
Radiology 218:176-182, 2001   2–16

Background.—Endoleaks are an important limiting factor on the success of endovascular stent-graft repair of abdominal aortic aneurysm (AAA). Few previous reports have addressed the association between patent branches feeding the aneurysmal sac and the risk of endoleak after stent-graft placement. A study was performed in a large group of patients to examine the relationship between patent sac branch vessels and early endoleak rate after endovascular AAA repair.

Methods.—The retrospective study included 158 patients with AAA who underwent endovascular stent-graft placement. Preprocedural and postprocedural CT angiograms were examined to assess the patency of the inferior mesenteric arteries (IMAs) and other sac branch "feeders," as well as the presence of endoleakage in the immediate postoperative period. The effects of total branch vessel, IMA, and lumbar artery patency on the endoleak rate were analyzed.

Results.—The total endoleak rate was 6% for patients with 0 to 3 total sac feeders, compared with 35% for patients with 4 to 6 feeders. The rate of type 2 endoleaks was 0% for patients with 0 to 3 sac feeders and 25% for patients with 4 to 6 feeders. Patency of the IMA was also associated with a total early endoleak rate. The total endoleak rate was 17% for patients with 0 to 3 patent lumbar arteries versus 60% for those with more than 6 patent lumbar arteries. Rates of type 2 endoleak were 13% and 60%, respectively.

Conclusion.—In patients undergoing endovascular stent-graft repair of AAA, the number of patent sac branch vessels is significantly related to the rate of early endoleak, especially type 2 endoleak. Patent sac branches may play an important role in the pathogenesis of endoleaks and may be a useful target for preventive measures.

▶ The presence of a patent IMA or multiple patent lumbar arteries increases the likelihood of endoleak after aortic stent-graft repair. That makes sense. What we really need to know is which endoleaks are dangerous. Just having a persistent leak is probably not enough. I doubt failure of the sac to shrink will even be enough if the AAA is not large. (See also previous comment.)

G. L. Moneta, MD

Eccentric Stent Graft Compression: An Indicator of Insecure Proximal Fixation of Aortic Stent Graft

Wolf YG, Hill BB, Lee WA, et al (Stanford Univ, Calif)
J Vasc Surg 33:481-487, 2001   2–17

Background.—Endovascular devices for the treatment of aortic aneurysms are usually constructed of metallic stents and fabric grafts. The effectiveness of the grafts in excluding aortic aneurysms from the circulation is usually determined by contrast CT angiography, MR angiography, or color-flow duplex US scanning. Fixation of the stent graft is dependent on radial expansion against the normal infrarenal aortic neck and iliac fixation and longitudinal columnar support. The stent graft is usually oversized by 10% to 20% in relation to the proximal aortic neck, which results in slight compression of the stent bodies within the infrarenal neck. The hypothesis that the contour of this compression deformity could provide clues to the status of proximal stent graft fixation on plain abdominal radiography was investigated.

Methods.—Stent graft structure was evaluated in a consecutive series of 100 patients with abdominal aortic aneurysms. The assessment included stent graft integrity, stent contour, angulation, compression, and position using plain abdominal radiography. These findings were correlated with contrast CT scanning, clinical findings, and outcomes. Repeated imaging was performed during follow-up of 3 to 38 months.

Results.—Stent graft repair was successful in all of the patients, and no stent fractures were identified. In 69% of the patients, there was visible evidence of concentric compression of the proximal portion of the stent graft, reflecting deliberate oversizing of the stent graft at implantation. In 5% of the patients, a short eccentric compression deformity of the proximal stent was observed in association with an increased risk of stent graft migration and an increased risk of development of a late proximal endoleak. Abdominal radiography was found to be less useful than CT scanning for assessment of short distances of migration (sensitivity 67% and specificity 79%). However, abdominal radiography provided better definition of the stent graft in relation to bony landmarks and better visualization of aortic calcification compared with CT.

Conclusions.—Plain abdominal radiographs have an important role in the postoperative evaluation of patients with aortic stent grafts. Compared with CT, plain radiographs allow more precise evaluation of the structural elements of the stent graft and thus may identify proximal fixation by demonstrating an eccentric compression deformity. However, plain abdominal radiographs are less useful than CT for the assessment of migration.

▶ Plain radiographs have been found useful for surveillance after endovascular repair to detect device material failure and intercomponent migration. Wolf et al have identified another utility of the device radiograph in a review of 100 consecutive patients. They found short eccentric compression deformity of the proximal end of the main trunk device in 5% of patients. When this finding was noted, 80% of the patients had caudal migration and 40% had a late type I endoleak. Reintervention was performed in this series, but the authors noted experience with 2 patients at other hospitals who had the same finding and had aneurysm rupture 9 and 14 months later. This is an excellent example of the continued stream of helpful information arising from astute observation by experienced investigators more than a dozen years after the endovascular repair was first introduced.

J. S. Matsumura, MD

Endoleaks Following Endovascular Repair of Abdominal Aortic Aneurysm: The Predictive Value of Preoperative Anatomic Factors—A Review of 100 Cases
Petrik PV, Moore WS (Univ of California, Los Angeles)
J Vasc Surg 33:739-744, 2001   2–18

Background.—The complication seemingly inherent in endovascular graft repair of abdominal aortic aneurysm is endoleak. Several anatomical conditions were assessed to see whether they were important predictors of the occurrence of endoleak.

Methods.—The first 100 infrarenal aneurysms treated with tube, bifurcated, and aortoiliac grafts were assessed. In 34 patients, endoleaks developed, either early or late in the postoperative course. All patients had preoperative CT scans and angiograms, which were reviewed for specific anatomical characteristics (number of patent lumbar arteries, presence of a patent inferior mesenteric artery, calcification and thrombus at proximal and distal attachment sites, proximal aortic angulation, and graft-vessel size discrepancy at both the proximal and distal attachment sites). Patients with endoleaks were compared with those without, based on these factors.

Results.—Overall, the endoleak rate was 39%, comparable to other studies. Six percent of patients had residual endoleaks at 1 year; in the other patients, endoleaks sealed spontaneously or by secondary intention. No graft type was associated with a higher risk of development of an endoleak. None of the anatomical factors showed a significant association with endoleak development.

Conclusion.—Endoleaks develop in a significant number of patients who have endovascular repair of abdominal aortic aneurysms, yet none of the anatomical characteristics assessed in this study showed a significant relationship to endoleak development. Thus, preoperative radiographs to identify these features are not necessary.

▶ In an effort to identify preoperative anatomy that predicts subsequent endoleak, Petrik and Moore have reviewed their first 100 cases of endorepair with tube, bifurcated, and aortomonoiliac repairs. They recorded neck characteristics of calcification, thrombus, angulation, and size mismatch as well as patency of aortic side branches on preoperative arteriograms and found no predictive risk factors for subsequent endoleak. Specifically, 44% of patients with and 43% without endoleaks have a patent inferior mesenteric artery, implying that many patients would be treated unnecessarily if embolized before stent-graft placement. Although sac thrombus has been correlated with risk of endoleak by others, no risk assessment system is strong enough to make pre-emptive embolization of endoleaks a useful strategy.

J. S. Matsumura, MD

Treatment of Type 2 Endoleaks After Endovascular Repair of Abdominal Aortic Aneurysms: Comparison of Transarterial and Translumbar Techniques

Baum RA, Carpenter JP, Golden MA, et al (Univ of Pennsylvania, Philadelphia)
J Vasc Surg 35:23-29, 2002   2–19

Introduction.—Because of uncertainty about the significance of collateral endoleaks, some physicians choose to follow up patients with serial imaging and to intervene only when there is enlargement of the aneurysm. Others repair collateral endoleaks as soon as they are identified. The efficacies of translumbar and transarterial embolization procedures in patients in whom type 2 endoleaks developed after endovascular aneurysm repair were evaluated and compared.

Methods.—Patients with 33 angiographically verified type 2 endoleaks underwent treatment with either transarterial inferior mesenteric artery embolization or direct translumbar embolization (20 and 13 patients, respectively) during an 18-month evaluation period. Embolization success was considered to be the resolution of the endoleak as seen on all subsequent CT angiograms. The likelihood of embolization failure between the 2 treatments was examined.

Results.—Sixteen of the 20 transarterial inferior mesenteric artery embolizations (80%) failed; the original endoleak cavity recanalized over time. One failure (8%) occurred in the direct translumbar embolization group in a patient who had a new attachment site leak. The remaining 12 translumbar endoleak embolizations (92%) were successful and long-lasting at a median follow-up of 254 days (Table 1). Patients who underwent transarterial inferior mesenteric artery embolization were significantly more likely to experience persistent endoleaks compared with those who underwent direct translumbar embolization (risk ratio, 4.6; 95% CI, 1.9-11.2; $P = .0001$).

TABLE 1.—Endoleak Embolization Treatment Results

| | Type of Embolization | |
	IMA	TLA
Success	4	12
Failure	16	1

Abbreviations: IMA, Inferior mesenteric artery; TLA, translumbar artery.
(Courtesy of Baum RA, Carpenter JP, Golden MA, et al: Treatment of type 2 endoleaks after endovascular repair of abdominal aortic aneurysms: Comparison of transarterial and translumbar techniques. *J Vasc Surg* 35:23-29, 2002.)

Conclusion.—Transarterial embolization of the inferior mesenteric arteries for the repair of type 2 endoleaks is not effective and should not be used. The therapy of choice is direct translumbar embolization when aggressive endoleak management is appropriate.

▶ Technical approaches for treatment of type II endoleaks include selective transfemoral catheterization of branches and direct translumbar puncture of the sac. Baum et al have reconsidered their previous technique in this review of 33 patients with proven branch endoleaks. They found an 80% (16 of 20) failure rate with microcoil embolization of the inferior mesenteric artery through subselective catheterization through the superior mesenteric artery. A translumbar approach with coiling of the sac "nidus" resulted in a 92% success rate with median follow-up of 254 days. To their credit, this is one of many experienced groups that have found and publicized critical reappraisals of impressive initial results with new endovascular treatments. The use of fluid embolic agents, particularly liquid thrombin, is a similar example described in the discussion of this article.

J. S. Matsumura, MD

3 Vascular Laboratory and Imaging

Low Levels of High-Density Lipoprotein Cholesterol Are Associated With Echolucent Carotid Artery Plaques: The Tromsø Study
Mathiesen EB, Bønaa KH, Joakimsen O (Univ of Tromsø, Norway)
Stroke 32:1960-1965, 2001

3–1

Background.—Plaque morphology seen on US independently predicts ischemic stroke. The risk factors associated with carotid plaque morphology were investigated.

Methods.—This population-based, cross-sectional, nested case-control study included 6727 participants in a population health survey. US of the right carotid artery was performed. Plaque echogenicity was defined as reflectance of the emitted US signal and was scored as echolucent, predominantly echolucent, predominately echogenic, or echogenic. Two hundred sixteen participants who had carotid stenosis were matched to 223 participants without stenosis by age and sex. Data on cardiovascular risk factors were obtained from measurements of blood pressure, weight, height, and nonfasting blood samples as well as a self-administered questionnaire.

Findings.—In univariate and multivariate analyses, low high-density lipoprotein (HDL) cholesterol levels and an increasing degree of stenosis correlated independently with an increased risk of an echolucent plaque. An HDL cholesterol increase of 1 standard deviation reduced the adjusted odds of being in a lower plaque echogenicity category by about 30%.

Conclusion.—Low levels of HDL cholesterol are associated with an increased risk of having echolucent, rupture-prone atherosclerotic plaques. Further research to verify these findings is needed.

▶ Carotid plaque echogenicity has long been a controversial predictor of ischemic neurologic events. The utility of plaque morphology in clinical practice has been limited because assessment of plaque morphology is inherently subjective. Nevertheless, there is increasing consensus that highly echogenic plaque, especially in association with high grade stenosis, is associated with an increased neurologic event rate. Investigators in this study were blinded to laboratory values of the patients undergoing carotid US. The association between low levels of HDL cholesterol and increased plaque echogenicity is therefore probably real. Improving HDL levels may therefore decrease the risk of cerebral as well as cardiac ischemic events.

G. L. Moneta, MD

Determinants of Carotid Plaque Instability: Echoicity Versus Heterogeneity
Tegos TJ, Stavropoulos P, Sabetai MM, et al (Imperial College of Science, Technology, and Medicine, London)
Eur J Vasc Endovasc Surg 22:22-30, 2001   3–2

Background.—Analysis of findings in the asymptomatic arm of the Cardiovascular Health Study in the United Kingdom found that at 3.3 years, hypoechoic carotid plaques were associated with a 3.5% incidence of stroke, isoechoic plaques were associated with a stroke incidence of 1.95%, and hyperechoic plaques with an incidence of 2.67%. A heterogeneous pattern was associated with a 5.4% prevalence rate for stroke, while a homogeneous pattern was associated with a 4.1% rate. Another study has found that in heterogeneous plaques, the prevalence of the hypoechoic plaque on the juxtaluminal region was higher in symptomatic plaques than in the asymptomatic plaques (67% vs 33%). In this study, the relative significance of the echogenicity and heterogeneity of carotid plaques in the development of ipsilateral neurovascular symptoms was investigated.

Methods.—The cross-sectional study consisted of 113 patients with 127 symptomatic and asymptomatic plaques. Duplex images of the plaques were analyzed echoically by computer that used Grey Scale Median (GSM) to describe plaque brightness, with low GSM denoting hypoechoic plaques and high GSM denoting hyperechoic plaques. Heterogeneous plaques were distinguished by a pattern of at least 2 regions in the plaque area being echoically uniform, occupying at least 10% of the plaque area, and having GSM difference greater than the overall plaque GSM. Plaques that did not demonstrate this pattern were considered homogeneous.

Results.—The symptomatic status was associated with plaques of low median GSM and 88% prevalence of the homogeneous pattern. In contrast, the asymptomatic status was associated with high median GSM and 65% prevalence of the homogeneous pattern.

Conclusions.—In this cohort, symptomatic plaques were associated with a hypoechoic and predominantly homogeneous echo pattern, while asymptomatic plaques were associated with a hyperechoic and less predominant homogeneous pattern.

▶ In this study, a quantitative method of measuring echogenicity of carotid plaques is utilized through a video capturing method in combination with an Adobe Photoshop program. The authors reach the same conclusion that other investigators have also reached using more qualitative methods: echolucent plaques are more likely to be associated with symptoms. What is of great interest is whether plaque morphology analysis will eventually allow better selection of patients with asymptomatic high grade stenoses for prophylactic carotid endarterectomy. In my opinion, this will be difficult to determine. The event rate in patients with asymptomatic lesions is sufficiently low that unless virtually all symptomatic patients have echolucent plaques, it will not be possible to separate the contribution of stenosis versus that of echogenicity in determining future neurologic events.

G. L. Moneta, MD

Progression and Clinical Recurrence of Symptomatic Middle Cerebral Artery Stenosis: A Long-term Follow-up Transcranial Doppler Ultrasound Study
Arenillas JF, Molina CA, Montaner J, et al (Hosp Vall d'Hebron, Barcelona)
Stroke 32:2898-2904, 2001   3–3

Background.—Recurrence after treatment of symptomatic intracranial atherosclerotic stenosis is common, yet little is known about what factors increase recurrence risk. Thus, a prospective study was undertaken in patients with symptomatic middle cerebral artery (MCA) atherosclerotic stenosis to identify which characteristics are associated with stenosis progression and to clarify how stenosis progression relates to the development of new ischemic events.

Methods.—The subjects were 40 patients (30 men and 10 women; mean age, 62.9 years) with a first transient ischemic attack (TIA) or stroke with an atherosclerotic symptomatic stenosis of the MCA. All patients underwent transcranial Doppler US (TCD) within 72 hours of symptom onset, and the source of the TIA or stroke was confirmed by angiography. Patients were treated with antiplatelet agents (aspirin or clopidogrel; 25 patients) or anticoagulant therapy (acenocoumarol; 15 patients), according to the decision of the neurologist in charge. Patients were followed up at regular intervals with TCD for a median of 26.55 months to determine MCA stenosis progression and clinical recurrence. Stenosis progression was defined as an increase of more than 30 cm/s in maximum mean flow velocity on TCD images.

Results.—During follow-up, MCA stenosis progressed in 13 patients (32.5%), regressed in 3 (7.5%), and remained stable in 24 (60%). Progression rates were significantly lower among patients treated with oral anticoagulants (2 of 15 patients, or 13.3%, had MCA stenosis progression) than in those treated with an antiplatelet agent (11 of 25 patients, or 44%). Progression rates were also significantly lower among patients without significant extracranial internal carotid artery stenosis; of 31 patients with a normal internal carotid artery, only 8 (25.8%) had disease progression. Logistic regression analysis identified treatment with oral anticoagulants as a significant independent predictor of a lower risk of MCA symptomatic atherosclerotic stenosis progression (odds ratio, 7.25).

During follow-up, a new ischemic event (6 TIAs and 2 strokes) developed in the territory supplied by the stenosed MCA in 8 patients (20%), for a re-

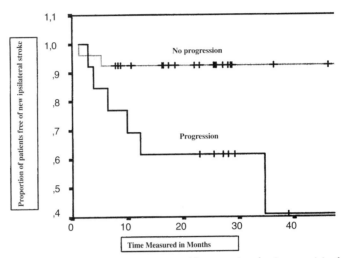

FIGURE 1.—Graph shows Kaplan-Meier estimates of the proportion of patients remaining free of new ischemic cerebrovascular events in the vascular territory dependent of the middle cerebral artery stenosis in those who showed progression of their stenosis (*lower curve*) compared with those whose stenosis did not progress (*upper curve*). $P = .0097$ (log-rank test). (Courtesy of Arenillas JF, Molina CA, Montaner J, et al: Progression and clinical recurrence of symptomatic middle cerebral artery stenosis: A long-term follow-up transcranial Doppler ultrasound study. *Stroke* 32:2898-2904, 2001. Reproduced with permission of *Stroke*. Copyright 2001, American Heart Association.)

currence rate of 9.05% per year. Overall, 13 patients experienced a major vascular event (TIA or stroke in any vascular territory, a coronary ischemic event, or the onset of intermittent claudication). Logistic regression analysis indicated that symptomatic MCA atherosclerotic stenosis progression was significantly and independently associated with a new ipsilateral ischemic event (odds ratio, 2.89) and with the occurrence of any major vascular event (odds ratio, 7.03). Survival was significantly higher in the patients whose MCA stenosis progressed than in those whose MCA stenosis regressed or remained stable (Fig 1).

Conclusion.—Symptomatic MCA atherosclerotic stenosis progression, as identified by serial TCD imaging, is a significant predictor of clinical recurrence. Treatment with oral anticoagulants significantly lowers the risk of progression compared with antiplatelet treatment.

▶ The development of symptoms associated with progression of symptomatic MCA is not all that surprising. The progression of cervical internal carotid artery stenosis is a well-known predictor of neurologic events as well. Those of us who operate on the cervical internal carotid artery often are unaware of the importance of intracranial lesions. While many studies suggest cervical internal carotid artery stenosis can be repaired without significant increased risk in patients with intracranial lesions, that does not mean intracranial lesions should be ignored. The data presented here suggest continued follow-up of intracranial MCA stenosis with transcranial Doppler is a good idea. I would not, however, make the leap to prophylactic treatment of asymptomatic MCA lesions from these data. The patients in this study apparently all had symptomatic lesions to begin with. Such lesions may be more prone to develop future symptoms than those that are asymptomatic at the time of their discovery.

G. L. Moneta, MD

Lack of Association Between Carotid Artery Volume Blood Flow and Cardiac Output
Eicke BM, von Schlichting J, Mohr-Kahaly S, et al (Johannes Gutenberg-Univ of Mainz, Germany)
J Ultrasound Med 20:1293-1298, 2001   3–4

Background.—The association between cardiac output and cerebral perfusion is not well understood. Cardiac output data were correlated with cerebral blood flow data to clarify this relationship.

Methods.—Forty-three patients with a range of cardiac performance were assessed by transthoracic echocardiography. Cerebral blood flow was determined by color M-mode measures of carotid artery blood flow.

Findings.—Heart minute volume ranged from 1.6 to 9.8 mL/min, with a mean of 4.65 mL/min. Ejection fraction ranged from 18% to 76%, with a mean of 48%. The subjects had a 15% relative fraction of carotid volume flow compared with heart minute volume. After adjustment for age, no association was found between ejection fraction, stroke volume, or heart minute volume and absolute volume flow in the carotid arteries. The relative fraction of the carotid volume flow was very significantly inversely associated with heart minute volume.

Conclusion.—Cerebral blood flow appears to be independent of cardiac output. Carotid volume flow was unassociated with the cardiac output parameters assessed in this study.

▶ In physiology, but clearly not in life, the brain overrules the heart.

G. L. Moneta, MD

Role of Conventional Angiography in Evaluation of Patients With Carotid Artery Stenosis Demonstrated by Doppler Ultrasound in General Practice
Qureshi AI, Suri FK, Ali Z, et al (State Univ of New York, Buffalo)
Stroke 32:2287-2291, 2001   3–5

Background.—Large trials have shown the effectiveness of carotid endarterectomy (CEA) in reducing the risk of stroke in patients with high-grade symptomatic and asymptomatic internal carotid artery stenosis. Candidates in these studies were selected on the basis of conventional angiographic results. Whether less invasive assessment with Doppler US could identify appropriate candidates for carotid intervention in general practice was prospectively examined.

Methods.—The subjects were 130 patients (59% men; mean age, 69 years) who were referred to the authors' endovascular service over a 12-month period to evaluate carotid stenosis. All patients were considered candidates for carotid intervention based on Doppler US; candidates were defined as symptomatic patients with 50% stenosis or greater (64 patients) or asymptomatic patients with 60% stenosis or greater (66 patients). All patients also underwent conventional cerebral angiography, and the severity of stenosis was assessed by an observer blinded to the results of the Doppler study. Results of Doppler US were compared with angiographic results to determine the former's value in identifying appropriate candidates for CEA or angioplasty with stent placement.

Results.—All patients met the Doppler US criteria for undergoing carotid intervention, but angiography showed that 22 patients (17%) had only 30% to 49% stenosis, and another 8 patients (6%) had less than 30% stenosis. In symptomatic patients, the positive predictive value of Doppler US was 80% and the false-positive rate was 20%. In asymptomatic patients, the positive predictive value was 59% and the false-positive rate was 41%. Ultimately, 60 patients (46%) underwent either CEA or angioplasty with stent placement.

No complications were observed in the 94 patients who underwent cerebral angiography alone. However, 11 of the 36 patients who underwent angiography followed by angioplasty and stent placement experienced vascular or neurologic complications. All of these complications were directly related to the larger catheters and delivery devices needed for angioplasty and stenting.

Conclusion.—At present, carotid Doppler US, as used in general practice, cannot be recommended as the sole method for identifying candidates for carotid intervention. Cerebral angiography is associated with low morbidity and high accuracy and should be performed in every patient being considered for carotid intervention.

▶ This study highlights the pitfalls of an oversimplistic approach to the use of duplex techniques to select patients for CEA. Everyone, including the authors of this study and the editors of *Stroke*, need to realize each combination of internal carotid artery peak systolic and end diastolic velocities is associated with a particular positive predictive value for predicting a specific level of angiographic stenosis. If one is going to operate for a degree of angiographic stenosis associated with marginal therapeutic benefit, a very high positive predictive value should be demanded. The combination of peak systolic and end diastolic velocities that places a patient barely into a particular category of stenosis will not be associated with an acceptable positive predictive value for operation without angiographic confirmation of an apparent lesion. On the other hand, peak systolic velocities and end diastolic velocities associated with very high positive predictive values should allow performance of CEA when the therapeutic index for the procedure is high and the complication rate for the procedure at that institution is sufficiently low.

G. L. Moneta, MD

Imaging of the Internal Carotid Artery: The Dilemma of Total Versus Near Total Occlusion

El-Saden SM, Grant EG, Hathout GM, et al (West Los Angeles VA Med Ctr)
Radiology 221:301-308, 2001   3–6

Background.—Accurately distinguishing between internal carotid artery (ICA) occlusion and near occlusion with duplex scanning is often difficult. The role of US and MR angiography in differentiating between ICA occlusion and near occlusion was investigated.

Methods and Findings.—Two hundred seventy-four patients with a total of 548 ICAs for which angiography was performed underwent catheter angiography, MR angiography, and US. Catheter angiography demonstrated 37 total occlusions and 21 near occlusions in 55 patients. US identified all total occlusions, and MR angiography depicted 92%. US showed 86% of 21 near occlusions, and MR angiography depicted 100%. Seventeen of 18 vessels judged to be patent at US were classified as having focal stenosis or diffuse disease. MR angiography was not useful for differentiating between focal and diffuse disease because flow gaps were demonstrated in vessels with both.

Conclusion.—When US is used as the initial imaging modality in the diagnosis of ICA occlusion, MR angiography can depict it. If occlusion is verified, no additional imaging is needed. US can help differentiate vessels with focal severe stenosis from those with diffuse disease. In this study, however, MR angiography contributed minimally. Catheter angiography continues to be useful for vessels with diffuse nonfocal narrowing.

▶ I agree with the implication of this study that an ICA occlusion diagnosed by US may not be an ICA occlusion—although, in fact, it usually is (37 out of 40 times in this study). A symptomatic patient with an ICA occlusion by duplex probably should have MR angiography to confirm occlusion of the internal carotid artery and avoid missing the occasional pseudo-occlusion falsely classified as occlusion by duplex. I would not extend this to asymptomatic patients with a new diagnosis of an ICA occlusion. Given the marginal therapeutic benefit of prophylactic carotid endarterectomy, I don't think the yield is high enough to justify confirmatory MR angiography in asymptomatic patients with a new diagnosis of carotid occlusion.

G. L. Moneta, MD

Transcranial Doppler in Carotid Endarterectomy

Dunne VG, Besser M, Ma WJ (Royal Prince Alfred Hosp, Camperdown, Australia)
J Clin Neurosci 8:140-145, 2001   3–7

Background.—The reduction of perioperative morbidity and mortality in patients with carotid endarterectomy (CEA) must focus on reducing the risk of ischemia, embolization, or both during the operative procedure and on preventing internal carotid artery thrombosis or embolization after surgery. Transcranial Doppler (TCD) can be used to monitor patients with CEA and detect potential problems before clinical symptoms develop, perhaps allowing surgical or pharmacologic interventions to be undertaken. The role of TCD was assessed with respect to the outcome of CEA by measuring perioperative intracerebral blood flow velocity, evaluating embolic load, and assessing the results after Dextran-40 treatment.

Methods.—In the 30 patients evaluated (age range, 46-82 years; 73.3% men), 32 CEAs were performed. Review of patients' medical records focused on flow velocities and embolic count as determined by continuous TCD monitoring of the ipsilateral middle cerebral artery. Changes in flow velocity were assessed in the light of electroencephalographic changes. When the postarteriotomy embolic load exceeded 50 counts/h, a Dextran-40 infusion was begun.

Results.—None of the patients died, but neurologic complications developed in 2 in the first 24 hours after surgery. The average drop in middle cerebral artery velocity when cross-clamping was used was 46% (percentage of the patient's 24-hour preoperative value). No uniform change in blood flow velocities from before to after surgery were found, but the mean change in absolute velocity was 16% (24 hours preoperatively to 24 hours postoperatively). Six patients required the administration of barbiturates based on electroencephalographic changes and/or TCD flow alterations. The embolic load distributions were similar in all patients until 20 to 40 minutes after closure of the arteriotomy.

When the clamps were released, patients fell into 2 groups: 1 had low or no emboli and maintained this for 24 hours; the other group had low embolic counts until 20 to 40 minutes after clamp release, then had a rapid rise until Dextran's effects began. In 29 cases, at least 1 embolus was detected, but in only 8 did the embolic counts exceed 50/h 1 to 2 hours after arteriotomy. These 8 patients received Dextran-40. With the Dextran protocol, the embolic count fell rapidly, with a mean drop of 92% (Table 4). Four of

TABLE 4.—Effect of Dextran-40 Infusion

CEA no.	Embolic Count (Per Hour)		
	60-120 Min Postarteriotomy	1 Day Postoperative After Dextran Infusion	% Decrease at 1 Day Postoperatively
1	252	12	95
2	188	14	93
3	96	9	91
4	140	10	93
5	360	12	97
6	112	20	82
7	648	12	98
8	146	16	89

Abbreviation: CEA, Carotid endarterectomy.
(Courtesy of Dunne VG, Besser M, Ma WJ: Transcranial Doppler in carotid endarterectomy. *J Clin Neurosci* 8:140-145, 2001. Copyright 2001 by permission of the publisher.)

the 8 patients placed on the Dextran protocol had systemic hemodynamic complications. All of the nonneurologic morbidity in this series was in these patients.

Conclusion.—TCD proved a useful adjunct to electroencephalographic monitoring in determining when barbiturates should be administered. The sample size is too small to make dependable estimates of any correlation between morbidity before and after TCD was used, but TCD may be able to indicate when reoperation is needed. The Dextran-40 protocol achieved rapid improvement in the embolic count but may be associated with an increased rate of complications.

▶ I admire the authors' objectivity in interpreting their results. In the conclusion of the article, they correctly acknowledge the results of this study "are of no assistance in the controversy over the best method of clamping (during CEA) for ischemic detection." Because of the difficulty and expense associated with TCD for intraoperative monitoring, its use in this regard will never be routine as long as the technology remains in its current state.

G. L. Moneta, MD

The Value of Transcranial Doppler in Predicting Cerebral Ischaemia During Carotid Endarterectomy

McCarthy RJ, McCabe AE, Walker R, et al (Royal United Hosp, Bath, England)
Eur J Vasc Endovasc Surg 21:408-412, 2001   3–8

Background.—When transcranial Doppler (TCD) is used, the need for a shunt during carotid endarterectomy (CEA) is indicated by finding a mean velocity in the middle cerebral artery (MCAV) less than 30 cm/s, a clamp/preclamp ratio less than 0.6, or a reduction in mean MCAV more than 50% on carotid clamping. TCD is used to measure MCAV, but awake-patient monitoring under local or regional anesthesia is the gold standard for intraoperative monitoring. The reliability of TCD criteria in predicting a need for shunting was assessed in patients having CEA under local/regional anesthesia, with the TCD method and awake-patient monitoring compared.

Methods.—With local/regional anesthesia used, 120 consecutive CEAs were done from July 1995 to May 2000. The patients were monitored by TCD and awake-patient monitoring, with shunts inserted if the patient experienced neurologic deterioration.

Results.—Twelve patients had cerebral ischemic symptoms develop, and the apparent neurologic deficit was reversed by the insertion of a shunt in all cases. Of the TCD criteria to predict the need for shunting, the most accurate results were obtained with the use of the mean MCAV reduction more than 50% criterion; this was 78% accurate. The sensitivity of using the mean MCAV less than 30 cm/s was 92% and that of the clamp/preclamp ratio less than 0.6 was 83%. None of the TCD criteria would have detected 1 patient.

Conclusions.—TCD appears to lack reliability in determining when shunting is required during CEA. The alert and cooperative patient remains the best and simplest indicator of intact cerebral function. TCD is not recommended for intraoperative monitoring during carotid endarterectomy.

▶ More evidence that the routine use of TCD in the operating room during carotid endarterectomy is essentially a waste of time, effort, and therefore money.

G. L. Moneta, MD

Routine Duplex Surveillance Does Not Improve the Outcome After Carotid Endarterectomy: A Decision and Cost Utility Analysis
Post PN, Kievit J, van Baalen JM, et al (Leiden Univ, The Netherlands)
Stroke 33:749-755, 2002   3–9

Background.—Recurrent stenosis may develop in patients undergoing carotid endarterectomy (CEA). Active follow-up of the operated artery therefore seems appropriate, so that repeat surgery can be done before complications occur. The costs and benefits of various follow-up strategies after CEA were evaluated.

Methods.—A Monte Carlo Markov model was designed by using a decision-analytic method. Costs and probabilities were established in a literature review. Empirical data on restenosis were used to construct a disease model to assess the efficacy of various follow-up strategies that involve duplex testing and angiography.

Findings.—For a 66-year-old patient, the mean quality-adjusted life expectancy was 6.3 years with the symptom-guided strategy, in which duplex scanning was done only when symptoms of cerebral ischemia were present. The average lifetime cost for this strategy was $5600. In this model, the cumulative stroke probability was 13%. Annual routine duplex tests performed for up to 5 years after surgery resulted in similar quality-adjusted life-years (QALYs) and probability of stroke. However, the cost was higher, at $7300. No other strategy increased QALYs.

Conclusions.—Routine duplex surveillance increases costs but not quality-adjusted life expectancy. A symptom-guided follow-up strategy is appropriate after successful CEA.

▶ This study only addresses follow-up of the operated carotid, and I think it misses 2 main points. One, it does not address follow-up of the opposite side. If the opposite side has a significant stenosis, it will be more prone to progression than if it does not, and therefore should be followed if the patient remains a candidate for prophylactic CEA. Two, the natural history of the late restenotic lesion may not be the same as for early restenosis, as late recurrent lesions are likely to be recurrence of atherosclerosis, and therefore have a more adverse natural history than an intimal hyperplastic lesion. Although this is not known for sure, it makes sense based on our knowledge of the natural history of primary lesions.

G. L. Moneta, MD

Carotid MR Angiography: Phase II Study of Safety and Efficacy for MS-325

Bluemke DA, Stillman AE, Bis KG, et al (Johns Hopkins Univ, Baltimore, Md; Cleveland Clinic, Ohio; William Beaumont Hosp, Royal Oak, Mich; et al)
Radiology 219:114-122, 2001   3–10

Background.—The properties of MS-325, an experimental IV MRI contrast agent, may make it useful for contrast-enhanced 3-dimensional MR angiography (MRA). The safety and efficacy of MS-325 for this purpose were evaluated in a phase II study.

Methods.—The study included a total of 50 arteries in 26 patients with suspected carotid artery occlusion. Patients were randomly assigned to receive IV MS-325 at a dose of 0.01, 0.03, or 0.05 mmol/kg, followed 5 to 50 minutes later by 3-dimensional spoiled gradient-recalled-echo MRA. Safety evaluation included laboratory tests and ECG monitoring for 3 days after contrast injection. The MS-325 and comparison images made with conventional contrast agents were reviewed in blinded fashion.

Results.—None of the patients experienced any serious adverse effects. At the 0.01 mmol/kg dose, the 5-minute MS-325 images were 100% sensitive in detecting greater than 70% carotid stenosis, with specificity and accuracy of 100%. Diagnostic values were lower for the other dose levels. A similar pattern was noted on the 50-minute images (Fig 1).

Conclusion.—The results suggest that contrast-enhanced carotid MRA with MS-325 is highly accurate for the diagnosis of carotid stenosis. Accuracy values of 88% to 100% are achieved by means of scans made 5 minutes

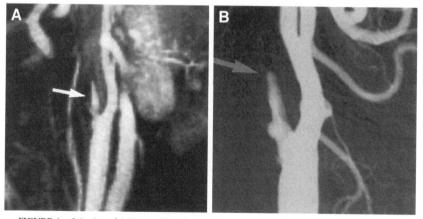

FIGURE 1.—Injection of 0.03 mmol/kg of MS-325 in a 52-year-old man. **A,** Lateral MR angiogram (21.2/2.2; 25° flip angle; 1 signal acquired; 0.7 × 0.9 mm pixel size) obtained 5 minutes after injection; anterior is to the *right*. There is complete occlusion of the internal carotid artery (*arrow*). The enhancing structure in the *left upper corner* is the submandibular gland. **B,** Corresponding lateral conventional angiogram shows similar anatomical findings; the *arrow* indicates the occluded internal carotid artery. (Courtesy of Bluemke DA, Stillman AE, Bis KG, et al: Carotid MR angiography: Phase II study of safety and efficacy for MS-325. *Radiology* 219:114-122, 2001. Radiological Society of North America.)

after injection of a 0.03 or 0.01 dose of MS-325. This contrast agent appears safe at all doses tested.

▶ Even though MRA is fairly useless in evaluating patients for possible carotid endarterectomy, that does not mean efforts should not be made to improve the procedure. Everything is potentially more useful if it is more reliable, and the MR contrast agents hold promise for providing significant improvement of all MRA images.

G. L. Moneta, MD

Contrast-Enhanced 3D MR Angiography of the Carotid Artery: Comparison With Conventional Digital Subtraction Angiography
Remonda L, Senn P, Barth A, et al (Univ of Bern, Switzerland)
AJNR Am J Neuroradiol 23:213-219, 2002   3–11

Background.—Several studies since 1996 have demonstrated the usefulness of contrast material–enhanced MR angiography for imaging supraaortic vessels. The accuracy of contrast-enhanced 3D MR angiography was compared with that of DSA for the evaluation of carotid artery stenosis.

Methods.—In a blinded comparison trial, 120 patients (240 arteries) underwent first-pass contrast-enhanced MR angiography and conventional DSA. The guidelines of the North American Symptomatic Carotid Endar-

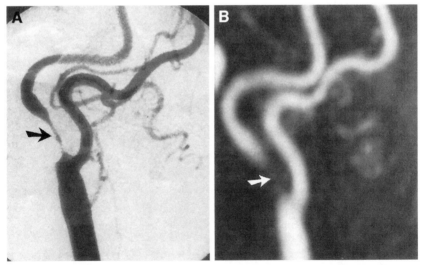

FIGURE 1.—Agreement between digital subtraction angiography (DSA) findings and those of MR angiography. DSA image of the right carotid bifurcation (**A**) shows a focal severe stenosis (*arrow*) of the internal carotid artery. The 3D contrast-enhanced MR angiographic maximum intensity projection image (magnification factor, 2) (**B**) shows the focal severe stenosis (*arrow*), correlating well with the DSA image. (Courtesy of Remonda L, Senn P, Barth A, et al: Contrast-enhanced 3D MR angiography of the carotid artery: Comparison with conventional digital subtraction angiography. *AJNR Am J Neuroradiol* 23:213-219, 2002. Copyright 2002 by American Society of Neuroradiology.)

terectomy Trial for the measurement of stenosis of the internal carotid artery were applied to maximum intensity projection images and conventional catheter angiograms.

Results.—There was agreement on the grading of stenosis on DSA images and MR angiograms in 89% of arteries (Fig 1). In the severe stenosis group, the rate of agreement was 93%. In addition, contrast-enhanced MR angiography accurately detected all 28 internal carotid occlusions and 7 of 9 pseudo-occlusions. The correlation between the 2 procedures for the determination of minimal, moderate, and severe stenosis and occlusion was statistically significant.

Conclusions.—These findings in a large group of patients confirm the value of contrast-enhanced MR angiography as a diagnostic tool in the treatment of patients with carotid artery disease.

▶ Again, contrast agents are helping with MR angiography (see comment for Abstract 3–10).

G. L. Moneta, MD

CT Angiography in Acute Ischemic Stroke: Preliminary Results
Verro P, Tanenbaum LN, Borden NM, et al (Univ of California at Davis, Sacramento; Seton Hall Univ, South Orange, NJ; New Jersey Neuroscience Inst; et al)
Stroke 33:276-278, 2002   3–12

Background.—A way is needed to rapidly, reliably confirm intracranial vessel occlusion before thrombolytic therapy. The ability of CT angiography (CTA) to determine vessel occlusion before acute stroke treatment was investigated.

Methods.—Fifty-four consecutive patients with acute focal neurologic deficits underwent immediate brain CTA. Findings of occlusion on CTA were correlated with the results of other neuroimaging assessments and clinical outcomes.

Findings.—Digital subtraction angiography verified CTA findings in 86% of 14 patients. Findings on CTA were consistent with at least 1 other neuroimaging assessment in 80% of 50 patients. Patients with CTA findings of occlusion had significantly worse National Institutes of Health Stroke Scale (NIHSS) scores at discharge than patients without these findings; the means were 14.3 and 4.5, respectively. Multivariate analyses showed that CTA findings of occlusion and admission NIHSS scores independently predicted clinical outcome.

Conclusion.—Acute CTA interpretation and subsequent imaging studies showed good agreement. Evidence of occlusion on CTA correlated strongly and independently with poor clinical outcomes. Thus, CTA provides relevant information on vessel patency in patients with acute stroke that may be of value in selecting patients for aggressive treatment.

▶ This study does not really allow for the assessment of accuracy of CTA, as there was no single standard for comparison: some CTA studies were compared with digital subtraction angiography and others with MR angiography. Nevertheless, I suspect CTA will become more widely used in the evaluation of acute stroke as CT scanners are readily accessible on an urgent basis in most hospitals.

G. L. Moneta, MD

Intermittent Claudication: An Objective Office-Based Assessment
McPhail IR, Spittell PC, Weston SA, et al (Mayo Clinic and Mayo Found, Rochester, Minn)
J Am Coll Cardiol 37:1381-1385, 2001   3–13

Background.—Palpation of the peripheral pulses is used to diagnose peripheral arterial occlusive disease (PAOD) in patients with intermittent claudication, but objective testing is more accurate. The most common noninvasive test, the ankle:brachial systolic blood pressure index (ABI), may fail to detect PAOD and may underestimate its severity unless performed with treadmill testing. Patients with suspected intermittent claudication participated in a study comparing traditional treadmill exercise with active pedal plantarflexion (APP), a simpler and more cost-effective alternative to treadmill testing.

Methods.—In a prospective, randomized, crossover study, 50 consecutive patients (100 lower extremities) were tested with both a treadmill exercise protocol and APP. The patients were 28 men and 22 women with a mean age of 71 years. Supine ABIs were measured immediately before and within the first minute after each form of exercise. The treadmill protocol consisted of a 5-minute walk on a 10% grade at 2 mph (reduced to 1.5 or 1.0 mph and symptom-limited, if necessary). The APP protocol, also symptom-limited, consisted of up to 50 consecutive repetitions of active ankle plantarflexion while standing.

Results.—The mean number of APP repetitions completed was 43, and the mean duration of treadmill walking was 3.5 minutes. Correlation was excellent ($r = 0.95$) between mean postexercise ABIs for treadmill exercise and APP. The outcome was not significantly affected by the order of testing or the severity of PAOD. Symptoms of angina or dyspnea occurred in 11 patients during treadmill exercise but in none during APP.

Conclusion.—Active pedal plantarflexion compared well with treadmill exercise for the noninvasive objective assessment of PAOD. In this series of patients, the mean pre-ABIs and post-ABIs were virtually identical (Fig 3)

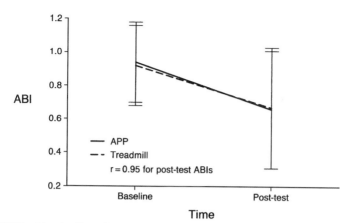

FIGURE 3.—Mean baseline and posttest ankle:brachial indexes (*ABIs*) ± 1 standard deviation for all subjects' active pedal plantarflexion (*APP*) and treadmill exercise. (Reprinted with permission from the American College of Cardiology courtesy of McPhail IR, Spittell PC, Weston SA, et al: Intermittent claudication: An objective office-based assessment. *J Am Coll Cardiol* 37:1381-1385, 2001.)

with the 2 tests. The complete APP test can be performed in less than 10 minutes and is significantly less costly than treadmill exercise testing.

▶ The authors have evaluated APP as an alternative to standard treadmill testing in assessment of lower extremity atherosclerotic occlusive disease. The test consists basically of repetitive tiptoe raises while standing. The authors imply that exercise-induced decreases in ABI may be a predictor of increased cardiovascular mortality and morbidity. While resting ABI is certainly such a predictor, there are no convincing data that exercise changes in ABI add anything to determination of resting ABIs in predicting future cardiovascular events. I therefore would not suggest pedal plantar raises as a routine part of determining the ABI. It may allow for exercise testing in a small group of patients who have normal or near normal resting ABIs, symptoms suggestive of claudication, but who are, for some reason, unable to tolerate treadmill walking.

G. L. Moneta, MD

The Value of Toe Pulse Waves in Determination of Risks for Limb Amputation and Death in Patients With Peripheral Arterial Disease and Skin Ulcers or Gangrene

Carter SA, Tate RB (Univ of Manitoba, Winnipeg, Canada)
J Vasc Surg 33:708-714, 2001   3–14

Background.—Toe pulse waves can be rapidly and easily checked with the use of photoplethysmography. Pulse wave amplitude is linked with blood flow and denotes distal perfusion. Whether there was a risk for later amputation and death in patients with arterial obstruction and skin lesions whose toe pulse wave amplitude was low was investigated. In addition, the ability

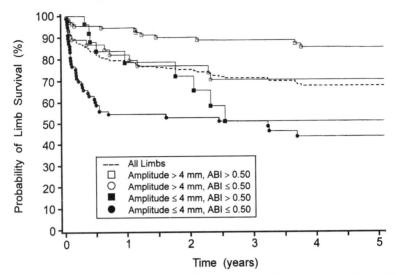

FIGURE 1.—Limb survival in whole group and in subgroups according to ankle/brachial index (*ABI*) and pulse wave amplitude. (Courtesy of Carter SA, Tate RB: The value of toe pulse waves in determination of risks for limb amputation and death in patients with peripheral arterial disease and skin ulcers or gangrene. *J Vasc Surg* 33:708-714, 2001.)

of combined pressure measurements and pulse wave amplitude to predict prognosis better than pressure measurements alone was assessed.

Methods.—Significant arterial disease was found in 309 patients (346 limbs). A subgroup of 217 patients (234 limbs) had toe pressures of 30 mm Hg or less. Follow-up ranged from 1 to 8 years (average, 5 years). Ankle and toe pressures, pressure indexes, and toe pulse wave amplitude measurements were related to risk of major amputation and total and cardiovascular death. In patients whose skin lesions affected both legs, data from the limb with more severe disease were used for death risk.

Results.—Valid measurements were obtained in 238 patients (266 limbs); 139 were men (mean age, 72 years) and 99 were women (mean age, 74 years). In 17% of the limbs, ankle pressures were 50 mm Hg or less, but more patients had low toe pressures, ankle/brachial indexes (ABIs), toe/brachial indexes (TBIs), and pulse wave amplitudes. Among the patients with severe disease, the proportions of the limbs below the cutoff values were larger in all cases. Toe pressures, ankle pressures, and pulse wave amplitudes were highly significantly correlated with an increased risk of cardiovascular death. Seventy-three limbs required major amputation, 69 required arterial reconstructive surgery, and 3 needed transcutaneous angioplasty. The total mortality rate was 66%, with 80% of the deaths attributable to cardiovascular causes.

Amputation risk was highest in limbs with ABI and pulse wave amplitude both below cutoff and lowest when both were above cutoff (Fig 1). Intermediate risk was noted when only 1 variable was below cutoff. Low wave amplitude was linked to a higher rate of amputation when the limbs had an ABI above or below 0.50. Increased risks of total death showed no significant relationship to ankle pressure, toe pressure, or ABI. A TBI of 0.10 or less and pulse wave amplitude of 4 mm was associated with an increased risk of total and cardiovascular death in all patients.

After 1 year, 62% of patients were alive without amputation, 23% had died, and 15% had had a major amputation. The mortality rate was 50% higher when the ABI was 0.50 or less and toe wave amplitude was 4 mm or less. The proportion of patients who had not died but had undergone a major amputation was approximately 3 times higher than for patients whose ABI was 0.50 or less but who had a higher wave amplitude. Similar 1-year outcomes were found among patients with an ABI of 0.50 or less and a high wave amplitude and those who had an ABI over 0.50.

Conclusion.—Recording toe pulse waves can yield prognostic information concerning both death and amputation in patients who have skin lesions and peripheral arterial disease. Combining pressure measurements and wave amplitude determinations improves the ability to estimate risks for the limb. Patients who have a high pulse wave amplitude with a low systolic pressure have a better prognosis than those with a low wave amplitude.

▶ Low amplitude toe waveforms correlate independently of ABI with risk of major (AK or BK) amputation. The authors postulate this may reflect some microcirculatory effect, but I suspect that it merely represents pedal artery disease that doesn't allow healing of local amputation.

G. L. Moneta, MD

TBI or Not TBI: That Is the Question. Is It Better to Measure Toe Pressure Than Ankle Pressure in Diabetic Patients?
Brooks B, Dean R, Patel S, et al (Royal Prince Alfred Hosp, Sydney, New South Wales, Australia; Univ of Sydney, New South Wales, Australia)
Diabetic Med 18:528-532, 2001   3–15

Introduction.—The measurement of ankle blood pressure is a simple method for determining lower limb arterial supply. Its use in patients with diabetes is questionable because of the presence of medial artery calcification. Determination of toe blood pressure has been suggested as an alternative; it is technically more difficult. The ankle brachial index (ABI) and toe brachial index (TBI) were compared in 174 patients with diabetes and in 52 healthy research subjects to guide clinicians as to when pressure measurements should be taken at the toe.

Methods.—Both the ABI and the TBI were measured by Doppler US or photoplethysmography. Agreement between the 2 methods was evaluated via the Bland and Altman method and the Cohen's method.

Results.—The mean differences between the ABI and the TBI in control subjects and in patients with diabetes were 0.40 and 0.37, respectively (Fig 2). Almost all patients with diabetes with an ABI lower than 1.3 had an ABI-TBI gradient falling within the normal range established from the nondia-

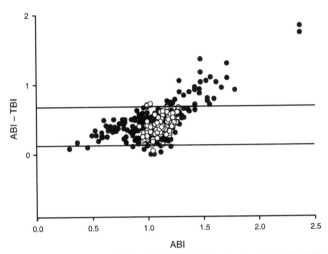

FIGURE 2.—Agreement between ankle brachial index (ABI) and toe brachial index (TBI) for diabetic patients and control subjects (control subjects: mean difference, 0.40; 2 SD, 0.14-0.67). *Closed circle*, Diabetic patients; *open circle*, control subjects. (Courtesy of Brooks B, Dean R, Patel S, et al: TBI or not TBI: That is the question. Is it better to measure toe pressure than ankle pressure in diabetic patients? *Diabetic Med* 18:528-532, 2001. Reprinted by permission of Blackwell Science, Inc.)

betic cohort. Most patients with diabetes who had an ABI of 1.3 or greater had ABI-TBI differences outside this range. When patients are categorized according to the ABI and the TBI, good agreement also exists between the tests when the ABI value is low or normal but not when the ABI is elevated.

Conclusion.—In most patients with diabetes, evaluation of the TBI has no advantage over the ABI in determining perfusion pressure of the lower limbs. Only in patients with overt calcification, which gives an ABI of 1.3 or higher, is the toe pressure measurement superior. This guideline should simplify evaluation and treatment of patients with diabetes who have disease of the lower limbs.

▶ Vascular surgeons are always amused when internists turn over an old rock and proclaim a great discovery. Proclaiming that toe pressures are most useful when the ankle vessels are completely incompressible or relatively incompressible suggests our more cerebral colleagues should spend less time thinking and more time reading vascular surgical textbooks.

G. L. Moneta, MD

Color-Flow Duplex Scanning of the Leg Arteries by Use of a New Echo-Enhancing Agent

Ubbink DT, Legemate DA, Llull J-B (Academic Med Ctr, Amsterdam; Bracco Research SA, Geneva)
J Vasc Surg 35:392-396, 2002

3–16

Background.—Color-flow duplex US is a valuable tool in the diagnosis of arterial disease of the lower limbs. The ideal contrast agent for these studies should be nontoxic, ready for IV use, capable of crossing the pulmonary capillaries, and stable enough to allow Doppler and gray-scale US enhancement. The effectiveness of sulfur hexafluoride (SF_6), an echo-enhancing contrast agent, was investigated for its possible use in color-flow duplex scanning of patients with peripheral arterial disease in whom assessment of vessel patency was difficult. Also assessed was the dosage required to give optimal images.

Methods.—The study was conducted as an open-label, randomized, dose-ranging, crossover investigation. The study group comprised 14 patients in whom assessment of vessel patency was difficult because of poor visibility or extensive calcification of the vessel wall. Contrast-enhanced duplex scanning was performed on the upper leg in 4 patients, the lower leg in 6 patients, and the pedal arteries in 4 patients after IV injection of 4 different dosages of SF_6. Findings in these patients were compared with findings from selective angiography of the vessel of interest. Contrast duration and agreement regarding the diagnosis and confidence in the diagnosis were obtained before and after administration of the contrast agent.

Results.—None of the patients experienced adverse effects from the contrast agent. A reasonable level of overall agreement (71%) between contrast-enhanced duplex scanning and angiography was reached regarding vessel patency. Nine of the 14 vessels (64%) appeared to be open when contrast was injected. This result could not be confirmed by angiography in 4 patients, and for 2 of these patients, the inability to confirm vessel status resulted from the presence of collateral vessels. All vessels that appeared to be occluded with the contrast agent were also occluded on the angiogram. The diagnostic confidence increased from 56% to 91% after contrast administration.

Conclusions.—The use of SF_6-enhanced color-flow duplex scanning can safely improve the assessment of the patency of leg arteries, particularly in settings of low flow. However, the visualization of collateral vessels on enhanced duplex scanning could be misleading because these vessels may be mistakenly identified as the vessel of interest.

▶ Contrast agents improve US visualization of vessels. I think that is reasonably well-established. The authors point out, however, that such agents also improve visualization of collaterals, and that collateral vessels may be mistaken for a "named" vessel. This is a "downside" of US contrast agents that I had not previously considered.

G. L. Moneta, MD

Should Duplex Ultrasonography Be Performed for Surveillance of Femoropopliteal and Femorotibial Arterial Prosthetic Bypasses?

Calligaro KD, Doerr K, McAffee-Bennett S, et al (Pennsylvania Hosp, Philadelphia)

Ann Vasc Surg 15:520-524, 2001   3–17

Introduction.—Duplex ultrasonography (DU) is beneficial for surveillance of lower extremity vein bypasses. Yet, DU is not widely used as part of a surveillance program for prosthetic grafts. DU was examined to determine whether it could reliably identify failing prosthetic infrainguinal arterial bypasses and whether there were differences in predictability of outcome between femoropopliteal (FP) and femorotibial (FT) prosthetic grafts.

Methods.—Between January 1992 and December 1997, 89 infrainguinal grafts in 66 patients were entered into the postoperative prosthetic graft surveillance protocol. This included clinical evaluation, segmental pressures, pulse volume recordings, and performance of DU every 3 months. Patients whose follow-up was less than 3 months were excluded unless the graft thrombosed.

Results.—Forty-seven of 89 prosthetic grafts thrombosed or failed during follow-up. Stenosis was observed most frequently in outflow arteries or at the distal anastomosis. The sensitivity for abnormal findings that accurately diagnosed a failing graft was 88% for FT bypasses and 57% for FP bypasses ($P = .04$). The positive predictive value was 95% for FT grafts compared with 65% for FP grafts ($P = .04$). The differences in specificity and negative predictive value between the 2 graft types did not reach statistical significance ($P > .05$).

Conclusion.—The routine use of DU as part of a graft surveillance protocol for FT but not FP prosthetic grafts is supported by these findings. DU should be a routine part of graft surveillance for FT prosthetic bypasses.

▶ I think this is an interesting article. I guess that's obvious, or I wouldn't have picked it for the YEAR BOOK. The authors found that prosthetic tibial bypasses usually have an identifiable anatomic reason for failure, while prosthetic popliteal bypasses often fail without obvious anatomic abnormality. There are many confounding variables in this study: the use of patches/cuffs for tibial bypasses, routine anticoagulation for tibial prosthetic bypasses, etc, that make it difficult to know whether the authors' conclusions regarding the effectiveness of surveillance as an independent variable in predicting patency of prosthetic grafts is valid. We could not do this study at our place, as we are more likely to discover oil on our medical school campus than do a prosthetic tibial bypass. Nevertheless, those performing such bypasses should at least consider surveillance in their patients with prosthetic tibial bypasses. It appears that you might actually find things to fix in these patients.

G. L. Moneta, MD

Effectiveness of Surveillance of Infrainguinal Grafts

Teo NB, Mamode N, Murtagh A, et al (Royal Infirmary, Glasgow, Scotland)
Eur J Surg 167:605-609, 2001   3–18

Introduction.—The effectiveness of surveillance programs for infrainguinal grafts has not been adequately tested. The graft surveillance program in a tertiary vascular unit was audited to determine its effectiveness in preventing occlusion of the grafts.

Methods.—Prospectively entered data of the graft surveillance database and all case notes of all patients involved in the surveillance program between June 1996 and June 1998 were examined. There were 59 consecutive patients who underwent 61 vein grafts during the evaluation period. Patients were evaluated at 1 week, 6 weeks, 3 months, and then every 3 months for a minimum of 1 year. The surveillance program included clinical examination with palpation of peripheral pulses, measurement of resting Doppler ankle/brachial pressure index, and color duplex scanning. The primary outcome measures were survival with an intact limb and patency of the graft.

Results.—Fifty-two patients (90%) were alive at follow-up, and 55 (90%) of the involved limbs were intact. Follow-up ranged from 180 to 1995 days (median, 660 days). Twenty-three stenoses were identified by the surveillance program. Of these, 17 grafts were revised and all were patent at follow-up. The other 8 grafts were occluded, necessitating 6 major amputations. The 1-year cumulative primary, primary-assisted, and secondary patency, and limb salvage rates were 63%, 88%, 88%, and 90%, respectively.

Conclusion.—Graft surveillance is useful in maintaining long-term patency of infrainguinal venous grafts. Surveillance should be performed for a minimum of 12 months and should be more frequent during the initial 6 months after the graft procedure. Aggressive revision may be helpful in grafts with stenoses.

▶ This is preaching to the choir.

G. L. Moneta, MD

Has Arteriography Gotten a Bad Name? Current Accuracy and Morbidity of Diagnostic Contrast Arteriography for Aortoiliac and Lower Extremity Arterial Disease

Schindler N, Calligaro KD, Lombardi J, et al (Pennsylvania Hosp, Philadelphia)
Ann Vasc Surg 15:417-420, 2001   3–19

Introduction.—Contrast arteriography has been challenged as the diagnostic test of choice for lower extremity arterial disease because of its related morbidity and questionable ability to identify acceptable distal outflow arteries. The experience with diagnostic contrast arteriography was examined to determine whether it should continue to be used as the diagnostic test of choice.

Methods.—Five hundred consecutive contrast arteriograms performed for aortoiliac and lower extremity arterial disease between November 1, 1994, and October 31, 1998, were reviewed retrospectively. Arteriograms combined with therapeutic procedures including balloon angioplasty, stent placement, and thrombolysis were excluded, leaving 244 diagnostic cases for analysis.

Results.—Of 244 patients, 112 (46%) had diabetes mellitus, 34 (14%) had an elevated baseline serum creatinine level, and 17 (7%) were dialysis dependent. Four (1.6%) of the 244 arteriograms failed to show an outflow vessel acceptable for bypass. Two of these patients underwent surgery, and no outflow vessel was detected. The other 2 underwent below-knee amputation without exploration for an outflow vessel. Pathology examination revealed diffusely diseased outflow arteries. One hundred twenty-nine patients underwent lower extremity infrainguinal bypass, and the remaining patients underwent procedures above the inguinal ligament, percutaneous procedures performed at a subsequent session, or no operative procedure. In all patients who underwent infrainguinal bypass, the artery identified as an acceptable outflow vessel by arteriography was suitable at surgery. There were 7 complications (2.9%).

Conclusion.—Diagnostic arteriography has an acceptably low morbidity, has an accuracy that is not likely to be surpassed by other modalities, and continues to be the diagnostic test of choice for lower extremity arterial disease.

▶ This group of Philadelphia surgeons says angiography is better than MR angiography in identifying vessels of interest. But another group of Philadelphia surgeons at the University of Pennsylvania, Dr Carpenter and colleagues, determined MR angiography is supposedly better than angiograms. I think both techniques can work well. One conclusion is that the angiographers are better at Dr Calligaro's hospital than at Dr Carpenter's. If Dr Carpenter would like to improve angiography at his facility, there is an angiographer in Portland whom I would gladly trade him for some baseball tickets.

G. L. Moneta, MD

Follow-up Evaluation of Endoluminally Treated Abdominal Aortic Aneurysms With Duplex Ultrasonography: Validation With Computed Tomography
d'Audiffret A, Desgranges P, Kobeiter H, et al (AP/HP Univ Paris XII)
J Vasc Surg 33:42-50, 2001   3–20

Background.—Endoluminal treatment for abdominal aortic aneurysms (AAAs) is being offered to an increasing number of patients. However, endoleaks, stenosis, and thrombosis occur in 25% to 30%. Thus, strict imaging surveillance after the procedure is needed. Duplex US (DU) and CT were compared in the follow-up of endoluminally treated AAAs.

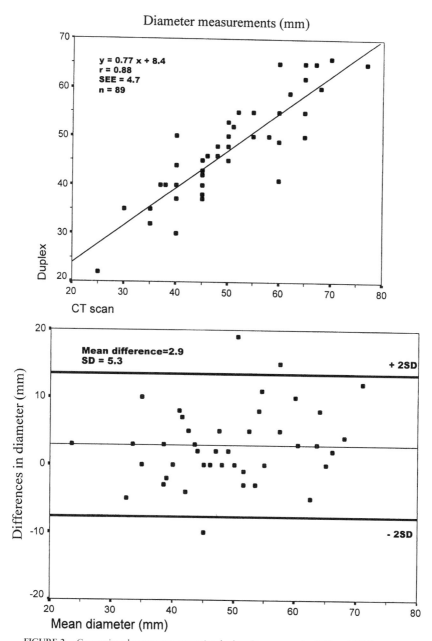

FIGURE 2.—Comparison between postoperative duplex ultrasonography (DU) and CT for aneurysm transverse diameters. (Courtesy d'Audiffret A, Desgrandes P, Kobeiter H, et al: Follow-up evaluation of endoluminally treated abdominal aortic aneurysms with duplex ultrasonography: Validation with computed tomography. *J Vasc Surg* 33:42-50, 2001.)

Methods and Findings.—Eighty-nine patients underwent CT and DU at 1, 3, 6, 12, and 24 months after endoluminal treatment. Fourteen type I and 21 type II endoleaks were identified with DU. In 1 patient, DU did not demonstrate a type II endoleak present on CT. In addition, CT did not confirm 3 type II leaks seen on DU. DU yielded 1 false-positive finding for type I endoleak. Compared with CT, DU had a 96% senstivity and a 94% specificity. The correlation between DU and CT was good according to linear regression analysis of the diameters. However, variability was high, suggesting poor agreement. The range of diameter evolution was identical in 45%, and the trend was similar in 73%. In 9% of patients, DU showed a decline in diameter, whereas CT demonstrated a significant increase (Fig 2).

Conclusions.—Compared with CT, DU is accurate in diagnosing endoleaks but less useful for measuring diameters. DU is currently a useful tool, but CT remains a key part of the postoperative assessment after endoluminal treatment of AAAs.

▶ I am not ready to recommend duplex rather than CT follow-up of aortic endografts. The trend seems to be a more conservative approach to management of type II endoleaks. This trend may be fueled more by difficulty of dealing with these leaks and their high frequency than accurate knowledge of the natural history. Nevertheless, the trend exists. Virtually everyone, however, would be concerned by an increase in sac diameter after endografting. If duplex doesn't give an accurate measurement of sac diameter trends as the authors found, better stick with CT scanning for follow-up of aortic endografts, at least for the time being.

G. L. Moneta, MD

Air Plethysmography: The Answer in Detecting Past Deep Venous Thrombosis

Kalodiki E, Calahoras LS, Delis KT, et al (St Mary's Hosp, London)
J Vasc Surg 33:715-720, 2001   3–21

Background.—In dealing with patients who have varicose veins and may be candidates for venous stripping, it is important to know the status of the deep veins. Air plethysmography (APG) offers a noninvasive and relatively inexpensive method for accurately measuring changes in the lower leg venous system (except the foot). The outflow fraction in the first second without occlusion (OF) or with occlusion of the superficial veins at the knee (OFs) can identify venous outflow obstruction, with reductions (especially the latter parameter) when deep venous thrombosis (DVT) is present. The usefulness of APG in detecting residual chronic outflow obstruction in patients who have symptoms characteristic of chronic venous insufficiency (CVI) was evaluated.

Methods.—A total of 202 patients (224 lower limbs) were referred to the vascular laboratory with indications of CVI; 41 patients (41 lower limbs) had signs and symptoms indicative of DVT but their deep veins were normal

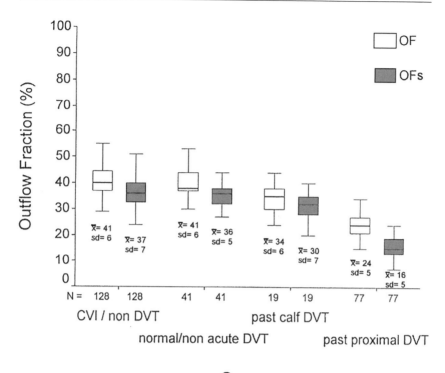

FIGURE 2.—Outflow fraction without (*OF*) and with superficial occlusion (*OFs*) at the first second. *Abbreviations: N,* Number of limbs; *CVI,* chronic venous insufficiency; *DVT,* deep venous thrombosis; *CVI/ non DVT,* patients with chronic venous insufficiency who had negative results on venograms; *normal/non acute DVT,* patients referred to the laboratory to exclude acute DVT; *CVI/non DVT* and *normal/non acute DVT,* non-DVT group; *x,* mean; *sd,* standard deviation. (Courtesy of Kalodiki E, Calahoras LS, Delis KT, et al: Air plethysmography: The answer in detecting past deep venous thrombosis. *J Vasc Surg* 33:715-720, 2001.)

on venography. All patients underwent venography and APG. The variables determined were OF; OFs; venous volume; and the minimum, median, maximum, mean, and standard deviation for each of these variables.

Results.—Venography identified past DVT in 96 patients with CVI; in 169 limbs, the results were negative for past DVT. Calf-only DVTs were found in 19 limbs; in 77 limbs, the DVTs were found at the popliteal level, or more proximally, or both. The results were significant for all 3 variables (Fig 2). The OFs was less than 28%. APG missed 4 limbs with past proximal DVT, and all of these were partially occluding the superficial femoral vein lumen. Seven of the 19 calf thrombi were detected. The sensitivity of APG in detecting past proximal DVT was 95%; specificity was 96%, positive predictive value was 92%, and negative predictive value was 98%.

Conclusion.—APG proved to be reliable and accurate in diagnosing hemodynamically significant DVT, even after recanalization of the involved vessels. This test is portable, inexpensive, and easy to perform.

▶ Not many vascular labs use APG despite tireless promotion by the St Mary's group. Most individuals doing high volume venous surgery do not use APG routinely in their preoperative assessment of patients with varicose veins. I would suggest to the authors that the next step in their work is to see if duplex can detect likely obstruction by visualization of collaterals, calcified thrombus, and contracted veins, etc. These findings could then be compared with APG values. After all, virtually every hospital has a duplex scanner, and APG machines are not that common outside of research settings.

G. L. Moneta, MD

4 Nonatherosclerotic Conditions

Residual Lifetime Risk for Developing Hypertension in Middle-Aged Women and Men: The Framingham Heart Study
Vasan RS, Beiser A, Seshadri S, et al (Natl Heart Lung and Blood Inst, Framingham, Mass; Boston Univ; Beth Israel Deaconess Med Ctr, Boston)
JAMA 287:1003-1010, 2002   4–1

Background.—Lifetime risk is the probability that a specific disease will develop in an individual over the course of his or her lifetime. Estimates of lifetime risk are available for a number of diseases, but not for hypertension. Data from the Framingham Heart Study were used to estimate the residual lifetime risk for hypertension in older adults living in the United States.

Methods.—Members of the Framingham Heart Study who were eligible for the study were free of hypertension in 1975 and underwent subsequent biennial examinations. Because the risk for hypertension increases markedly during and after the sixth decade of life, the residual lifetime risk was evaluated at the baseline age of 55 and 65 years. Blood pressure was recorded during the course of each examination, and participants were asked whether they used antihypertensive medications to lower blood pressure. Stage I high blood pressure was defined as 140/90 mm Hg or higher, and stage 2 high blood pressure as 160/100 mm Hg or higher.

Results.—During the study period (1976-1998), 1298 participants (589 men, 709 women) provided 8469 person-years of observation. The residual lifetime risk for development of hypertension was 90%. Within 10 years, hypertension developed in more than half of the 55-year-old participants and about two thirds of those who were 65 years. The lifetime probability of receiving antihypertensive medication was 60%. Compared with men in an earlier period (1952-1975), men in the 1976 to 1998 period were at approximately 60% higher risk for hypertension. Risk was similar for women during the 2 periods. A potential cause for this gender difference is the tendency for increased body mass index among men in the sample. In the more recent period, however, the residual lifetime risk for stage 2 high blood pressure was considerably lower in both sexes, a change attributed to an increased use of antihypertensive medications.

Conclusions.—The residual lifetime risk for hypertension among middle-aged and elderly individuals is 90%. The incidence of stage 2 high blood pressure has been reduced, but hypertension remains a major public health issue, which should be addressed through encouragement of lifestyle changes.

▶ Once again, the Framingham Heart Study has produced truly fascinating information. Healthy 55- and 65-year-old individuals without hypertension have, over the remaining years of their life, about a 90% chance of hypertension. It appears that virtually none of us will escape this disease as we age. Old age appears to be bad for your health.

G. L. Moneta, MD

Moyamoya: Indiana University Medical Center Experience

Yilmaz EY, Pritz MB, Bruno A, et al (Indiana Univ, Indianapolis)
Arch Neurol 58:1274-1278, 2001   4–2

Background.—Moyamoya disease (MMD), a nonatherosclerotic, noninflammatory, nonamyloid vasculopathy, is usually seen with cerebral ischemia in children and intracranial hemorrhage in adults. Optimal treatment for this disorder has still not been established. One experience was reported.

Patients and Findings.—Twenty adults and children given a diagnosis angiographically of MMD between 1995 and 1999 were included in the review. Patient age at symptom onset ranged from 2 to 54 years (mean, 17 years). Thirteen patients were younger than 18 years (group 1), and 7 were 18 years or older (group 2). In both groups, ischemic stroke or transient ischemic attack was the predominant initial manifestation. One group 2 patient had an intraparenchymal brain hemorrhage. Treatment consisted of medical therapy in 5 patients and surgical revascularization in 15. The mean duration of time between symptom onset and surgery was significantly longer for group 1 than for group 2 patients. Patients were followed up for a mean of 36 months. One group 1 patient had an ischemic stroke. Whether treated medically or surgically, patients did not differ in stroke recurrence, mortality, or modified Rankin scale score.

Conclusion.—These findings underscore the need to better understand the natural history of MMD and the clinical benefits of various treatments. Structured, multicenter, randomized clinical studies are needed to determine optimal treatment for patients with MMD in the United States.

▶ This study tries to draw conclusions about the epidemiology and severity of Moyamoya disease in the United States. The article is based on observations of patients seen at the University of Indiana, and a review of other studies of US populations. Moyamoya disease is a noninflammatory and nonatherosclerotic arteriopathy. It results in progressive stenosis or occlusion of the terminal internal carotid artery and/or proximal, middle, and anterior cerebral arteries. It is occasionally the source of a high resistance pattern in an internal carotid artery waveform obtained with duplex scanning. The authors' speculation that the disease has a different set of demographics and a different spectrum of morbidity in the United States versus Asia is interesting, although I have no idea why this should be the case.

G. L. Moneta, MD

Outcome of Surgical Treatment for Carotid Body Paraganglioma
Plukker JTM, Brongers EP, Vermey A, et al (Univ Hosp Groningen, The Netherlands)
Br J Surg 88:1382-1386, 2001   4–3

Background.—Carotid body paragangliomas (CBPs), which encroach on and gradually encase the carotid bulb, may extend along the carotid artery and involve adjacent cranial nerves— including the vagus, hypoglossal and glossopharyngeal nerves—and the sympathetic chain. The most effective treatment is surgery. A 30-year experience in managing CBPs was presented.

Methods.—All 39 patients with CBP seen between 1966 and 1997 were included in the review. The patients had a total of 45 tumors. The median follow-up was 10 years. Complication rates and long-term operative outcomes were classified by means of the Chamblin system.

Findings.—Preoperative information obtained from MR angiography and color Doppler imaging was similar to that obtained from standard 4-vessel arteriography. The median duration of surgery and blood loss was markedly greater for patients with Shamblin type III tumors. Four patients had major vascular complications, and 3 had permanent neurologic complications; all 7 had type III tumors.

Conclusion.—Staging based on MR angiography and color Doppler imaging plays an important role in surgical planning and prediction of perioperative complications in patients with CBPs. In this series, serious complications occurred mainly in patients with type III CBPs.

▶ Studies such as this are useful as pseudo textbook chapters. It is too bad that even mildly unusual conditions such as carotid body tumor can only be studied using what Dr Porter described as the "Mayo Clinic" technique of surgical research: large numbers of operations performed over many years by many different surgeons, with no consistent approach. The conclusions in this study are that good planning in the resection of carotid body tumors helps the conduct of the operation and that complications are more common in difficult operations. Who can argue with such genius?

G. L. Moneta, MD

A Clinical Trial of Estrogen-Replacement Therapy After Ischemic Stroke

Viscoli CM, Brass LM, Kernan WN, et al (Yale Univ, New Haven, Conn; McGill Univ, Montreal)
N Engl J Med 345:1243-1249, 2001   4–4

Background.—Many observational studies have linked postmenopausal estrogen therapy with a reduced risk of vascular disease, particularly morbidity and mortality from cardiovascular causes. There is concern, however, that these findings may result not from estrogen therapy but from other differences between users and nonusers of such therapy. Estrogen therapy may have beneficial effects on lipid metabolism, coagulation, and vascular tone but also may have adverse prothrombotic and proinflammatory effects. Because of contradictory epidemiologic evidence on whether estrogen use protected against stroke, increased the risk of stroke, or had no effect, estrogen replacement for the secondary prevention of cerebrovascular disease was studied in a randomized, double-blind, placebo-controlled trial.

Methods.—The subjects were 664 postmenopausal women with a mean age of 71 years. All had recently suffered an ischemic stroke or transient ischemic attack. The women were recruited from 21 hospitals in the United States and were monitored for the occurrence of stroke or death.

Results.—There were 99 strokes or deaths among the women in the estradiol group, compared with 93 in the placebo group, over a mean follow-up period of 2.8 years (Fig 2). Estrogen therapy was not effective in reducing the risk of either death or nonfatal stroke. Women who were randomly chosen for estrogen therapy had a higher risk of fatal stroke, and nonfatal strokes among these women were associated with slightly worse neurologic and functional deficits.

Conclusions.—Mortality or stroke recurrence in postmenopausal women with cerebrovascular disease is not reduced by estradiol therapy. Estradiol should not be prescribed for the secondary prevention of cerebrovascular disease.

▶ A crusty, retired anesthesiologist friend of mine endeared himself to the female operating room staff one day by declaring estrogen to be a cerebral toxin. In this study, he is proven wrong. In postmenopausal women, estrogen does not adversely affect outcome in patients with transient ischemic attack or stroke. The authors make a good case that it doesn't help either.

G. L. Moneta, MD

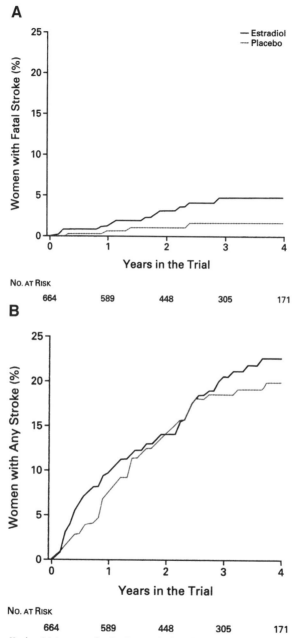

FIGURE 2.—Kaplan–Meier curves for the times to fatal stroke **A** and to any stroke **B**. $P = .05$ by the log-rank test for the analysis of time to fatal stroke; $P = .57$ by the log-rank test for the analysis of time to any stroke. (Reprinted by permission of *The New England Journal of Medicine* from Viscoli CM, Brass LM, Kernan WN, et al: A clinical trial of estrogen-replacement therapy after ischemic stroke. *N Engl J Med* 345:1243-1249, 2001. Copyright 2001, Massachusetts Medical Society. All rights reserved.)

Plasma Homocysteine Concentration, C677T *MTHFR* Genotype, and 844ins68bp *CBS* Genotype in Young Adults With Spontaneous Cervical Artery Dissection and Atherothrombotic Stroke

Pezzini A, Del Zotto E, Archetti S, et al (Università degli Studi di Brescia, Italy; Università degli Studi di Pavia, Italy)

Stroke 33:664-669, 2002   4–5

Background.—Mild hyperhomocysteinemia has been found to be a risk factor for cerebral ischemia. However, its role may depend on stroke subtype. This hypothesis was tested.

Methods.—Twenty-five patients with spontaneous cervical artery dissection (sCAD), 31 patients younger than 45 years with atherothrombotic stroke (non-CAD), and 36 control subjects were studied in the prospective, case-control investigation. Fasting total plasma homocysteine (tHcy) concentration, C677T *MTHFR* genotype, and 844ins68bp *CBS* genotype were determined. In the patient groups, biochemical data were acquired in the first 72 hours after stroke onset.

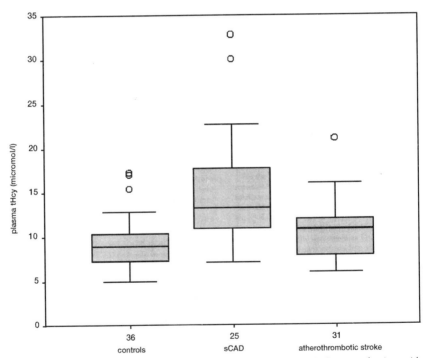

BOX.—Box plot of fasting total plasma homocysteine (*tHcy*) concentration in the group of patients with spontaneous cervical artery dissection (*sCAD*), patients with atherothrombotic ischemic stroke, and control subjects. (Courtesy of Pezzini A, Del Zotto E, Archetti S, et al: Plasma homocysteine concentration, C677T *MTHFR* genotype, and 844ins68bp *CBS* genotype in young adults with spontaneous cervical artery dissection and atherothrombotic stroke. *Stroke* 33: 664-669, 2002. Reproduced with permission of *Stroke*. Copyright 2002, American Heart Association.)

Findings.—The median tHcy concentrations were significantly greater in patients with sCAD than in control subjects. Significantly more patients in the sCAD group than in the control group had tHcy levels exceeding 12 µmol/L (Box). In addition, the *MTHFR TT* genotype was significantly associated with sCAD. The 3 groups did not differ significantly in tHcy levels or in the prevalence of thermolabile *MTHFR*. The groups also did not differ in the distribution of the 844ins68bp *CBS* genotype or in the prevalence of *TT MTHFR* and 844ins68bp carriers.

Conclusion.—These findings support the hypothesis that increased plasma tHcy concentrations and the *TT MTHFR* genotype are risk factors for sCAD. However, their role in atherothrombotic stroke remains uncertain.

▶ While human beings think, some better than others, and clearly surgeons better than radiologists, we are all ultimately a soup of biochemical reactions determined in large part by genetics. This study points out many cases of carotid artery dissection are associated with increased homocysteine levels and a genotype leading to elevated levels of homocysteine. I had always regarded carotid artery dissection as a purely anatomic problem. Clearly, there is some interesting biochemistry here as well.

G. L. Moneta, MD

Coagulation Abnormalities in Pediatric and Adult Patients After Sclerotherapy or Embolization of Vascular Anomalies
Mason KP, Neufeld EJ, Karian VE, et al (Children's Hosp, Boston)
AJR 177:1359-1363, 2001   4–6

Background.—Extensive limb venous malformations and some hemangiomas may manifest coagulation disturbances. However, no one to date has reported detailed coagulation profiles of patients with vascular anomalies at baseline and 24 hours after sclerotherapy or embolization. The coagulation status in patients with vascular anomalies who had had sclerotherapy or embolization was examined.

Methods.—Twenty-nine patients were included in the prospective pilot study. All had had sclerotherapy or embolization of large vascular anomalies. Before, immediately after, and 1 day after the procedure, measures of fibrinogen, platelet, and d-dimer levels and prothrombin time were obtained.

Findings.—Before their procedure, 5 patients with venous malformations had positive d-dimer concentrations. A subgroup analysis demonstrated an association with the type of agent used and change in coagulation status. The use of dehydrated alcohol or sodium tetradecyl sulfate was positively associated with a disruption in coagulation profiles, as evidenced by reduced platelets and fibrinogen, increased prothrombin time, and conversion from negative to positive d-dimers. However, coagulation disturbances were not associated with sclerotherapy or embolization with cyanoacrylic, polyvinyl alcohol foam particles, or platinum microcoils.

Conclusions.—The coagulation disturbances associated with dehydrated alcohol or sodium tetradecyl sulfate sclerotherapy or embolization may compromise clotting ability. Patients receiving these agents with sclerotherapy or embolization may have coagulation disturbances that could increase their risk of bleeding, thrombosis, or hematoma. Glue, foam, or coils may be substituted for these agents.

▶ Arteriovenous malformations have traditionally been treated with compression therapy alone. Increasing experience with sclerotherapy techniques and sclerotherapeutic agents has led, however, to more aggressive treatment for arteriovenous malformations. This article serves to remind us that not all sclerotherapy agents are the same, and some may actually be harmful in the treatment of arteriovenous malformations. The use of the agents described in this article that adversely affect coagulation problems should be avoided in the treatment of arteriovenous malformations.

G. L. Moneta, MD

External Beam Irradiation for Inhibition of Intimal Hyperplasia Following Prosthetic Bypass: Preliminary Results
Illig KA, Williams JP, Lyden SP, et al (Univ of Rochester, NY)
Ann Vasc Surg 15:533-538, 2001   4–7

Background.—Initimal hyperplasia (IH), a proliferative response to injury, occurs after nearly any manipulation of a blood vessel interior. Whether external beam irradiation administered immediately after graft implantation can inhibit anastomotic IH 1 month after polytetrafluoroethylene (PTFE) bypass in a sheep carotid artery model was determined.

Methods.—Bilateral bypass of the ligated common carotid artery with 8-mm PTFE in 23 sheep was followed immediately by a single dose of irradiation of 15, 21, or 30 Gy to one side. Fifteen sheep with bilaterally patent

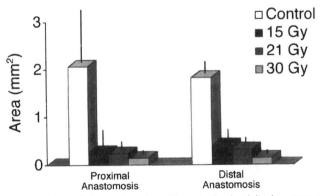

FIGURE 2.—Intimal hyperplasia area, in mm², at mid-proximal and mid-distal anastomoses. (Courtesy of Illig KA, Williams JP, Lyden SP, et al: External beam irradiation for inhibition of intimal hyperplasia following prosthetic bypass: Preliminary results. *Ann Vasc Surg* 15:533-538, 2001.)

grafts were killed at 1 month, and graft-arterial anastomoses were harvested. Computer-aided image analysis was used to measure IH areas and thicknesses.

Findings.—Graft patency was 83% at 1 month. Patency did not differ among treatments delivered. In the control sheep, IH was greatest at mid anastomosis and minimal in the native vessel. At the proximal anastomosis, 30 Gy decreased the IH region 20-fold, from 2.06 to 0.14 mm² (Fig 2). Thickness was reduced 70-fold, from 29 to 0.4 μm. Effects at the distal anastomosis were similar. Radiation treatment did not produce adverse effects.

Conclusions.—In this animal model, modest doses of radiation administered immediately after surgery in a single fraction profoundly inhibited IH 1 month after end-to-side arterial-PTFE anastomoses. No apparent toxicity resulted.

▶ Radiation inhibits anastomotic intimal hyperplasia but also results in degeneration of PTFE grafts. Since the September 11 tragedy, the US Post Office has been x-raying packages sent through the mail. Because of this, some manufacturers of PTFE grafts avoid using the US Postal Service for distribution of their grafts fearing radiation damage to the grafts. Radiation, of course, could also be toxic to the arterial wall as well. Studies such as this are interesting but demand further follow-up. Hopefully, we are not trading decreased intimal hyperplasia for an increased incidence of late anastomotic disruption.

G. L. Moneta, MD

Risk Factors Associated With Thrombosis in Patients With Antiphospholipid Antibodies
Hansen KE, Kong DF, Moore KD, et al (Duke Univ, Durham, NC)
J Rheumatol 28:2018-2024, 2001   4–8

Background.—A few theories have been proposed to explain why in some patients with antiphospholipid antibodies (aPL) thrombosis develops, but in others it does not. Among these is the 2-hit hypothesis, which holds that other acquired or inherited factors contribute to the prothrombotic state in these patients. Both acquired and inherited factors were examined to determine their association with the development of arterial or venous thrombosis in patients with aPL.

Methods.—The subjects were 99 patients (average age, 40 years; 58% women; 79% white) with primary aPL syndrome (58 patients), systemic lupus erythematosus (25 patients), or other connective tissue disease (6 patients). Medical records were reviewed to identify thrombosis and events associated with aPL, and to determine acquired risk factors for thrombosis, including estrogen use, tobacco use, hypertension, diabetes mellitus, hyperlipidemia, and obesity. Blood samples were obtained to determine inherited risk factors for thrombosis, including factor V Leiden (factor V_{R506Q}), methylene tetrahydrofolate reductase (MTHFR), and the 3' prothrombin gene (PTG) polymorphisms.

Results.—Seventy-eight patients had experienced 1 or more prior thromboembolic events, including 41 patients with venous events, 25 with arterial events, and 12 with both arterial and venous events. Acquired risk factors for thrombosis were prevalent, including obesity (body mass index of 27 kg/m² or greater) in 63% of patients, hypertension in 39%, hyperlipidemia in 38%, tobacco use in 34%, estrogen use in 19%, and diabetes mellitus in 10%. Acquired risk factors that were significantly associated with the development of arterial thrombosis were diabetes mellitus, hypertension, hyperlipidemia, and tobacco use. The latter 3 factors were also significantly associated with venous thrombosis.

Inherited thrombophilic disorders included factor V_{R506Q} in 8 patients, MTHFR homozygosity in 9 patients, and 3' PTG polymorphisms in 3 patients. None of these inherited factors was significantly associated with the development of arterial thrombosis. However, the presence of factor V_{R506Q} or 3' PTG polymorphism was significantly associated with the development of venous thrombosis.

Conclusion.—Acquired risk factors—including diabetes mellitus, hypertension, hyperlipidemia, and tobacco use—are associated with the development of arterial thrombosis in patients with aPL. In contrast, inherited (factor V_{R506Q} and 3' PTG polymorphisms) are more important in the development of venous thrombosis in patients with aPL.

▶ It makes sense that there must be other reasons besides chance that patients with antiphospholipid antibodies should have thrombosis involve the arteries in some cases and veins in others. This is an interesting first step in identifying features that may result in venous or arterial thrombi in the antiphospholipid antibody syndrome. The authors purport to be involved in a prospective study to answer the interesting questions performed by the current report. We await their results with interest, but caution as well. After all, when all is said and done, there is usually more said than done.

G. L. Moneta, MD

Early Detection of Microcirculatory Impairment in Diabetic Patients With Foot at Risk
Zimny S, Pfohl M, Dessel F, et al (Ruhr-Universität Bochum, Germany)
Diabetes Care 24:1810-1814, 2001   4–9

Background.—Foot ulcerations in patients with diabetes can be a major health problem, leading to amputation of the lower limb and lower survival rates. The mechanisms involved in producing foot ulcerations include diabetic neuropathy, mechanical stress, and alterations of blood flow, all of which interact with the microcirculation to cause a decrease in skin capillary flow. The resulting decline in skin oxygenation and the accompanying sensory and autonomic neuropathy increases the risk of developing foot ulcerations. Information about the microcirculation can be obtained by measuring transcutaneous oxygen pressure ($TcPO_2$) even in the absence of any signs of tissue hypoxia. How autonomic neuropathy, skin blood flow, and $TcPO_2$ interact remains unclear, as does the relevance of $TcPO_2$ in detecting impaired microcirculation in the earliest stages of diabetic foot syndrome. To determine potential indicators of peripheral or autonomic neuropathy, the skin oxygen supply and alterations in $TcPO_2$ for patients with type 2 diabetes with a foot at risk were assessed.

Methods.—The study included the following 3 groups: (1) 21 patients (11 men, 10 women; mean age, 65.8 years) who had type 2 diabetes and a foot that had neuropathy but no present or past ulceration (foot-at-risk group); (2) 20 patients (9 men, 11 women; mean age, 63.4 years) with type 2 diabetes and no foot lesions or neuropathy (no-foot-at-risk group; and (3) 21 normal individuals (9 men, 12 women; mean age, 59.9 years) as a control group. The $TcPO_2$ was measured at the dorsum of the foot while the patient was first supine and then sitting to determine skin blood flow. Doppler US was used to determine whether peripheral vascular disease was present. Peripheral diabetic neuropathy was evaluated with the use of vibration perception threshold, and autonomic neuropathy was detected with the use of heart rate variation at rest (supine), deep respiration, and Valsalva maneuvers, then confirmed when at least 2 positive test results were present.

Results.—Patients in the foot-at-risk group had a significantly reduced $TcPO_2$ when supine compared with those without neuropathy (no-foot-at-risk) and the control group. In the sitting position, however, no significant differences were noted between the 3 groups. A significantly higher difference between measurements of $TcPO_2$ at rest and sitting marked the foot-at-risk group. The mean sitting/supine $TcPO_2$ ratio for those with a foot at risk was 0.12, that in the group without neuropathy was 1.32, and that in the control group was 1.25. Significant differences were found between the foot-at-risk group and the other 2 groups in the vibration perception threshold and the heart rate variation coefficient at rest and at deep respiration. Patients without neuropathy and the control group showed no significant differences on these measures except the heart rate variation coefficient at deep respiration. No differences in Valsalva test results were found. The sitting/supine ratio of $TcPO_2$ was inversely correlated with heart rate variation coefficient at rest and deep respiration for patients with a foot at risk.

Conclusions.—A significant reduction of the $TcPO_2$ is found in patients with type 2 diabetes who have peripheral diabetic neuropathy when compared with patients without neuropathy and control subjects. Thus, impaired vessel autoregulation may play a principal role in producing diabetic foot ulcers. Measuring the $TcPO_2$ can identify patients whose foot is at risk of developing foot ulcerations.

▶ The message is that neuropathy associated with diabetes may place patients at risk for infectious complications through decreased sensation, but also through impaired autoregulation of skin and cutaneous blood flow. Clearly, the microvascular disease of diabetic foot problems has been difficult to prove on an anatomic basis. Functionally, however, it appears to be a real thing.

G. L. Moneta, MD

Polyarteritis Nodosa and Churg-Strauss Angiitis: Characteristics and Outcome in 38 Patients Over 65 Years

Mouthon L, Le Toumelin P, Andre MH, et al (Université Paris-Nord, Bobigny, France; Institut Mutualiste Montsouris, Paris)

Medicine 81:27-40, 2002   4–10

Background.—The clinical characteristics and outcomes of elderly patients with polyarteritis nodosa (PAN) were compared with those of younger patients to investigate whether the increased morbidity and mortality in older patients with PAN are associated with treatment or with decreased life expectancy.

Methods.—The authors retrospectively reviewed the files of 38 patients with PAN or Churg-Strauss angiitis (CSA) who were 65 years of age or older at diagnosis (20 men and 18 women; median age, 72 years), and 60 patients with PAN/CSA who were less than 65 years of age at diagnosis (38 men and 22 women; median age, 47 years). All diagnoses were made between 1978 and 1998. Patients were treated with corticosteroids and, if necessary, immunosuppressive drugs and were followed for a mean of 95 months. The type of vasculitis, clinical and laboratory characteristics, response to treatment (including treatment-related side effects), and survival were compared between the 2 groups.

Results.—Microscopic polyangiitis was significantly more common in the elderly group (44.7% vs 23.3%), while CSA was significantly more common in the younger group (26.7% vs 5.3%). Elderly patients were significantly more likely to have a history of hypertension (28.9% vs 8.3%) or atheromatous disease (21.1% vs 1.7%) and to be first seen with peripheral neuropathy (77.7% vs 56.7%). They were significantly less likely than younger patients to be seen with asthma (25% vs 5.3%). The 2 age groups did not differ significantly in laboratory test results.

Corticosteroid therapy rapidly controlled disease activity in all but 1 patient (an elderly woman with hepatitis B virus infection). Treatment-related side effects were significantly more common in the elderly patients (68.4% vs 13.3%), and many elderly patients experienced more than 1 adverse event. In particular, elderly patients were significantly more likely to experience severe infection (34.2% vs 8.3%), probably as a result of immunosuppression by corticosteroids or immunotherapy.

Elderly patients had significantly worse survival than younger patients, as 50% of the elderly patients died during follow-up, compared with 26.7% of the younger patients. Five-year survival rates for elderly and younger patients were 69.8% and 85.5%, respectively, and 10-year survival rates were 39.1% and 75.5%. Shorter survival was significantly associated with age 65 years and older and with gastrointestinal tract involvement. However, death did not occur earlier for elderly patients than for the younger patients.

Conclusion.—Elderly patients with PAN are more likely to experience microscopic polyangiitis and less likely to experience CSA than are younger patients. Elderly patients are also more likely to be seen with peripheral neuropathy and to have a history of hypertension and atheromatous disease.

Much of the morbidity experienced by elderly patients was caused by treatment-related side effects, especially severe infection. The poorer survival of the elderly patients reflected their decreased life expectancy more than an accelerated course of disease.

▶ The authors point out that elderly patients with PAN do poorly compared with younger patients, and that aging is associated with immune system deterioration. I appreciate the information regarding the prognosis of PAN patients, but I already knew from a personal series of 1 that aging is associated with deterioration of just about everything.

G. L. Moneta, MD

Risk Factors for Visual Loss in Giant Cell (Temporal) Arteritis: A Prospective Study of 174 Patients
Liozon E, Herrmann F, Ly K, et al (Dupuytren's Univ, Limoges, France; Univ Hosps of Geneva)
Am J Med 111:211-217, 2001   4–11

Background.—Patients with temporal or giant cell arteritis can have permanent visual loss, but the risk factors associated with this complication are not known. The relationship between thrombocytosis and visual loss was examined in a large group of patients with temporal arteritis.

Study Design.—The study group consisted 147 patients with biopsy-proven giant cell arteritis. At diagnosis, pretreatment clinical, laboratory, and pathology data were recorded. All patients were treated according to the same protocol. Only visual events that occurred either before or within 2 weeks after therapy initiation were included. Multivariate logistic regression analysis was used to explore the relationship between pretreatment characteristics and visual loss.

Findings.—Visual ischemic complications of giant cell arteritis developed in 28% of patients, and permanent visual loss occurred in 13%. Independent factors associated with an increased risk of permanent visual loss included transient visual ischemic symptoms and high platelet counts. Constitutional symptoms, polymyalgia rheumatica, and C-reactive protein level were associated with a decreased risk of permanent visual loss. No patients with upper limb artery involvement had permanent visual loss. Of the 87 patients with thrombocytosis, 37% had ischemic visual complications compared with 18% of those without thrombocytosis.

Conclusions.—A large group of patients with temporal arteritis were evaluated to identify prognostic factors for the development of permanent visual loss. An elevated platelet count was strongly associated with a risk of permanent visual loss in this group of patients. This suggests that standard treatment with glucocorticoids may not be sufficient for patients with giant cell arteritis and thrombocytosis. Further studies should be performed to examine whether additional therapy with anticoagulants or platelet inhibitor agents would be useful for these patients.

▶ There are 2 take-home points in this article: (1) Patients with giant cell arteritis and thrombocytosis more than 400,000 have an increased risk of visual deficits. (2) Steroids are not completely protective of the dreaded complication of blindness in patients with giant cell arteritis. The authors also point out no patients with giant cell arteritis and upper extremity ischemia had visual deficits develop. There is no reason to believe upper extremity ischemia should be protective of visual deficits in patients with giant cell arteritis. The authors' observation that no patient with upper extremity ischemia had ocular difficulties with giant cell arteritis may be merely a function of the relatively small numbers of patients studied. I still believe upper extremity ischemia secondary to giant cell arteritis deserves prompt steroid therapy in a maximal effort to mitigate the dreaded complication of blindness that can be associated with this disease.

G. L. Moneta, MD

Spontaneous Dissection of the Superior Mesenteric Artery Diagnosed on Multidetector Helical CT
Furukawa H, Moriyama N (Natl Cancer Ctr Hosp, Tokyo)
J Comput Assist Tomogr 26:143-144, 2002   4–12

Introduction.—Several conditions cause acute back pain. Described is a patient with sudden onset back pain caused by dissection of the superior mesenteric artery.

Case Report.—Male, 52, was seen for sudden onset back pain that was followed by watery diarrhea. These symptoms continued for several days, then spontaneously disappeared. Physical examination findings were normal. His history was unremarkable, and he had no history of alcohol abuse or hypertension. His white blood cell count ($11,000 \times 10^3/\mu L$) and C-reactive protein level (1.3 mg/dL) were elevated. Contrast-enhanced multidetector helical CT (MDHCT) revealed a contrast material–filled double channel with an intervening intimal flap in the superior mesenteric artery (Fig 1). The dissection extended from the axis of the superior mesenteric artery to the bifurcation of the first jejunal artery, which was verified by CT arteriography that was reconstructed by transaxial images taken with MDHCT. The initial conventional US examination was not remarkable. Repeated color Doppler US after the MDHCT examination identified the intimal flap and double channel. Dissection of the superior mesenteric artery was the diagnosis given to the patient. Because the caliber of the lesion was not severely dilated, the blood supply to the intestine was well preserved. He had no cardiovascular risk factors and was followed up conservatively without any interven-

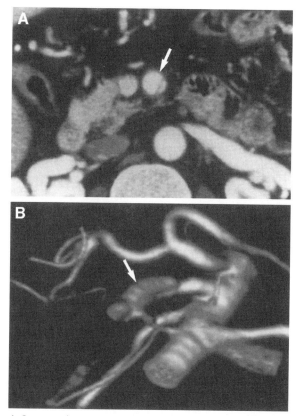

FIGURE 1.—**A**, Contrast-enhanced CT shows dissected superior mesenteric artery (*arrow*). Intimal flap is seen in the arterial lumen. **B**, CT arteriography shows the thickening of the root of the superior mesenteric artery. (Courtesy of Furukawa H, Moriyama N: Spontaneous dissection of the superior mesenteric artery diagnosed on multidetector helical CT. *J Comput Assist Tomogr* 26:143-144, 2002.)

tional treatment. At a 1-year follow-up, he had no further problems, and a CT scan showed no changes.

Conclusion.—Conservative observation can be an option in patients with arterial dissection. MDHCT can have an important role in diagnosing the acute abdomen and in guiding treatment.

► We have encountered 2 patients with isolated dissection of the superior mesenteric artery. Both of our patients, however, were symptomatic. Repair was accomplished with local resection of the flap and vein patch closure of the artery.

G. L. Moneta, MD

5 Perioperative Considerations

Hospital Volume and Surgical Mortality in the United States
Birkmeyer JD, Siewers AE, Finlayson EVA, et al (Dept of Veterans Affairs Med Ctr, White River Junction, Vt; Dartmouth-Hitchcock Med Ctr, Lebanon, NH; Dartmouth Med School, Hanover, NH; et al)
N Engl J Med 346:1128-1137, 2002   5–1

Background.—Patients undergoing certain elective but high-risk surgeries have been encouraged to choose high-volume hospitals, but the relevance of the data on which this is based has been questioned. Limitations on applicability include the use of outdated studies, the focus on state-level data bases or regional populations whose results cannot be broadly generalized, and the fact that not all procedures have been studied widely enough to yield meaningful data. Current national data (1994 through 1999) were assessed for the impact of hospital volume on operative mortality rates, focusing on 6 types of cardiovascular procedures and 8 types of major cancer resections.

Methods.—Data were collected from the national Medicare claims data base and the Nationwide Inpatients Sample. Mortality rates for 1994 through 1999 for 2.5 million cardiovascular or cancer-related procedures were analyzed using regression techniques relating hospital volume and mortality rates and adjusted for patient characteristics. Thus, the total number of procedures performed annually was linked to mortality rates in the hospital or within 30 days of hospital admission.

Results.—For the 14 procedures, Medicare claims and total volume were highly correlated (overall correlation coefficient of 0.97). Patient age and sex did not vary consistently among the levels of hospital volume, but for most procedures African American patients were more likely to undergo surgery at a lower-volume hospital than other patients. The likelihood that a patient would be admitted nonelectively at a lower-volume hospital was more pronounced in some cancer-related procedures than in cardiovascular ones. Both observed and adjusted operative mortality rates for all procedures were linked to hospital volume. A moderate attenuation of the link between volume and patient outcome was shown when the odds ratios for death were adjusted for patient characteristics for carotid endarterectomy, colectomy, gastrectomy, esophagectomy, and pulmonary lobectomy, but other procedures showed little effect. The importance of volume varied significantly with the type of procedure. The absolute differences in adjusted mortality rates between hospitals with very low volumes and those with very high volumes ranged from 2% to 5% for gastrectomy, cystectomy, nonruptured abdominal aortic aneurysm repair, and replacement of the aortic and mitral valve. For coronary artery bypass grafting, lower-extremity bypass, colectomy, lobectomy, and nephrectomy, differences did not reach 2%. The least absolute difference in mortality rates between the 2 extremes of volume was found for carotid endarterectomy, determined at 1.7% for very-low-volume hospitals and 1.5% for very-high-volume hospitals. In intermediate-volume hospitals, widely varying relationships were noted between volume and patient outcome. For several procedures (coronary artery bypass grafting, valve replacement, and pancreatic resection), mortality rates decreased with each level of increased volume; for others (elective repair of abdominal aortic aneurysm, gastrectomy, and pneumonectomy), mortality rate differences showed more variation at volume extremes.

Conclusions.—Hospitals performing a higher volume of the cardiovascular or cancer-related procedures tended to have lower operative mortality rates. Variations were notable between the absolute magnitude of the relationship and the type of procedure targeted. The quality of surgery appears to vary significantly between high-volume and low-volume hospitals for specific procedures, and patients should seek a high-volume hospital when undergoing the identified procedures.

▶ Not surprisingly, high-risk surgical procedures have lower mortality rates in hospitals performing higher volumes of the procedure in question. With respect to vascular procedures, the differences between low- and high-volume hospitals were small with respect to carotid endarterectomy (1.7% vs 1.5%), moderate for lower-extremity bypass (5.1% vs 4.1%), and more impressive for abdominal aortic aneurysm (6.5% vs 3.5%). The analysis focused only on mortality. Morbidity differences may be more dramatic. While surgeons who practice in small hospitals may find such analyses difficult to accept, the very large majority of studies examining volume/outcome relationships have similar findings. Patients and, increasingly, payers are also aware of such data.

G. L. Moneta, MD

Exercise Capacity and Mortality Among Men Referred for Exercise Testing
Myers J, Prakash M, Froelicher V, et al (Stanford Univ, Palo Alto, Calif; Veterans Affairs Palo Alto Health Care System, Calif)
N Engl J Med 346:793-801, 2002   5–2

Background.—Exercise capacity is known to be an important prognostic indicator in patients with cardiovascular disease, but whether it also predicts mortality in healthy persons is unclear. The predictive power of exercise ca-

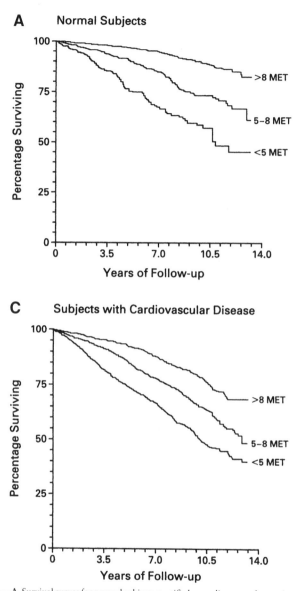

FIGURE 3.—-A, Survival curves for normal subjects stratified according to peak exercise capacity and C, survival curves for subjects with cardiovascular disease stratified according to peak exercise capacity. In all the analyses, the stratification according to exercise capacity discriminated among groups of subjects with significantly different mortality rates—that is, the survival rate was lower as exercise capacity decreased ($P <$ .001). (Reprinted by permission of *The New England Journal of Medicine* from Myers J, Prakash M, Froelicher V, et al: Exercise capacity and mortality among men referred for exercise testing. *N Engl J Med* 346: 793-801, 2002. Copyright 2002, Massachusetts Medical Society. All rights reserved.)

pacity compared with other clinical and exercise-test variables is also unknown.

Methods.—A total of 6213 consecutive men referred for treadmill exercise testing for clinical indications were followed up for a mean of 6.2 years. Of these subjects, 3679 had abnormal exercise test findings or a history of cardiovascular disease, and 2534 had normal exercise test results and no history of cardiovascular disease.

Findings.—During follow-up, 1256 men died, for an average annual mortality rate of 2.6%. Nonsurvivors were older than survivors and had a lower maximal heart rate, lower maximal systolic and diastolic blood pressure, and lower exercise capacity. After adjustment for age, the strongest predictor of risk of death in men with and without cardiovascular disease was peak exercise capacity measured in metabolic equivalents. Absolute peak exercise capacity was a better predictor of risk of death than the percentage of the age-predicted value obtained. The use or nonuse of β-blockade showed no interaction with the predictive power of exercise capacity. Each 1–metabolic equivalent increase in exercise capacity was associated with a 12% improvement in survival (Fig 3).

Conclusion.—These data confirm the prognostic value of exercise capacity for men. Exercise capacity proved to be a better predictor of mortality in this group than other established risk factors for cardiovascular disease.

▶ The ability to exercise to moderately strenuous levels is associated with increased survival, even among patients who are medically "normal." Even if you seem healthy, if you cannot exercise (ie, you are not fit), statistically you will not live as long as your neighbor, the cyclist or runner. "Just do it."

G. L. Moneta, MD

Identifying Patient Preoperative Risk Factors and Postoperative Adverse Events in Administrative Databases: Results From the Department of Veterans Afffairs National Surgical Quality Improvement Program
Best WR, Khuri SF, Phelan M, et al (Hines VA Midwest Ctr for Health Services and Policy Research, Ill; Loyola Univ, Maywood, Ill; Veterans Affairs Boston Health Care System, West Roxbury, Mass; et al)
J Am Coll Surg 194:257-266, 2002   5–3

Background.—Health care networks, payers, and other groups are increasingly requesting information on the comparative quality of care provided by various institutions and clinicians. As part of the Department of Veterans Affairs National Surgical Quality Improvement Program (NSQIP), trained data collectors prospectively gather preoperative patient charactersitics and 30-day postoperative outcomes for most major operations performed at 123 Department of Veterans Affairs hospitals. Some authorities have suggested that routine hospital discharge abstracts could be used to provide the same information at a much lower cost. This possibility was investigated.

Methods.—Using preoperative risks and 30-day outcomes recorded by the data collectors as criteria standards, the authors tested the sensitivity and positive predictive value of ICD-9-CM hospital discharge diagnosis codes in the patient treatment file. The ICD-9-CM codes for 61 preoperative patient characteristics and 21 postoperative adverse events were analyzed.

Findings.—Thirty-seven NSQIP preoperative patient characteristics (61%) were judged to have moderately good ICD-9-CM matches of descriptions. For another 25%, good data were available from other automated sources. However, ICD-9-CM coding was available for only 45% of the top 29 predictors. The sensitivity and positive predictive value exceeded 50% in only 23% and 31% of the variables, respectively. All 21 NSQIP postoperative adverse events had ICD-9-CM matches. Multiple matches were appropriate for most of these. Postoperative occurrence was implied in 41%. The same breadth of clinical description was noted in only 23%. Sensitivity and positive predictive value exceeded 50% in only 7% and 4%, respectively.

Conclusion.—Compared with NSQIP data, administrative data had a low sensitivity and positive predictive value. The substitution of administrative data for NSQIP data methods is not recommended.

▶ As surgeons, our outcomes are constantly being evaluated, questioned, and criticized. This article points out that gathering data to evaluate medical outcomes can be very problematic. "Garbage in, garbage out" certainly applies to assessing complications and risk factors in surgery. We should not accept the results of surgical outcome studies without demanding the authors prove the validity of their methods.

G. L. Moneta, MD

ACC/AHA Guideline Update for Perioperative Cardiovascular Evaluation for Noncardiac Surgery—Executive Summary: A Report of the American College of Cardiology/American Heart Association Task Force on Practice Guidelines (Committee to Update the 1996 Guidelines on Perioperative Cardiovascular Evaluation for Noncardiac Surgery)
Eagle KA, Berger PB, Calkins H, et al (American College of Cardiology, Bethesda, Md)
Circulation 105:1257-1267, 2002   5–4

Background.—The American College of Cardiology and the American Heart Association Task Force on Practice Guidelines has updated the 1996 guidelines on perioperative cardiovascular evaluation for noncardiac surgery. These guidelines—which are intended for physicians involved in the preoperative, operative, and postoperative care of patients undergoing noncardiac surgery—provide a framework for assessing the cardiac risk associated with noncardiac surgery in various patient groups and surgical situations. A detailed overview of these guidelines is provided.

Overview of Guidelines.—The guidelines emphasize that preoperative intervention is rarely needed simply to lower the risk of such surgery, unless intervention is indicated irrespective of the preoperative context. The objectives of preoperative assessment are to determine the patient's current medical status, rather than just giving medical clearance; to make recommendations about the evaluation, management, and risk of cardiac problems over the whole perioperative period; and to provide a clinical risk profile for treatment decision making that may influence short- and long-term cardiac outcomes. During consultation, the goal is to identify the most appropriate testing and treatment strategies, evaluate short- and long-term cardiac risk, and avoid unnecessary testing.

The guidelines classify evidence into 1 of 3 groups. Class I includes conditions for which there is evidence or general agreement that a particular treatment will be useful and effective. Class II includes conditions for which evidence or opinions of the usefulness of the treatment are conflicting. The "class IIa" designation is applied when the weight of evidence or opinion is in favor of a treatment's usefulness, and "class IIb" is applied when the usefulness of the treatment is less well established. Finally, class III includes conditions for which there is evidence or general agreement that a particular treatment would not be useful and would possibly even be harmful.

▶ This article is a "must read" for all vascular surgeons. It provides a logical outline of assessment of preoperative cardiac risk and, most importantly, emphasizes that coronary artery bypass grafts and coronary artery angioplasty are only rarely indicated solely "to get a patient through" noncardiac vascular surgery. Coronary procedures are indicated when the patient's long-term outcome would be improved by coronary revascularization.

G. L. Moneta, MD

Predictors of Cardiac Events After Major Vascular Surgery: Role of Clinical Characteristics, Dobutamine Echocardiography, and β-Blocker Therapy

Poldermans D, for the DECREASE Study Group (Univ Hosp Rotterdam, The Netherlands; et al)
JAMA 285:1865-1873, 2001   5–5

Introduction.—Because peripheral vascular disease is commonly associated with coronary artery disease, there is a substantial risk of perioperative cardiac complications in patients undergoing major vascular surgical procedures. Certain clinical variables and the results of noninvasive cardiac tests, such as dobutamine stress echocardiography (DSE), can identify patients at high risk. However, routine DSE is associated with high costs, among other disadvantages. One recent report suggested that the rate of cardiac complication in high-risk patients can be reduced by perioperative β-blocker treatment. The effects of clinical variables, DSE results, and β-blocker therapy on cardiac event risk were evaluated in a large group of patients undergoing major vascular surgery.

Methods.—A total of 1351 patients at 8 European centers were included in the study. Eighty-one percent of patients underwent DSE, and 27% received β-blockers. Thirty-day rates of cardiac mortality or nonfatal myocardial infarction were assessed.

Findings.—The rate of perioperative cardiac death or nonfatal infarction was 3.3%. Several clinical risk factors were identified on multivariate analysis: age 70 years or older; current or previous angina pectoris; and a history of myocardial infarction, heart failure, or stroke. Among patients with 0 to 2 clinical risk factors, the rate of cardiac complications was 0.8% for those receiving β-blockers and 2.3% for untreated patients. The results of DSE provided additional information of value only in patients with 3 or more clinical risk factors. The cardiac event rate was significantly lower for patients who did not have stress-induced ischemia on DSE. Among patients treated with β-blockers, the event rate was 10.6% for patients with stress-induced ischemia compared with 2.0% for those without. The cardiac event rate increased from 2.8% for patients with stress-induced ischemia in 1 to 4 segments to 36% for those with more extensive ischemia.

Conclusion.—For patients undergoing major vascular surgery, DSE can provide useful information on the risk of perioperative cardiac events. However, DSE offers little additional prognostic data among patients at low clinical risk who are receiving β-blockers. Thus, for most patients, DSE can be avoided and vascular surgery can be performed without delay. For patients at intermediate to high clinical risk who are taking β-blockers, preoperative DSE can identify those who may proceed to vascular surgery versus those who are candidates for cardiac revascularization.

▶ The authors have identified myocardial infarction, prior congestive heart failure, cerebrovascular accident, angina, and age greater than 70 as determinants of an increased risk of a cardiac event in patients undergoing vascular surgery. However, when such patients are treated with β-blockers, their risk of perioperative cardiac complications appears negligible. This article further confirms the value of β-blockers in vascular surgical patients. Unless there is a specific contraindication, all patients undergoing vascular surgery should be on perioperative β-blocker therapy.

G. L. Moneta, MD

Effects of an Angiotensin-Converting-Enzyme Inhibitor, Ramipril, on Cardiovascular Events in High-Risk Patients
Yusuf S, for the Heart Outcomes Prevention Evaluation Study Investigators (Hamilton Gen Hosp, Ont, Canada)
N Engl J Med 342:145-153, 2000   5–6

Objective.—For patients with a low ejection fraction, with or without heart failure, treatment with angiotensin-converting enzyme (ACE) inhibitors can reduce the risk of myocardial infarction. It is unknown whether these drugs may be beneficial in other groups of patients. The effects of ramipril for patients at high risk for cardiovascular events but without left ventricular dysfunction or heart failure were evaluated.

Methods.—The study included 9297 patients, aged 55 years or older, considered at high risk for cardiovascular events, although they did not have a low ejection fraction or heart failure. The patients did have vascular disease or diabetes as well as 1 other cardiovascular risk factor, including either hypertension, high total cholesterol, low high-density-lipoprotein cholesterol, or microalbuminuria. They were randomly assigned to receive either the ACE inhibitor ramipril or placebo; both treatments continued for a mean of 5 years. The patients were followed up for a composite outcome of myocardial infarction, stroke, or cardiovascular death.

Results.—The percentage of patients reaching the composite outcome was 14.0% in the ramipril group and 17.8% in the placebo group (relative risk [RR], 0.78). This reduction became apparent after the first year of treatment and persisted thereafter. Cardiovascular mortality was 6.1% with ramipril vs 8.1% with placebo. The myocardial infarction rates were 9.9% and 12.3%, respectively (RR, 0.74), while the stroke rates were 3.4% and 4.9% (RR, 0.68). Patients receiving ramipril also at lower risk for all-cause mortality (RR, 0.84), revascularization procedures (RR, 0.85), cardiac arrest (RR, 0.63), heart failure (RR, 0.77), and diabetic complications (RR, 0.84).

Conclusions.—Treatment with the ACE inhibitor ramipril significantly reduces the cardiovascular event rate in a broad range of high-risk patients. This study found significant reductions in the risk of myocardial infarction, stroke, and death in a group of patients without left ventricular dysfunction or heart failure. In a 2-by-2 factorial design, the study also evaluated the effects of vitamin E supplementation; vitamin E had no beneficial effects on cardiovascular outcomes.

▶ In a large prospective, randomized study, an ACE inhibitor provided reduction in morbid events in high-risk patients with a magnitude of effect similar to β-blockers, lipid-lowering therapy, and aspirin. So far, routine treatment of vascular surgical patients with ACE inhibitors is not common practice. The results of this article and early retrospective analyses, however, suggest that a daily cocktail of aspirin, a β-blocker, a lipid-lowering agent, and an ACE inhibitor may not be far off for the patient with arterial disease.

G. L. Moneta, MD

The Use of a Questionnaire and Simple Exercise Test in the Preoperative Assessment of Vascular Surgery Patients
McGlade DP, Poon AB, Davies MJ (St Vincent's Hosp, Melbourne, Australia)
Anaesth Intensive Care 29:520-526, 2001   5–7

Background.—The history constitutes a principal ingredient of a patient's preoperative clinical assessment. To evaluate cardiovascular status, both objective and subjective data are gathered concerning exercise tolerance and functional capacity. A questionnaire can be used as part of this evaluation, and the Duke Activity Status Index (DASI) serves this purpose, covering several broad areas of daily activity. Subjective assessments rely on the patient to give accurate data. The ease and applicability of administering the DASI to determine functional capacity were tested, the reliability of the responses was evaluated by seeking the opinion of someone who knew the patient well, the applicability of a simple ward exercise test to the participants was assessed, and the results of the patient's questionnaire were compared with his or her ability to perform the test.

Methods.—Preoperative interviews were conducted with 100 consecutive elective vascular surgery patients using a modified DASI questionnaire. Reliability was assessed by administering the questionnaire to the patient's closest available relative. Next, the patient walked up 2 flights of stairs, with time to complete the task or reason for failing noted.

Results.—Language difficulties prevented 2 patients from completing the questionnaire, and no next-of-kin questionnaires were available for 7 patients. A statistically significant correlation was found between the scores obtained from the patients and those from the next of kin. Forty-one patients did not attempt the ward test, and 15 discontinued it after only a single flight of stairs. For the 3 groups (able to perform test, ceasing test, and not attempting test), DASI scores from the patient and the next of kin were statistically different. Time to perform the task and score on the DASI showed an inverse correlation. Thirteen of 68 patients who said they could climb a flight of stairs could not do so; many patients could not perform exercise at a Metabolic Equivalent (MET) value of 4 METS. This threshold has been used to indicate when further noninvasive cardiac testing is required before a patient undergoes various surgical procedures.

Conclusions.—The DASI was considered fairly easy to administer and showed good correlation between patient and next-of-kin responses. Scores in response to the exercise test were statistically different between the groups. There were major differences found between what an individual claimed to be able to do and what they could actually do.

▶ Questionnaires purporting to assess functional assessment in vascular surgical patients are popping up like toadstools in spring. By and large, the results of this study suggest that while the Duke Activity Status Index is easily administered to patients, the results are not very reliable in vascular patients. A lot of questions remain about questionnaires.

G. L. Moneta, MD

Advantages of Exercise Echocardiography in Comparison to Dobutamine Echocardiography in the Diagnosis of Coronary Artery Disease in Hypertensive Subjects

Pasierski T, Szwed H, Malczewska B, et al (Natl Inst of Cardiology, Warszawa, Poland)
J Hum Hypertens 15:805-809, 2001   5–8

Background.—Diagnosing coronary artery disease in hypertensive persons is often difficult. The efficacy and safety of 2 stress echocardiography methods—exercise and dobutamine—for this purpose were reported.

Methods.—One hundred ninety-seven treated hypertensive patients (mean age, 53 years) were included in the prospective study. None had a history of myocardial infarction. All had been referred for coronary angiography and underwent exercise ECG, exercise, and dobutamine echocardiography.

Findings.—The sensitivies of exercise ECG, exercise echocardiography, and dobutamine echocardiography were 77%, 82%, and 75%, respectively. These values did not differ significantly. The negative predictive value of exercise ECG was 64%, significantly lower than that of exercise echocardiography, at 79%. The specificity and positive predictive value of exercise ECG were substantially lower than those of exercise and dobutamine echocardiography. Echocardiographic left ventricular hypertrophy did not influence the specificity or sensitivity of these diagnostic methods. Dobutamine infusion was more frequently associated with marked arterial blood pressure increase or decline than was exercise (7% and 2%, respectively) and with simple ventricular ectopy (15.7% and 6.1%, respectively).

Conclusion.—Both stress echo methods were significantly more specific than was exercise ECG in these hypertensive patients. Maximal exercise produces fewer adverse effects than dobutamine infusion. Thus, exercise echocardiography may be preferred for diagnosing angina in hypertensive patients.

▶ We continue to believe that the use of exercise testing and echocardiography to detect the presence of coronary artery disease in vascular surgical patients is a waste of time and money. An approach of assuming all vascular patients have coronary artery disease and treating them as such, reserving detailed evaluation for specific clinical markers of coronary artery disease (see Abstracts 5–4 and 5–5) seems to make the most sense.

G. L. Moneta, MD

Tolerability of β-Blocker Initiation and Titration in the Metoprolol CR/XL Randomized Intervention Trial in Congestive Heart Failure (MERIT-HF)

Gottlieb SS, and the MERIT-HF Investigators (Univ of Maryland, Baltimore; et al)

Circulation 105:1182-1188, 2002

5–9

Introduction.—β-Blockade improves survival, decreases hospitalizations for heart failure, and improves left ventricular function when administered over a long period of time to patients with heart failure. Concern exists that β-blockade may cause a deterioration in a patient's heart condition when the therapy is initiated. It is recommended that drugs be initiated at low doses and slowly titrated to effective doses.

Methods and Findings.—Data from the Metoprolol CR/XL Randomized Intervention Trial in Congestive Heart Failure, a randomized, double-blind, placebo-controlled trial of the controlled-release/extended release (CR/XL) formulation of metoprolol succinate in 3993 patients with heart failure, were used to ascertain which patients were at risk of deterioration and for what period after β-blocker initiation. The events and symptoms during the initial 90 days were examined. When the 5 subgroups were analyzed (patients with New York Heart Association [NYHA] class II status, III/IV status, or III/IV status with an ejection fraction below 0.25; patients with a heart rate of 76 beats/min or lower; and patients with systolic blood pressure of 120 mm Hg or lower), the Kaplan-Meier curves for the combined end point of all-cause mortality/all-cause hospitalization were similar in all patients; no significant differences were found in favor of placebo at any visit or in any of the analyzed subgroups. At 60 days, the curves began to diverge in favor of β-blockade. A low heart rate was the most common factor that limited titration. In NYHA class III/IV, 5.9% of patients randomly assigned to placebo discontinued the study medication during the initial 90 days versus 8.1% of those who received metoprolol CR/XL ($P = .037$ unadjusted); for those with NYHA class III/IV and an ejection fraction lower than 0.25, these rates were 7.1% and 8.0%, respectively ($P = $ NS). From 90 days until completion of the trial, more patients in the placebo group discontinued the study medication in all subgroups. No changes occurred in diuretic or angiotensin-converting enzyme inhibitor dosing with β-blocker titration. Most patients did not experience a change in the symptoms of breathlessness or fatigue during the titration phase.

Conclusion.—When carefully titrated, metoprolol CR/XL can be safely administered to most patients with stable to moderate heart failure, and minimal deterioration and few side effects occur.

▶ Since the benefits of perioperative β-blocker therapy are well-established in vascular surgical patients, this study should reassure us that extension of such therapy to patients with stable to moderate congestive heart failure is reasonable in an effort to prevent perioperative cardiac complications.

G. L. Moneta, MD

Association Between Heart Rate Variability Recorded on Postoperative Day 1 and Length of Stay in Abdominal Aortic Surgery Patients

Stein PK, Schmieg RE Jr, El-Fouly A, et al (Washington Univ, St Louis; Barnes-Jewish Hosp, St Louis)
Crit Care Med 29:1738-1743, 2001   5–10

Background.—Researchers have investigated the role of heart rate variability (HRV) as a marker of clinical status and as a predictor of outcomes in the ICU. The ability of HRV measured in the surgical ICU on the first postoperative day to predict clinical outcome in patients undergoing abdominal aortic surgery was investigated.

Methods.—One hundred six patients admitted to the ICU after abdominal aortic surgery were included in the prospective study. Twenty-four-hour Holter recordings were analyzed. Clinical and demographic data from medical records were also analyzed. A short length of stay (LOS) was defined as 7 days or fewer, and a long LOS as more than 7 days.

Findings.—Patients with a long LOS had increased heart rates and reduced short- and intermediate-term HRV. However, there was no difference in overall HRV, which primarily reflects circadian rhythm. Factors independently predicting LOS were advanced age, insulin-dependent diabetes, and reduced HRV.

Conclusion.—Increased heart rate and reduced intermediate-term HRV indexes determined on postoperative day 1 independently predicted complicated recovery. The strongest HRV predictors of outcome were natural logarithm very low frequency power assessed for 24 hours and during the day.

▶ This is an example of a study that is outdated prior to publication. Apparently patients were not routinely β-blocked before operation, a standard in our practice.

G. L. Moneta, MD

The Clinical Course of New-Onset Atrial Fibrillation After Elective Aortic Operations

Valentine RJ, Rosen SF, Cigarroa JE, et al (Univ of Texas, Dallas)
J Am Coll Surg 193:499-504, 2001   5–11

Introduction.—The onset of atrial fibrillation (AFIB) postoperatively has been linked with increased morbidity and mortality for patients undergoing noncardiothoracic surgeries. The incidence, associated complications, and outcomes of AFIB after aortic surgeries were analyzed in 211 consecutive patients.

Methods.—The medical records of all patients undergoing elective aortic surgeries between 1994 and 2000 were analyzed retrospectively. All patients underwent postoperative continuous ECG monitoring and routine cardiac enzyme determinations in the ICU for a mean of 6 days after onset. Follow-up data were collected from a review of both outpatient office visit records and the computerized medical center database system.

Results.—Of 211 patients who underwent elective procedures, 22 (10%) developed AFIB at a mean of 2 days after surgery, and the AFIB lasted for a mean of 4 days after onset. Of these 22 patients, 16 reverted back to normal sinus rhythm, 3 needed cardioversion (2 chemical, 1 electrical), and 3 continued to experience AFIB at discharge. Four patients experienced additional cardiac complications: antecedent myocardial infarction (MI) in 3 (14%) and sustained cardiogenic shock necessitating electrical cardioversion in 1. The incidence of MI in the 189 remaining patients was 4% (nonsignificant). No deaths in the AFIB group occurred, and none suffered embolization. All patients had normal sinus rhythm on ECG obtained at a mean of 14 months after discharge. Patients with and without AFIB did not differ in the mean duration of ICU stay (6 days), total length of hospital stay (10 days), or hospital mortality rate. Patients with AFIB were older (71 vs 66 years; $P = .016$). No significant between-group differences were noted in sex or use of β-blockers.

Conclusion.—Atrial fibrillation is not uncommon after aortic surgery. It is not correlated with increased morbidity, mortality, or length of hospital stay. A minority of affected patients may experience other cardiac complications, including MI; these complications are typically recognized before the onset of AFIB. The outcome of aortic surgery is not affected by AFIB. Most patients revert spontaneously to normal sinus rhythm and do not need long-term anticoagulation to prevent thromboembolic complications.

▶ I have never regarded new-onset AFIB occurring in the perioperative period as a significant problem, provided it was not associated with ischemic changes, hemodynamic instability, or significant tachycardia. Results of this study do not, however, mean that perioperative AFIB should not be treated, only that the long-term prognosis for eventual sinus rhythm is excellent.

G. L. Moneta, MD

Routine Perioperative Pulmonary Artery Catheterization Has No Effect on Rate of Complications in Vascular Surgery: A Meta-analysis

Barone JE, Tucker JB, Rassias D, et al (Stamford Hosp, Conn; Columbia Univ, New York)
Am Surg 67:674-679, 2001   5–12

Background.—Despite 3 decades of experience with the pulmonary artery (PA) catheter, there is no agreement regarding its appropriate use. A meta-analysis was undertaken to determine whether preoperative PA catheters reduce complications or mortality after vascular surgery.

Methods.—The authors reviewed MEDLINE and relevant bibliographies to identify appropriate articles regarding PA catheters. Only randomized prospective studies with specific therapeutic goals that involved patients undergoing vascular surgery and that were published in English were eligible for inclusion. The primary outcomes of interest were mortality and complications that were caused by or could have been prevented by a preoperative PA catheter.

Results.—Only 4 articles met the inclusion criteria; these 4 articles comprised 211 patients who received a preoperative PA catheter. There were 174 controls. All 4 studies excluded patients who had had a myocardial infarction within 3 months, who had undergone coronary artery bypass grafting within 6 months, or who had uncompensated congestive heart failure or unstable angina. Meta-analysis indicated that the PA catheter and control groups did not differ significantly in either mortality rates or in complications related to the PA catheter.

In a separate analysis, the authors extracted data from 3 of these 4 studies and from 2 others that did not meet the strict inclusion criteria for the meta-analysis but did include information on IV fluid administration. In 3 of these 5 studies, the amount of IV fluid administered was significantly higher in patients who underwent PA catheterization than it was in the controls.

Conclusion.—This meta-analysis could find no significant benefit of routine preoperative PA catheterization for either mortality or complications when used with moderate-risk patients undergoing vascular surgery. PA catheterization does, however, appear to increase the need for IV fluids in these patients. Based on these findings, the routine use of preoperative PA catheterization in moderate-risk patients undergoing vascular surgery is not justified.

"You cannot ask us to take sides against arithmetic."

Winston Churchill

G. L. Moneta, MD

Impact of Perioperative Haemodynamic Monitoring on Cardiac Morbidity After Major Vascular Surgery in Low Risk Patients: A Randomised Pilot Trial

Bonazzi M, Gentile F, Biasi GM, et al (Bassini Hosp, Milano, Italy; Univ of Milano-Bicocca, Italy)

Eur J Vasc Surg 23:445-451, 2002   5–13

Introduction.—The use of perioperative hemodynamic optimization through pulmonary artery catheter (PAC) monitoring to improve patient outcome from infrarenal abdominal aortic surgery is limited by available ICU resources and the lack of supportive evidence. The rate of major cardiac complications after abdominal aneurysmectomy for patients without clinical and echocardiographic evidence of coronary artery disease was investigated.

Methods.—The study included 100 consecutive patients younger than 75 years who were asymptomatic for angina and arrhythmias and had an ejection fraction of 50% or more. In addition, the patients had no evidence of left ventricular wall motion abnormalities at preoperative transthoracic echocardiography at rest. Patients were randomly assigned to either hemodynamic optimization through the use of a PAC (cardiac index > 3.01 L/min per m², pulmonary wedge pressure > 10 and < 18 mm Hg, systemic vascular resistance < 1450 dyne/s/cm⁻⁵, oxygen delivery > 600 mL/min per m²), or conventional treatment. The Acute Physiology and Chronic Health Evaluation was used to assess preoperative illness severity, and the Sequential Organ Failure Assessment was used to describe postoperative individual organ dysfunction/failure in a continuous form. Both groups underwent periodic postoperative ECGs and measurements of lactic dehydrogenase, creatine phosphokinase, MB isoenzyme, AST, and ALT. The primary outcome variable was cardiovascular morbidity rate.

Results.—At preoperative hemodynamic assessment, 35 patients did not need any intervention, 10 patients on chronic diuretic therapy for hypertension underwent volume loading alone, and 5 needed additional inotropic treatment at low doses. After declamping, no episodes of arterial hypotension that needed pharmacologic treatment in the patient group occurred; 6 control subjects required volume load and/or inotropic drugs ($P < .05$). For both groups, no in-hospital death, non-fatal myocardial infarction, or postoperative renal failure occurred. Groups were similar in duration of hospital stay. Patients in the control group tended to have a slightly higher rate (nonsignificant) of individual cardiac events.

Conclusion.—This pilot investigation showed no benefit to hemodynamic optimization for patients who were free of cardiac artery disease.

▶ I regard this article as "old news." Just because a study is randomized and prospective does not mean it is useful. It must have been a slow month at the *European Journal of Surgery.*

G. L. Moneta, MD

Normal Saline Versus Lactated Ringer's Solution for Intraoperative Fluid Management in Patients Undergoing Abdominal Aortic Aneurysm Repair: An Outcome Study
Waters JH, Gottlieb A, Schoenwald P, et al (Cleveland Clinic Found, Ohio)
Anesth Analg 93:817-822, 2001   5–14

Background.—The only previous study of differences in patients resuscitated with normal saline (NS) infusion compared with those resuscitated with lactated Ringer's (LR) solution was done in a patient population of young, previously healthy soldiers, which represents a group quite different from those usually seen in hospitals. An infusion containing 0.9% NS has been shown to lead to the development of metabolic hyperchloremic acidosis, promoting the hypothesis that NS may adversely affect patient outcome. The validity of this hypothesis was tested.

Methods.—The test included 2 groups of patients (33 in each group) who were undergoing aortic surgery and were considered particularly vulnerable to the detrimental effects of NS solutions. The patients were randomly assigned to receive either LR or NS as the primary resuscitating agent. The 2 groups showed no differences in demographic data or incidence of chronic disease (except hypertension). Of those receiving NS solutions, 29 had infrarenal repairs; 1, suprarenal; and 3, thoracoabdominal. Of the LR group, 30 repairs were infrarenal; 1, suprarenal; and 2, thoracoabdominal. All patients were monitored with arterial and central venous catheters, and pulmonary arterial catheters were placed as needed. Standard anesthetic and fluid management protocols were followed, and patient outcome was determined according to several measures (ventilation time, ICU length of stay, hospital stay).

Results.—No differences were noted in the volume of crystalloid fluids administered to the 2 groups, but the NS group required more transfused platelets than the LR group. Overall, the LR group had significantly less blood product exposure than the NS group. The preoperative values for pH, base excess, serum bicarbonate concentration, Na^+, and Cl^- differed significantly from those obtained postoperatively. No differences were noted between the 2 groups for postoperative complications, death, ventilator time, time in the intensive care unit (ICU), or hospital stay. The amount of furosemide used operatively and postoperatively was also the same for both groups. A significant difference in volume of bicarbonate was noted for the groups during the operative time, but this did not extend to the postoperative period. Ventilation time was predicted by amount of diuretic use, β-adrenergic blocker use, and patient age; surgical ICU time was predicted only by the presence of chronic obstructive pulmonary disease; and hospital length of stay was predicted by asthma and age more than 65 years. These times showed no correlation with type of crystalloid fluid used.

Conclusions.—Hyperchloremic metabolic acidosis developed in patients in the NS group, whereas it did not occur in patients in the LR group; however, few differences were noted in clinical outcome measures. More blood products were transfused in those receiving the NS solution than the LR solution, suggesting that NS should not be the first choice for procedures producing a large blood loss.

▶ The problem of NS-induced hyperkalemic acidosis is well recognized by virtually any surgical intern. I don't understand why the NS-treated patients had more use of blood products than the LR-treated patients; but apparently they did. Overall, LR appears superior to NS for fluid management in patients undergoing open abdominal aortic aneurysm repair.

G. L. Moneta, MD

Autologous Versus Allogeneic Transfusion in Aortic Surgery: A Multicenter Randomized Clinical Trial

McCollum CN, for the ATIS Investigators (Wythenshawe Hosp, Manchester, England)

Ann Surg 235:145-151, 2002

5–15

Background.—The costs of blood preparations have risen sharply in the United Kingdom in recent years as a result of concerns over the risks of transfusion-related infection, including transmission of HIV, hepatitis C, and spongiform encephalopathies. As a result of these concerns, British donor plasma is no longer used for fractionation, and nucleic acid testing for hepatitis C is required for all plasma components, with leukodepletion for all cellular products. The rising costs associated with the use of allogeneic blood, as well as immune consequences and risks of surgical bleeding associated with allogeneic blood transfusion, have made autologous transfusion more attractive. This study evaluated the efficacy of acute normovolemic hemodilution (ANH) and intraoperative cell salvage (ICS) in blood-conservation strategies for infrarenal aortic surgery.

Methods.—In a multicenter prospective randomized trial, standard transfusion practice was compared with autologous transfusion that combined ANH with ICS. The study group comprised 145 patients undergoing elective aortic surgery. The primary outcome measures were the proportion of patients who required allogeneic blood and the volume of allogeneic transfusion. The secondary outcome measures were the frequency of complications, including postoperative infection, and the length of hospital stay postoperatively. Fifty-six percent of patients underwent allogeneic transfusion, and 43% underwent autologous transfusion.

Results.—The use of a combination of ANH and ICS reduced the volume of allogeneic blood transfused from a median of 2 units to a median of 0 units. There were no differences between the 2 groups in terms of complications or the length of postoperative hospital stay.

Conclusion.—Both acute ANH and ICS were found to be safe and effective in reducing the requirement for allogeneic blood in patients undergoing elective infrarenal aortic surgery.

► Allogeneic blood transfusion can be reduced in aortic surgery patients with a combination of acute hemodilution and intraoperative cell salvage. The details of this article are, however, important. Patients with large blood volumes and high preoperative hemoglobin levels and those undergoing surgery for occlusive disease are less likely to benefit from hemodilution and cell salvage. On our vascular surgical service, we use cell savers primarily for more complex aortic aneurysm procedures.

G. L. Moneta, MD

The Effect of Changing Transfusion Practice On Rates of Perioperative Stroke and Myocardial Infarction in Patients Undergoing Carotid Endarterectomy: A Retrospective Analysis of 1114 Mayo Clinic Patients

Waggoner JR III, for the Mayo Perioperative Outcomes Group (Mayo Clinic, Rochester, Minn)

Mayo Clin Proc 76:376-383, 2001   5–16

Background.—Both stroke and myocardial infarction (MI) can occur in patients who undergo carotid endarterectomy (CEA). Patients who undergo perioperative blood transfusions are also at risk of hemolytic, allergic, or febrile reactions; immunomodulation; and the transmission of infectious microorganisms (eg, HIV). To avoid these potential complications, changes in transfusion practices have been made for patients undergoing CEA at the Mayo Clinic in Rochester, Minn. To evaluate the effectiveness of these changes and their effect on neurologic and cardiac morbidity rates, a retrospective study was done.

Methods.—The association between perioperative transfusion practice and the occurrence of stroke or MI in an early practice group of 552 patients who had CEA between 1980 and 1985, a period before HIV screening, was compared with the same association in a recent-practice group of 562 patients having CEA between 1990 and 1995. The χ^2 test for categorical variables and a rank sum test for continuous variables were used, together with logistic regression to evaluate any relationship between perioperative transfusion practice and the occurrence of stroke or MI.

Results.—Significantly older patients (mean age, 69.6 years) were among those in the recent-practice group than in the early practice group (mean age, 65.9 years). Patients scoring a Sundt neurologic grade 3 or 4 were found more often in the recent-practice group than in the early practice group. In addition, the recent-practice group had a significantly higher frequency of patients with American Society of Anesthesiologists (ASA) physical status scores of 3 or 4, diabetes mellitus, mitral valve disease, ischemic heart disease, and previous cardiac revascularization procedures. A significantly lower frequency of current smokers and heparin use before surgery along with significantly lower hemoglobin concentrations measured perioperatively were also noted among the recent-practice patients. The recent-practice group received significantly fewer transfusions of red blood cells (RBCs) at all phases of the CEA. Preoperatively, these patients had a 75% decrease in percentage transfused; intraoperatively, they had a 96% decrease; postoperatively, they had a 64% decrease; and overall, they had an 88% decrease. No significant differences, however, in the rates of stroke or MI occurring perioperatively were found between the 2 groups. On both univariate and multivariate analysis, higher preoperative Sundt grade, preoperative heparin use, and RBC transfusion perioperatively were significantly associated with perioperative stroke. Those factors associated with perioperative MI on univariate analysis were older age, higher Sundt grade, higher ASA physical status score, and use of preoperative heparin. Older age, higher Sundt grade, and current smoking status were linked with perioperative MI on multivariate analysis.

Conclusions.—Despite the change in transfusion practice and the performance of CEA in older patients with more significant comorbidity rates, patients in both the recent-practice and early practice groups had similar frequencies of perioperative stroke and MI. The majority of those in the early practice group received RBC transfusions in the intraoperative period, whereas the majority of those in the recent-practice group received the transfusions postoperatively. Overall, no increased risk of cerebral or cardiac ischemia accompanied modest perioperative anemia for patients having CEA.

▶ Another argument for less blood transfusions in our vascular surgical patients (see also Abstract 5–15).

G. L. Moneta, MD

Daily Hemodialysis and the Outcome of Acute Renal Failure
Schiffl H, Lang SM, Fischer R (Universität München, Munich)
N Engl J Med 346:305-310, 2002   5–17

Background.—Although intermittent hemodialysis is commonly used as a renal-replacement therapy for acute renal failure, an adequate dose has not been established. The effect of daily intermittent hemodialysis was compared with that of conventional, alternate-day intermittent hemodialysis for patients with acute renal failure in a prospective study.

Methods.—The study included 160 patients with acute renal failure who were randomly assigned to daily or conventional intermittent hemodialysis. The 2 groups were comparable in age, sex, cause, severity of acute renal failure, medical or surgical intensive care setting, and Acute Physiology, Age, and Chronic Health Evaluation scores.

Findings.—Compared with conventional hemodialysis, daily hemodialysis produced better control of uremia, fewer hypotensive episodes during hemodialysis, and faster resolution of acute renal failure. According to the intention-to-treat analysis, the mortality rate for patients receiving daily dialysis was 28%, compared with 46% for those receiving alternate-day dialysis. Multiple regression analysis identified less frequent hemodialysis as an independent risk factor for death.

Conclusions.—Critically ill patients with acute renal failure requiring renal-replacement therapy have a high death rate. This high mortality rate is associated with coexisting conditions and uremic damage to other organ systems. Intensive hemodialysis decreases the mortality rate in this patient population without increasing hemodynamically induced morbidity.

▶ This is another in a series of articles in this year's YEAR BOOK that should have a profound impact on the care of our patients in the ICU. The authors have found patients with acute renal failure who require dialysis that daily dialysis improves outcomes without increasing hemodynamic instability. These results should be taken seriously. Any improvement in the care of these seriously ill patients is welcome.

G. L. Moneta, MD

Intensive Insulin Therapy in Critically Ill Patients
Van den Berghe G, Wouters P, Weekers F, et al (Catholic Univ of Leuven, Belgium)
N Engl J Med 345:1359-1367, 2001   5–18

Background.—Hyperglycemia and insulin resistance will develop in many ICU patients, even if they have no previous history of diabetes. Insulin therapy can return blood glucose levels to normal, although the prognostic impact of this treatment is uncertain. The effects of intensive insulin therapy to correct blood glucose levels on the outcomes of ICU patients were studied.

Methods.—Participants were 1548 patients in a surgical ICU who were receiving mechanical ventilation. They were randomly assigned to receive intensive insulin therapy or conventional treatment. In the intervention group, insulin was given to maintain blood glucose levels within a target range of 80 to 110 mg/dL; in the control group, insulin infusion was given only if blood glucose levels rose above 215 mg/dL, with a target range of 180 to 200 mg/dL. Morbidity and mortality rates were compared between groups.

Results.—The mortality rate in the ICU was 4.6% in the intensive insulin group, compared with 8.0% in the conventional therapy group. Much of the prognostic impact of intensive insulin therapy came in the reduction of deaths from multiple organ failure with a confirmed septic focus. Intensive insulin therapy was effective in almost all subgroups of patients defined according to the Acute Physiology and Chronic Health Evaluation (APACHE II) score and the Simplifed Therapeutic Intervention Scoring System (TISS-28) score during the first 24 hours after admission. Patients receiving intensive insulin therapy also had a 34% reduction in in-hospital mortality. Significant reductions in morbidity were noted as well, including a 46% reduction in bloodstream infections, a 41% decrease in acute renal failure requiring dialysis or hemofiltration, a 50% reduction in red blood cell transfusion, and a 44% reduction in critical illness polyneuropathy.

Conclusion.—For surgical ICU patients, intensive insulin therapy to maintain good control of blood glucose levels is associated with significant improvement in measures of morbidity and mortality. Blood glucose levels should be maintained at 110 mg/dL or below, whether or not the patient has a history of diabetes.

▶ Another important study. Hyperglycemia has been postulated to predispose to many adverse events, including impaired wound healing, multiorgan failure, sepsis, and death. It therefore makes sense that attention to glycemic control should improve outcomes in ICU patients. The results of this study clearly indicate that we must do better at controlling blood sugar levels in critically ill patients.

G. L. Moneta, MD

Double-Masked Randomized Trial Comparing Alternate Combinations of Intraoperative Anesthesia and Postoperative Analgesia in Abdominal Aortic Surgery
Norris EJ, Beattie C, Perler BA, et al (Johns Hopkins Med Institutions, Baltimore, Md; Vanderbilt Univ, Nashville, Tenn; Johns Hopkins Univ, Baltimore, Md; et al)
Anesthesiology 95:1054-1067, 2001   5–19

Background.—The use of epidural anesthesia and analgesia may result in better patient outcomes and utilization of medical resources than the use of general anesthesia and IV opioids. However, the relative importance of intraoperative compared with postoperative technique has not been investigated. Alternate combinations of intraoperative anesthesia and postoperative analgesia were compared.

Methods.—One hundred sixty-eight patients undergoing abdominal aorta surgery were included. By random assignment, patients received thoracic epidural anesthesia combined with a light general anesthesia or general anesthesia alone intraoperatively and either IV or epidural patient-controlled analgesia (PCA) postoperatively. The PCA was continued for 72 hours or longer.

Findings.—The 4 treatment groups were similar in length of stay and direct medical costs. The groups were also similar in mortality and rates of myocardial infarction, myocardial ischemia, reoperation, pneumonia, and renal failure. Epidural PCA correlated with a significantly shorter time to extubation. The treatment groups had comparable times to ICU discharge, ward admission, first bowel sounds, first flatus, tolerance of clear liquids and regular diet, and independent ambulation. Postoperative pain scores were also comparable.

Conclusion.—In patients undergoing abdominal aorta surgery, thoracic epidural anesthesia combined with a light general anesthesia followed by IV or epidural PCA appears to have no major advantages or disadvantages, compared with general anesthesia alone followed by IV or epidural PCA. The rates of complications, pain scores, and length of stay were comparable among the treatment groups.

▶ I guess what matters is that the patients lie still during the operation. How you get them to lie still doesn't really matter much.

G. L. Moneta, MD

Variation in Surgical and Anaesthetic Technique and Associations With Operative Risk in the European Carotid Surgery Trial: Implications for Trials of Ancillary Techniques

Rothwell PM, for the European Carotid Surgery Trialists' Collaborative Group (Radcliffe Infirmary, Oxford, England; et al)
Eur J Vasc Endovasc Surg 23:117-126, 2002   5–20

Background.—Some baseline risk factors for patients undergoing carotid endarterectomy cannot be modified, but quality control focuses on those that can, such as surgical and anesthetic technique. The study of clinical practice should involve a cohort of patients established prospectively in which the decisions to analyze and report the results do not depend on the data obtained. The European Carotid Surgery Trial (ECST) patients form the largest published cohort of patients with symptomatic carotid stenosis, and the complications that developed in them in response to certain ancillary techniques used with endarterectomy were evaluated.

Methods.—Carotid endarterectomy was done in 1729 patients within 1 year of randomization. The ancillary procedures assessed included carotid shunts and patches, with the 147 participating surgeons also documenting their use of intraoperative anticoagulation and EEG monitoring, length of the operation, and the total carotid artery occlusion time, when no blood was flowing distally into the internal carotid artery. The principal surgical outcome measure was death from any cause or stroke that lasted longer than 7 days within 30 days of the procedure. Other surgical complications also were noted.

Results.—During the 30 days after carotid endarterectomy, 17 patients died, 11 because of stroke, and 105 nonfatal strokes lasting more than 7 days occurred. The risk of death or stroke lasting more than 7 days was 7.1%. Surgeons varied significantly, including among countries, as to which ancillary operative techniques they used. Techniques were sometimes used selectively, and patient characteristics differed depending on the techniques used. The use of some techniques was significantly related to the use of other techniques. Initially, increased surgical risk attended the use of a shunt and failure to use anticoagulation, surgeons' perception of greater operative difficulty, and lower stump pressure. Better surgical outcome tended to be associated with the use of local anesthetic and EEG monitoring, but this was not shown to be significant. On final analysis, the use of intraoperative anticoagulants and a duration of operation over 1.5 hours were significantly associated with surgical outcome, the other variables ceasing to be relevant in the light of case mix and other surgical technique variables.

Conclusions.—The risk associated with operation showed more significant relationships with patient characteristics, length of surgery, and surgeons' perception of the surgery's difficulty than with any particular ancillary operative technique. Neither stroke nor death risk was increased with the use of a particular ancillary technique. In addition, the study proved the importance of assessing nonrandomized retrospective analyses of surgical results with caution because of the many confounding variables that arise.

▶ Basically, it doesn't matter about the specifics of doing a carotid endarterectomy as long as you do it well. Surgeons achieving good results with their technique of carotid endarterectomy should keep on using that technique. Don't change just because some guy in a suit with a laptop gives a slick presentation.

G. L. Moneta, MD

Three Cases of Hyperperfusion Syndrome Identified by Daily Transcranial Doppler Investigation After Carotid Surgery
Schaafsma A, Veen L, Vos JPM (Martini Ziekenhuis Groningen, The Netherlands)
Eur J Vasc Endovasc Surg 23:17-22, 2002   5–21

Introduction.—The hyperperfusion syndrome (HS) is infrequent and serious, but it is a potentially treatable complication of carotid endarterectomy (CEA). Postoperative transcranial Doppler (TCD) was assessed to determine whether its routine use during the first 4 days after CEA would be beneficial in the identification of HS.

Methods.—Between July 1998 and January 2001, TCD was used for 4 days postoperatively to monitor 104 of 112 patients who underwent CEA. The TCD measurements were obtained by means of US equipment with a 2 MHz-pulsed Doppler transducer.

Results.—During the evaluation period, 3 patients had HS. All 3 demonstrated TCD abnormalities hours before exhibiting symptoms. One patient experienced a full-blown HS. It is possible that symptoms in the other 2 patients could have been prevented by the timely initiation or restoration of antihypertensive therapy.

Conclusion.—HS should be considered for any patient with abnormally high middle cerebral artery flow velocities during the first few days after CEA, particularly when high flow velocities occur before or after postoperative day 1. These patients need to be transferred to the ICU for monitoring of arterial blood pressure (ABP). Antihypertensive treatment should attempt to keep systolic ABPs below 150 mm Hg and diastolic ABPs below 90 mm Hg.

▶ TCD may be able to detect changes consistent with hyperperfusion before the onset of actual clinical symptoms. However, it seems extremely unlikely that asymptomatic patients will be monitored routinely for 4 days postoperatively with TCD. It would be interesting, however, to consider a TCD study in a patient after CEA with headache and treat for hyperperfusion syndrome if middle cerebral artery velocities are significantly elevated.

G. L. Moneta, MD

Coagulopathy as a Result of Factor V Inhibitor After Exposure to Bovine Topical Thrombin

Neschis DG, Heyman MR, Cheanvechai V, et al (Univ of Maryland, Baltimore)
J Vasc Surg 35:400-402, 2002   5–22

Background.—Postoperative coagulopathy may be secondary to supra-therapeutic levels of heparin or warfarin sodium, malnutrition, sepsis, or hypothermia. A less-frequent cause of postoperative coagulopathy is the development of inhibitors to factor V. A case of severe coagulopathy after mesenteric revascularization is discussed in which laboratory investigation discovered the presence of plasma inhibitors of factor V, which were believed to result from exposure to bovine thrombin used for intraoperative hemostasis.

Case Report.—Woman, 75, had undergone multiple lower-extremity revascularization procedures in the past and now underwent mesenteric revascularization with a bifurcated polytetrafluoroethylene graft from the supraceliac aorta. Bovine thrombin (about 5000 U) was used as a topical hemostatic agent. The patient's initial postoperative course was uncomplicated. On the ninth postoperative day, however, daily coagulation studies showed significant elevation in the patient's prothrombin time (PT) and activated partial thromboplastin time (aPTT), peaking on the 11th postoperative day at an aPTT of 102 seconds and a PT of 46.9 seconds. The administration of vitamin K and fresh frozen plasma (FFP) did not resolve the abnormal readings. Coagulation study results showed that the patient had circulating inhibitors of human factor V, most likely stimulated by the patient's prior exposure to bovine thrombin. Little cross reactivity of the antibody with human thrombin was present, but a marked cross reactivity was noted with human factor V, resulting in a profound inhibition of factor V activity.

Conclusions.—Topical thrombin preparations are widely used in various forms, including sprays, paste, fibrin, glue, or other dry procoagulant materials soaked in the topical thrombin. In the United States, most of these preparations are prepared from bovine thrombin. It is likely that the incidence of patients developing factor V inhibitors is higher than has previously been realized, which may account for some otherwise unexplained postoperative coagulation disorders.

▶ We use thrombin-soaked gelfoam routinely in our arterial reconstructions and have not recognized this complication, despite many reoperative procedures. Perhaps we have been lucky. Perhaps we haven't looked hard enough. Perhaps both.

G. L. Moneta, MD

Combination Therapy in Peripheral Vascular Disease: The Rationale of Using Both Thrombolytic and Antiplatelet Drugs

Shlansky-Goldberg R (Univ of Pennsylvania, Philadelphia)

J Am Coll Surg 194:S103-S113, 2002   5–23

Background.—Local thrombolysis is a well-established technique for the treatment of arterial and venous thromboembolic disease and graft occlusions. The technique is, however, limited by dose and the duration of treatment, the need for intensive care monitoring, and exposure of patients to the risk of bleeding. Since the main elements of a thrombus include fibrin, thrombin, and platelets, this review focused on the combined use of thrombolytic and antiplatelet agents in the treatment of peripheral arterial occlusions.

Overview.—An understanding of how antiplatelet drugs work must begin with an understanding of how platelet activation and aggregation begin. Investigations in the 1970s showed that platelets in patients with Glanzmann thrombasthenia were devoid of fibrinogen and had a deficiency of 2 different platelet glycoproteins (GPs), designated GP IIb and GP IIIa, that combine to form a complex. It was not until the late 1970s that it was determined that the interaction of fibrinogen with the platelet surface was needed for platelet aggregation, and that the site of this interaction was the GP IIb/IIIa receptor. Three parenteral GP IIb/IIIa inhibitors currently have FDA approval for coronary use for the treatment of coronary syndromes and percutaneous interventions. The rationale for combining thrombolytic and antiplatelet drugs is rooted in the fact that, although the fibrin component of an occlusive thrombus is sensitive to dissolution by fibrinolytics, platelets are not, and thus they can cause "thrombolytic resistance." In addition, GP IIb/IIIa antagonists have the ability to dissolve platelet-rich clots, resulting in dethrombosis, which refers to clot dissolution caused by antagonism of the IIb/IIIa platelet receptor that results in disaggregation rather than fibrinolysis. Current experience with the combination of IIb/IIIa inhibitors and thrombolytic therapy in peripheral arteries is limited to case series. Results, however, suggest the combination of a IIb/IIIa inhibitor and thrombolytic therapy results in more complete and more rapid lysis than the use of thrombolytic therapy alone.

Conclusions.—There are many unknowns to be explored regarding the use of combination therapy, including determination of the correct lytic and heparin doses. This therapy may represent a powerful technique for the improvement of outcomes and efficiency of locally delivered catheter thrombolysis.

▶ This article reviews the rationale and mechanism of action of IIb/IIIa inhibitors of platelet aggregation. The authors postulate, based on a few small studies, that IIb/IIIa inhibitors, which are very useful in coronary artery catheter-based interventions, may also be useful in peripheral arterial thrombolytic procedures. Certainly, one cannot ignore the fact that these agents are very useful in the coronary circulation, and that there have often been unsatisfactory results with peripheral thrombolysis. Careful trials evaluating IIb/IIIa inhibitors as adjuncts to thrombolytic agents in the performance of peripheral catheter-based intervention seem warranted.

G. L. Moneta, MD

6 Thoracic Aorta

Staged Repair of Extensive Aortic Aneurysms: Morbidity and Mortality in the Elephant Trunk Technique
Safi HJ, Miller CC III, Estrera AL, et al (Univ of Texas, Houston)
Circulation 104:2938-2942, 2001

6–1

Background.—Graft replacement of the ascending aorta, arch, and descending thoracic aorta in a single operation increases the surgical risks to patients with extensive aortic aneurysms. Staged repair is an alternative. The patients reported here all had first-stage or second-stage elephant trunk procedures for elective repair of extensive aortic aneurysms.

Methods.—Between February 1991 and May 2000, 1146 operations for aortic aneurysms were performed at the study institution. A total of 117 patients underwent 182 first- or second-stage elephant trunk procedures (15.9% of all aortic aneurysm operations). The patients were 61 men and 56 women with a mean age of 62.9 years. Aortic dissection, present in 49 patients, was chronic in 42. Stage 1 was completed in all 117 patients and stage 2 (Fig 3) in 65.

Results.—Twenty (17.1%) first-stage patients had significant coagulopathy during surgery, and 2 postoperative strokes occurred in the period before

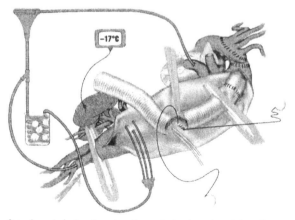

FIGURE 3.—Stage 2 repair during visceral cooling and reimplantation of visceral arteries after proximal anastomosis of second stage graft to "elephant trunk." (Courtesy of Safi HJ, Miller CC III, Estrera AL, et al: Staged repair of extensive aortic aneurysms: Morbidity and mortality in the elephant trunk technique. *Circulation* 104:2398-2942, 2001.)

1991, when retrograde perfusion became part of the standard operating procedure. The 30-day mortality rate was 5.1% for the first stage and 6.2% for the second stage. During the interval between operations, 4 (3.6%) patients died (3 of aneurysm rupture). Among the 43 patients who did not return for second-stage repair, 13 (30.2%) died within an average of 3.4 years; 4 of these deaths were the result of rupture.

Conclusion.—The elephant technique uses measures that provide protection to the brain and guard against stroke in the first stage of the procedure and provide protection to the spinal cord during the second stage. Extensive aortic aneurysms can thus be repaired with acceptable morbidity and mortality rates. Prompt treatment of the remaining segment in stage 2 is crucial to the success of the elephant trunk procedure.

▶ This is obviously a very large experience with a relatively infrequently performed procedure. About 40% of the patients failed to complete the second stage of the procedure. However, only 4 of the 43 patients (approximately 9%) who did not complete the second stage died of aneurysm rupture at an average follow-up of 3.4 years. Given the authors' 30-day mortality of 6.2% with the second stage of the elephant trunk technique, one wonders a little about the risk/benefit balance in this procedure.

G. L. Moneta, MD

Morbidity and Mortality After Extent II Thoracoabdominal Aortic Aneurysm Repair
Coselli JS, LeMaire SA, Conklin LD, et al (Baylor College of Medicine, Houston)
Ann Thorac Surg 73:1107-1116, 2002   6–2

Introduction.—Surgical repair of Crawford type II thoracoabdominal aortic aneurysm (TAAAs) is associated with significant morbidity and mortality. The outcome of a large consecutive series of type II TAAA repairs (Fig 1) was analyzed. Risk factors that affect morbidity and mortality were assessed.

Methods.—The study included 1415 consecutive patients who underwent graft repair of TAAAs between January 11, 1986, and December 31, 1999. Of these, 442 (31.2%) were type II TAAAs. Data from a prospectively maintained database were examined to ascertain which factors were correlated with death and major complications.

Results.—The operative mortality rate was 10.0% (44 patients). Postoperative complications were as follows: 33 (7.5%) patients, paraplegia/paraparesis; 158 (35.7%) patients, pulmonary complications; and 69 patients (15.9%), renal failure. Multivariable analysis showed that renal insufficiency (odds ratio [OR], 2.6), increasing age (OR, 1.1/y), and increasing red blood cell transfusion requirements (OR, 1.1/U) were predictive of mortality; renal insufficiency (OR, 2.8) and peptic ulcer disease (OR, 9.3) were predictive of renal failure; and rupture (OR, 6.3) was predictive of

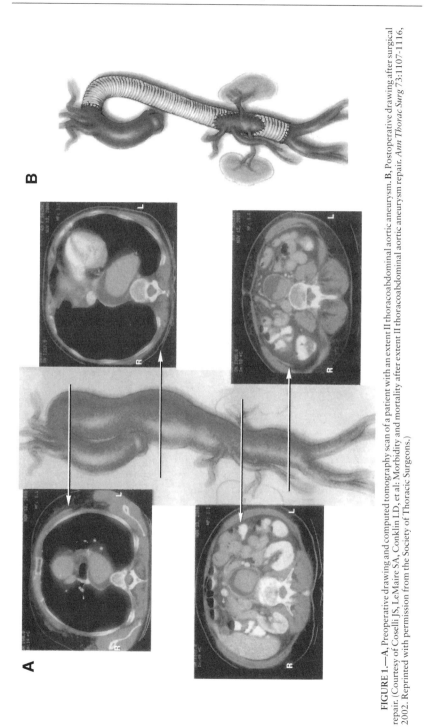

FIGURE 1.—A, Preoperative drawing and computed tomography scan of a patient with an extent II thoracoabdominal aortic aneurysm. B, Postoperative drawing after surgical repair. (Courtesy of Coselli JS, LeMaire SA, Conklin LD, et al: Morbidity and mortality after extent II thoracoabdominal aortic aneurysm repair. *Ann Thorac Surg* 73:1107-1116, 2002. Reprinted with permission from the Society of Thoracic Surgeons.)

paraplegia. Left heart bypass was an independently protective factor against paraplegia (OR, 0.4).

Conclusion.—Acceptable levels of morbidity and mortality rates were observed in this high-risk cohort. Left heart bypass provided protection against paraplegia.

▶ Repair of type II TAAAs is a high-risk operation for a high-risk disease. Surgeons wishing to perform this operation need to consider the mortality rate and complication rate presented in this series. They must be honest enough with themselves to realize they are likely not to do as well as Coselli and colleagues.

G. L. Moneta, MD

A New Predictive Model for Adverse Outcomes After Elective Thoracoabdominal Aortic Aneurysm Repair

LeMaire SA, Miller CC III, Conklin LD, et al (Baylor College of Medicine, Houston)

Ann Thorac Surg 71:1233-1238, 2001   6–3

Background.—An individual patient's risk of thoracoabdominal aortic aneurysm rupture must be balanced against the risk of adverse outcomes after surgical repair. Which preoperative risk factors currently predict adverse outcomes after elective thoracoabdominal aortic aneurysm repair was studied.

Methods.—Data were obtained on 1108 patients. An adverse outcome was defined as stroke, paraplegia, paraparesis, death within 30 days of surgery, death before hospital discharge, or acute renal failure necessitating dialysis.

Findings.—The incidence of adverse outcomes was 13%. Factors that predicted adverse outcomes were preoperative renal insufficiency, increasing age, symptomatic aneurysms, and extent II aneurysms (Fig 2). An equation based on these risk factors was constructed to estimate the probability of an adverse outcome for an individual patient.

Conclusions.—The predictive model developed may be useful for making decisions about elective thoracoabdominal aortic aneurysm repair. Contemporary surgical techniques yield favorable outcomes in suitable candidates.

▶ If you do a lot of high-risk operations, you have plenty of material to write about complications.

G. L. Moneta, MD

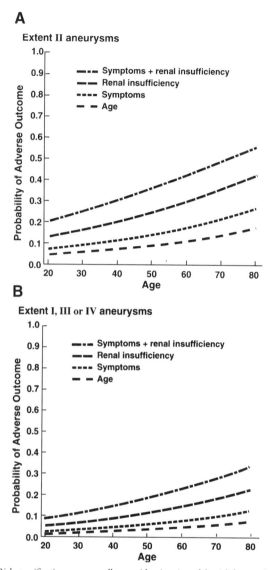

A

Extent II aneurysms

- — ·· — Symptoms + renal insufficiency
- — — Renal insufficiency
- ····· Symptoms
- — — Age

B

Extent I, III or IV aneurysms

- — ·· — Symptoms + renal insufficiency
- — — Renal insufficiency
- ····· Symptoms
- — — Age

FIGURE 2.—Risk stratification curves to allow rapid estimation of the risk for an adverse outcome after elective surgical repair of a thoracoabdominal aortic aneurysm is used for patients who require an extent II repair (**A**), and is used for patients who undergo an extent I, III, or IV repair (**B**). (Reprinted with permission from the Society of Thoracic Surgeons from LeMaire SA, Miller CC III, Conklin LD, et al: A new predictive model for adverse outcomes after elective thoracoabdominal aortic aneurysm repair. *Ann Thorac Surg* 71:1233-1238, 2001.)

Safety and Efficacy of Hypothermic Cardiopulmonary Bypass and Circulatory Arrest for Operations on the Descending Thoracic and Thoracoabdominal Aorta

Kouchoukos NT, Masetti P, Rokkas CK, et al (Missouri Baptist Med Ctr, St Louis; Cleveland Clinic Found, Ohio)
Ann Thorac Surg 72:699-708, 2001   6–4

Background.—Hypothermic cardiopulmonary bypass with circulatory arrest is increasingly being used for operations on the distal aortic arch and the descending thoracic and thoracoabdominal aorta. This approach has many advantages over other techniques, but there have been concerns that early mortality and complication rates are higher. One center's experience with the safety and efficacy of hypothermic cardiopulmonary bypass with circulatory arrest for operations on the distal aortic arch and descending thoracic and thoracoabdominal aorta was described.

Methods.—The subjects were 161 patients (60% men; mean age, 61 years) with disease of the distal aortic arch, the descending thoracic aorta, or the thoracoabdominal aorta. Comorbid conditions were common; 71% of patients had hypertension and 65% had a history of smoking. Marfan's syndrome was present in 22 patients (14%). About one third had previously undergone proximal aortic repair (36%) or an aortic valve procedure (31%). Seventeen patients (11%) had a rupture or an acute type B aortic dissection that required emergent surgery. All patients underwent resection of the diseased segment and graft replacement while receiving hypothermic cardiopulmonary bypass, usually in combination with circulatory arrest. Outcomes and complications up to 90 days after surgery were identified and examined to determine the safety and efficacy of the operation.

Results.—Ten patients died before hospital discharge, for a 30-day mortality rate of 6.2%. Thirty-day mortality rates were significantly higher among patients requiring emergent surgery (7 of 17 patients, or 41%) than among the other patients (3 of 144, or 2.1%). By 90 days, an additional 9 patients had died (11.8% overall). Actual survival rates at 1, 3, and 5 years were 85%, 76%, and 63%, respectively.

All but 1 of the 157 patients who survived the operation were assessed postoperatively to determine neurologic function. Four of these 156 operative survivors experienced paraplegia and 1 experienced paraparesis (3.2% overall), 15 patients (9.6%) had transient neurologic dysfunction, and 3 patients (1.9%) had a stroke. The 4 patients with early paraplegia had thoracoabdominal aortic disease; this included 1 of 33 patients (3.0%) with Crawford type I disease, 1 of 34 patients (2.9%) with type II disease, and 2 of 24 patients (8.3%) with type III disease. In the entire series, 50 patients had aortic dissection; none of these patients experienced paralysis. The duration of spinal cord ischemia was not significantly related to the development of paraplegia or paraparesis.

Four of the 157 operative survivors (2.5%) required renal dialysis; 3 of these died in the early postoperative period, and renal function recovered completely in 1. None of these 4 patients had preoperative renal dysfunction as determined by serum creatinine levels, and they had both kidneys at the time of surgery. Thirty-one operative survivors (20%) required prolonged mechanical ventilation (more than 48 hours), 17 survivors (11%) required prolonged inotropic support (more than 48 hours), 13 survivors (8%) required tracheostomy, and 10 survivors (6.4%) experienced gastrointestinal complications. In 9 survivors (6%), deep venous thrombosis developed; 8 survivors (5%) required reoperation for bleeding; 7 survivors (4%) sustained wound complications; and in 7 survivors (4%), sepsis developed.

Conclusion.—Hypothermic cardiopulmonary bypass with circulatory arrest is a safe and effective method for protecting patients with distal aortic arch and descending thoracic and thoracoabdominal aorta dissection or rupture against neurologic, renal, cardiac, and visceral organ system failure. The safety and efficacy of this technique rival those of simple aortic clamping, partial cardiac or total cardiopulmonary bypass, and regional hypothermia, and it does not require other adjuncts.

▶ Turning patients into popsicles to facilitate thoracic and thoracoabdominal aneurysm repair apparently works quite well in terms of preserving spinal cord and renal function in these high-risk operations. The authors make a reasonable case that the technique should be used more widely. This of course would effectively take peripheral vascular surgeons out of the thoracoabdominal aneurysm business. However, for most of us, the infrequency in which we perform these procedures and the high complication rates reported by those with extensive experience with these operations suggest that this may not be such a bad idea (see Abstract 6–3).

G. L. Moneta, MD

Risk of Spinal Cord Ischemia After Endograft Repair of Thoracic Aortic Aneurysms
Gravereaux EC, Faries PL, Burks JA, et al (Mount Sinai School of Medicine, New York)
J Vasc Surg 34:997-1003, 2001   6–5

Background.—The surgical repair of thoracoabdominal aneurysm is associated with a high risk of spinal cord ischemia. An endovascular approach to thoracic aortic aneurysm (TAA) repair has many benefits over open surgery, but endovascular treatment has been associated with this devastating complication as well. The incidence of spinal cord ischemia at a single center and the risk factors for its development were studied in patients undergoing endovascular TAA exclusion.

Methods.—The subjects were 53 patients who underwent endoluminal exclusion of their TAA during a 4-year period. All patients underwent preoperative CT and angiography to determine endograft sizing. Endografts were inserted in the operating room under C-arm fluoroscopic guidance. Patients were followed up at discharge and at regular intervals thereafter to identify neurologic deficits caused by spinal cord ischemia.

Results.—During follow-up, spinal cord ischemia developed in 3 of these 53 patients (5.7%). All 3 patients had comorbid conditions that put them at high risk for open surgery. Neurologic deficit (left leg weakness) occurred early in 1 patient with chronic obstructive lung disease after concomitant open infrarenal abdominal aortic aneurysm (AAA) and endovascular TAA repair. CSF drainage and a steroid bolus were instituted, and mean arterial pressure was maintained at approximately 90 mm Hg. The neurologic deficit had improved markedly by 12 hours after treatment and resolved completely by postoperative day 3. The other 2 patients experienced delayed-onset paralysis, either on postoperative day 2 or at 1 month after endovascular TAA repair. Both of these patients had 3 or more comorbid conditions (including hypertension and chronic obstructive pulmonary disease), and both had previously undergone AAA repair. Both patients had an extensive area of TAA involvement (aneurysms were 235 and 275 mm long), and thus required long endografts. Spinal cord ischemia and paralysis were irreversible in these 2 cases.

Conclusion.—About 6% of these patients undergoing endovascular repair of TAA experienced spinal cord ischemia, which was reversible in 1 case but permanent in the other 2 cases. Factors that contributed to spinal cord ischemia in these patients included prior or concomitant AAA repair and a long-segment thoracic aortic exclusion. Spinal cord protective measures should be instituted for patients with these risk factors who are undergoing endovascular TAA exclusion, including CSF drainage, steroids, and the prevention of hypotension.

▶ Note that spinal cord ischemia in thoracic aneurysms repaired with endografts occurs just like open repair and may occur at variable times postoperatively. We also recently had a patient who had paraparesis develop 2 weeks after TAA repair with an endograft; she did not have a previous aortic repair or a long segment graft, and fortunately recovered full function. Based on this "n of 1," I am not sure the authors' conclusions regarding risk factors for this complication are necessarily correct. The main risk factor is probably having the procedure.

G. L. Moneta, MD

Reduction of Ischemic Spinal Cord Injury by Dextrorphan: Comparison of Several Methods of Administration
Terada H, Kazui T, Takinami M, et al (Hamamatsu Univ, Japan)
J Thorac Cardiovasc Surg 122:979-985, 2001   6–6

Introduction.—Dextrorphan and other noncompetitive antagonists of N-methyl-D-aspartate (NMDA) reduce paraplegia after spinal cord ischemia, a severe complication of surgery on the descending aorta and thoracoabdominal aorta. The effect of dextrorphan on reduction of ischemic spinal cord injury and safe aortic clamping time achieved by various drug delivery methods were examined in an animal study.

Methods.—Spinal cord ischemia was induced in 5 groups of New Zealand White rabbits: group A received simple clamping; groups B and C received dextrorphan pretreatment (10 mg/kg) followed by continuous IV or intra-aortic infusion (1 mg/min), respectively; group D received the same dextrorphan pretreatment and bolus intra-aortic injection at clamping (1 mg per minute of clamping time); and group E received bolus intrathecal injection of dextrorphan (0.2 mg/kg). A small number of untreated control animals were included in each of the 4 treatment groups. Neurologic status was evaluated 48 hours after unclamping, and the animals were then killed for histopathologic examination.

Results.—Neurologic status at 48 hours was recorded on a scale ranging from 0 to 5 (0, hind limb paralysis); 1, severe paraparesis; 2, functional movement, no hopping; 3, ataxic hopping; 4, minimal ataxia; 5, normal). Neurologic function was better in all dextrorphan-treated groups than in the respective control animals, all of which showed paraplegia after 30 minutes of clamping. Among dextrorphan-treated animals, those in group C exhibited the best neurologic function (neurologic score of 5.0 after 30, 35, 40, 45, 50, and 55 minutes of clamping). Few obvious differences were observed in spinal cord histologic features in animals with scores between 2 and 4.

Conclusion.—In animals with induced spinal cord ischemia, dextrorphan reduced the severity of neurologic injury. Continuous intra-aortic infusion of the drug prolonged the safe clamping time significantly more than other delivery routes.

▶ This is a rat study. I am personally not very interested in rat research (I have never killed a rat in my academic career). However, everything has to start somewhere, and rats are a frequent starting point. Spinal cord protection in thoracic aortic surgery is currently based primarily on cooling and/or presumed control of perfusion pressure to the cord during aortic clamping. Targeting the biochemical response of the neuron to ischemia may eventually offer an additional and/or additive means of avoiding spinal cord injury associated with thoracic or thoracoabdominal aneurysm surgery.

G. L. Moneta, MD

Yearly Rupture or Dissection Rates for Thoracic Aortic Aneurysms: Simple Prediction Based on Size
Davies RR, Goldstein LJ, Coady MA, et al (Yale Univ, New Haven, Conn)
Ann Thorac Surg 73:17-28, 2002   6–7

Background.—The surgical treatment of patients who have thoracic aortic aneurysms has been dependent on the patients' individual clinical condition, and few guidelines are based on statistical data. If patients are to be offered the best treatment, the risk of complications related to the thoracic aortic aneurysm should be weighed against the risk of complications from the operative intervention. A database was developed to aid in evaluating the annual rate of rupture or dissection of thoracic aneurysms, thereby facilitating a better decision-making process.

Methods.—The database was developed at the Yale Center for Thoracic Aortic Disease, into which were entered 721 patients ranging in age from 8 to 95 years (median age, 65.8 years) over the course of 9 years. A total of 3115 imaging studies were included, of which 570 had sufficient follow-up to offer a basis for survival analysis. In 304 patients, no dissections were present at the initial examination; these were followed up to determine the natural history of the disorder, including rupture, dissection, and death information. When surgery was performed, the patient was eliminated from the analysis.

Results.—Aneurysms of substantial size were found more often in the ascending aorta, and patients with Marfan syndrome had smaller mean aortic sizes than patients without Marfan syndrome. Compared with ascending aortic aneurysms, those of the aortic arch and thoracoabdominal aorta were significantly larger. The growth rate in aneurysms of the descending or thoracoabdominal regions was markedly higher than that in ascending aorta or aortic arch aneurysms; dissected versus nondissected aortas had a similar differential between growth rates. Higher growth rates accompanied Marfan syndrome and a history of pulmonary disease. Size, specifically an initial aortic size of 6.0 cm or greater, was a strong predictor of a rupture or dissection (Fig 1). Males were significantly less likely to have a rupture or dissection. On multivariate regression analysis, increasing aortic size strongly predicted a rupture or dissection, and a size of 6.0 cm or more carried a fivefold higher cumulative risk of complications. Male sex was protective, and Marfan disease carried a relative risk of 3.7; a history of stroke was

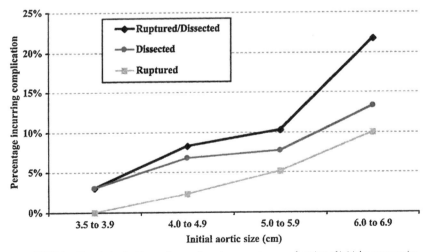

FIGURE 1.—Cumulative incidence of acute dissection or rupture as a function of initial aneurysm size. The increase in the rate of a rupture or dissection with increasing size is statistically significant ($P = .003$), as is the increase in the incidence of a rupture ($P = .006$). (Courtesy of Davies RR, Goldstein LJ, Coady MA, et al: Yearly rupture or dissection rates for thoracic aortic aneurysms: Simple prediction based on size. *Ann Thorac Surg* 73:17-28, 2002. Reprinted with permission from the Society of Thoracic Surgeons.)

accompanied by an increased rate of complications. The yearly rates of complications increased significantly when the aneurysm measured 6 cm or greater, and rates were more than 4 times higher than those for patients with smaller aneurysms. The 5-year survival rate when surgery was not done was 54%; 55 patients died, 13 had ruptures, and 24 had dissections. The annual rate of a rupture or dissection was 6.9%; the annual death rate was 11.8%. Life expectancy was restored to normal by preemptive elective surgical repair.

Conclusions.—Thoracic aneurysms can be fatal, and the size of the aneurysm plays a major predictive role with respect to risk of a rupture, dissection, or death. Patients whose aneurysms are more than 6 cm have a yearly rate of a rupture or dissection of at least 6.9% and a death rate of 11.8%. Repairing the aneurysm electively is associated with a survival rate that is nearly normal.

▶ Getting hard data on rupture rates of aneurysms is surprisingly difficult. Many studies tend to overestimate true rupture rates. If anything, however, based on their methods of analysis, the authors' data (see Fig 1) may be a bit of an underestimate. Not in the abstract, but in the body of the article is information indicating females may have even higher risk of rupture as will patients with other manifestations of vascular disease. Surprisingly, aneurysm growth averaged only 0.1 cm per year.

G. L. Moneta, MD

Useful CT Findings for Predicting the Progression of Aortic Intramural Hematoma to Overt Aortic Dissection

Choi SH, Choi S-J, Kim JH, et al (Univ of Ulsan, Seoul, Korea)
J Comput Assist Tomogr 25:295-299, 2001   6–8

Background.—Aortic intramural hematoma is being reported more frequently with the increased application of CT, MRI, and transesophageal echocardiography. The relationship of aortic intramural hematoma to aortic dissection has not been defined, and treatment strategies are unclear. The CT findings for 29 patients were analyzed for variables that might predict the progression of aortic intramural hematoma to aortic dissection.

Methods.—The patients were 17 men and 12 women with a mean age of 65 years. All experienced symptoms of abrupt chest pain, back pain, or abdominal pain. An initial CT scan was obtained an average of 2.24 days after disease onset. Criteria for aortic intramural hematoma were (1) crescent-shaped or concentric high-attenuated aortic wall thickening on nonenhanced scan, (2) no definable intimal flap, and (3) no enhancement of thickened aortic wall after contrast agent injection. The scans were analyzed for involved site, maximum thickness of hematoma, the presence or absence of compression of true lumen, and pericardial and pleural effusion. All patients had 2 to 8 follow-up CT scans. Follow-up was by MRI in 5 patients.

Results.—Eight patients had type A aortic intramural hematoma (with involvement of the ascending aorta) and 21 had type B (limited to the descending aorta). Progression to aortic dissection occurred in 7 of 8 type A patients and in 3 of 21 type B patients, a significant difference in frequency. Progression occurred at periods ranging from 7 days to 790 days after diagnosis (mean, 223 days). The CT findings predictive of progression to overt aortic

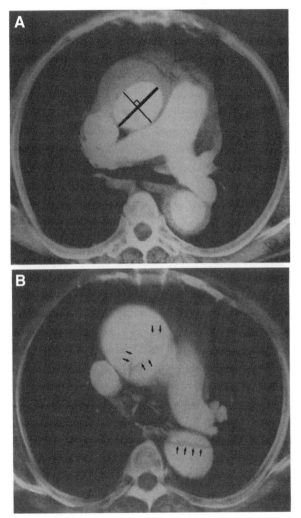

FIGURE 1.—Compression of the true lumen. **A,** The minimum (*thin line*) and maximum (*thick line*) transverse diameters of the true lumen were measured in the axial plane so that the thickness of the hematoma was maximum. The ratio of the minimum and maximum transverse diameters was calculated. Compression of the true lumen was defined as when the ratio was less than 0.75. In this patient, the ratio was 0.68. **B,** After 2 months, a follow-up CT scan showed overt aortic dissection in the ascending and descending thoracic aorta (*arrows*). (Courtesy of Choi SH, Choi S-J, Kim JH, et al: Useful CT findings for predicting the progression of aortic intramural hematoma to overt aortic dissection. *J Comput Assist Tomogr* 25:295-299, 2001.)

dissection included type A intramural hematoma, thick hematoma, compression (Fig 1) of the true lumen, and the presence of pericardial or pleural effusion.

Conclusion.—A number of CT findings are useful in predicting the progression of aortic intramural hematoma to overt aortic dissection. An objective new finding, compression of the true lumen, was associated with a high probability of progression.

▶ Aortic intramural hematomas, although first recognized more than 80 years ago, are only recently receiving significant attention. An intramural hematoma is characterized by thrombosis of the "false lumen" and no recognized intimal flap. It is thought to be caused by rupture of the aortic vaso vasorum with subintimal hemorrhage. Type A involves the ascending aorta, and type B is limited to the descending aorta, same as the Stanford classification for aortic dissection. Some acute intramural hematomas resolve and some do not. Risk factors for those that don't are delineated in this article. The basic point of the article is that one should worry about type A intramural hematomas and big type B intramural hematomas, and that the natural history of small type B intramural hematomas appears relatively benign.

G. L. Moneta, MD

False Lumen Patency as a Predictor of Late Outcome in Aortic Dissection
Bernard Y, Zimmermann H, Chocron S, et al (Univ Hosp Jean-Minjoz, Besançon, France)
Am J Cardiol 87:1378-1382, 2001   6–9

Background.—Patients with aortic dissection (AD) are at high risk of death, often as a result of complications involving nonoperated segments of the aorta. The course of nonoperated aortic segments in patients with AD was analyzed by a retrospective serial imaging study.

Methods.—The analysis included 109 patients, 81 men and 28 women, (mean age, 61 years) who were operated on for AD between January 1984 and August 1996. All available imaging studies were reviewed, including transthoracic and transesophageal echocardiograms, aortograms, and MRI scans. The mean follow-up was 44 months, and when possible, a new MRI scan was obtained. Predictors of mortality were assessed by univariate and multivariate analysis.

Results.—One-year actuarial survival was 52% for patients with type A AD and 76% for those with type B AD (Fig 1). The 5-year survival rate was 46% for type A and 72% for type B; the 10-year survival rates for types A and B were 37% and 46%, respectively. Patients aged more than 70 years were at higher risk of late mortality (relative risk [RR], 1.08) as were also those with a false lumen patency of the thoracic descending aorta postoperatively (RR, 3.4). The presence of false lumen patency was associated with increased diameter of the descending aorta (31 vs 44 mm). For patients with type A AD, surgery extending to the aortic arch was associated with a lower rate of patency.

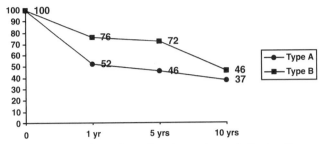

FIGURE 1.—Actuarial survival according to dissection type (percent). (Reprinted by permission of the publisher from Bernard Y, Zimmerman H, Chocon S, et al: False lumen patency as a predictor of late outcome in aortic dissection. *Am J Cardiol* 87:1378-1382, 2001. Copyright 2001, by Excerpta Medica, Inc.)

Conclusions.—For patients with AD, long-term progression of aortic dilatation is related to patency of the false lumen of the descending aorta. The results suggest that patients with type A AD should undergo open distal repair of the aorta. This allows the surgeon to check and replace the aortic arch when necessary, reducing the risk of false lumen patency and enhancing late survival.

▶ Type A dissections, as expected, have higher mortality than type B. However, if patients survive emergency surgery for type A dissection, their long-term mortality will be no different than that of type B dissection. Most late operations are, in fact, in patients with type B dissection and relate to continued patency of the false lumen leading to aortic enlargement. Close follow-up of patients with type B dissections and patent false lumens, therefore, seems mandatory.

G. L. Moneta, MD

Predicting Death in Patients With Acute Type A Aortic Dissection
Mehta RH, for the International Registry of Acute Aortic Dissection (IRAD) Investigators (Univ of Michigan, Ann Arbor; et al)
Circulation 105:200-206, 2002   6–10

Background.—Patients with acute type A aortic dissection are at increased risk for death. Other studies have identified predictors of death in this population, but those studies have generally been performed in selected (surgical) patients from a single institution and have not distinguished acute from chronic stable dissection, nor type A from type B dissection. The International Registry of Acute Aortic Dissection (IRAD) Investigators studied a large group of unselected patients with acute type A aortic dissection and described predictors of death in these patients.

Methods.—The subjects were 547 patients with type A aortic dissection (65.5% men; mean age, 61.9 years) seen within 14 days of symptom onset and who were enrolled in 1 of 18 centers in 6 countries between 1996 and

1999. Patient demographics, clinical histories, and in-hospital complications were examined to identify predictors of in-hospital mortality.

Results.—Of the 547 patients studied, 178 (32.5%) died while hospitalized. The mortality rate among patients treated without surgery was almost twice that of patients who underwent surgery (56.2% vs 26.9%). Compared with patients who survived, patients who died were significantly older and were significantly more likely to be men and to have a history of prior aortic dissection. Patients who died were also significantly more likely to experience hypotension, myocardial or mesenteric ischemia, kidney failure, cardiac tamponade, limb ischemia, neurologic deficits, or altered mental status while in-hospital. Logistic regression analysis identified 6 significant independent presenting characteristics that were associated with an increased risk of in-hospital mortality: kidney failure (odds ratio [OR], 4.77); hypotension, shock, or tamponade (OR, 2.97); abrupt onset of chest pain (OR, 2.60); pulse deficit (OR, 2.03); abnormal electrocardiograph results (OR, 1.77); and age 70 years or older (OR, 1.70). A predictive model based on these risk factors was presented.

Conclusion.—Almost one third of these patients with acute type A aortic dissection did not survive to hospital discharge, including about one fourth of those who were treated surgically. Several presenting characteristics can be used to identify patients who are at highest risk of in-hospital death.

▶ Old people in shock with renal insufficiency are more likely to die of acute type A aortic dissection than younger people with normal renal function and no shock. This comes under the category "basically stating the obvious."

G. L. Moneta, MD

Preoperative Risk Factors for Hospital Mortality in Acute Type A Aortic Dissection

Kawahito K, Adachi H, Yamaguchi A, et al (Jichi Med School, Saitama, Japan)
Ann Thorac Surg 71:1239-1243, 2001   6–11

Background.—Acute type A aortic dissection is associated with high rates of postoperative complications and mortality. To determine preoperative and perioperative risk factors for hospital death, 122 patients with acute type A dissections were retrospectively reviewed.

Methods.—Patients were 72 men and 50 women with a mean age of 63 years (range, 25 to 92 years). Emergency surgery was performed within 48 hours of acute onset. The operation was limited to the ascending aorta in 85 patients; 31 required partial or total replacement of the aortic arch. A total of 32 perioperative risk factors, including preoperative and operative variables, were analyzed for prediction of mortality.

Results.—Fifteen patients (12.3%) died in-hospital, with heart failure the most common cause of death. Twelve patients died after discharge at intervals ranging from 2 months to 8 years postoperatively. The actuarial survival rate (including in-hospital death) was 72% at 5 years. In univariate analysis, 10 factors were statistically significant predictors of hospital death: age, year of operation, Marfan syndrome, preoperative ST segment elevation, heart failure from aortic regurgitation, preoperative shock, preoperative coma, operative time exceeding 6 hours, cardiopulmonary bypass time longer than 4 hours, and massive (more than 20 units) blood transfusion. In multiple logistic regression analysis, both preoperative ST-T segment elevation and massive blood transfusion during operation were statistically significant independent risk factors for hospital death.

Conclusion.—Strong predictors of operative death among patients with acute type A aortic dissection were ST segment elevation on the ECG before the operation and massive blood transfusion during the operation.

▶ Unlike the previous article (Abstract 6–10), which looked at all comers with acute type A aortic dissection, this one examines only patients treated surgically. Not much in the way of new information is presented here. At least 8 previous publications on this subject have reached pretty much the same conclusions. I guess it is good to know that Japanese surgeons have the same problems as everyone else.

G. L. Moneta, MD

Transluminal Placement of Endovascular Stent-Grafts for the Treatment of Type A Aortic Dissection With an Entry Tear in the Descending Thoracic Aorta
Kato N, Shimono T, Hirano T, et al (Mie Univ, Japan; Matsusaka Gen Hosp, Mie, Japan)
J Vasc Surg 34:1023-1028, 2001   6–12

Background.—Ascending aortic replacement is the current treatment for type A aortic dissection. Recent advances in surgical technique and anesthesiology have resulted in marked improvements in operative mortality and morbidity. However, because of the need for extensive aortic replacement, type A aortic dissection with an entry tear in the descending thoracic aorta is still difficult. An experience with stent graft repair of type A aortic dissection with the entry point in the descending thoracic aorta was reported.

Methods.—Ten patients with type A aortic dissection (and an entry point in the descending thoracic aorta) received endovascular stent grafts to cover the entry point. The false lumen of the ascending aorta was patent in 5 patients and thrombosed in 5. Dissection was acute in 7 patients and subacute in 3. Pericardial effusion was present in 4 patients. Stent grafts were made from expanded polytetrafluoroethylene and Z-stents.

Findings.—In all patients, entry closure was achieved, and complete thrombosis of the false lumen of the ascending aorta was noted after stent grafting (Figure). Two patients needed a second stent graft to obtain complete thrombosis of the false lumen of the descending thoracic aorta. A minor stroke in 1 patient was the only procedure-related complication. There were no aortic ruptures or aneurysm formations in either the ascending or

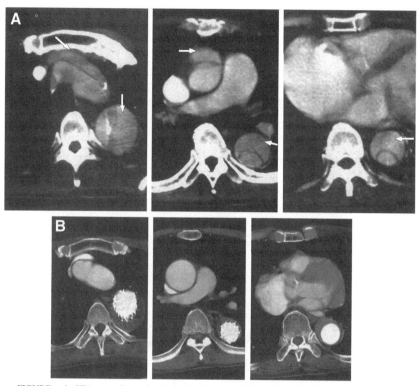

FIGURE.—**A,** CT images obtained at the levels of the proximal, mid, and distal segments of the descending aorta before stent grafting. The false lumen (*arrow*) can be identified at all levels. **B,** CT images obtained at each level 1 year after stent grafting. The false lumen is completely thrombosed and shrunk. (Courtesy of Kato N, Shimono T, Hirano T, et al: Transluminal placement of endovascular stent-grafts for the treatment of type A aortic dissection with an entry tear in the descending thoracic aorta. *J Vasc Surg* 34:1023-1028, 2001.)

descending thoracic aorta during a mean follow-up of 20 months. All patients were alive and well at the most recent follow-up. In 1 patient, an abdominal aortic aneurysm was enlarged after stent grafting and was treated by closing the fenestrations of the abdominal aorta with stent grafts.

Conclusion.—Stent graft repair of aortic dissection with an entry tear in the descending thoracic aorta appears to be safe and effective. In carefully selected patients, this approach may be an alternative to surgical graft replacement.

▶ There is a subgroup of patients with type A dissection in which the dissection of the arch and/or ascending aorta is secondary to retrograde dissection from a tear in the descending thoracic aorta. In this study, patients without complications of retrograde dissection of the aorta (ie, no tamponade, no regurgitation, and no signs of cardiac ischemia) were successfully treated with obliteration of the entry site via a transfemorally placed aortic stent graft. Obviously, this technique is only applicable to a small number of type A dissections, but it probably should be considered in appropriate patients.

G. L. Moneta, MD

Endovascular Repair of Thoracic Aortic Aneurysms: Stent-Graft Fixation Across the Aortic Arch Vessels
Burks JA Jr, Faries PL, Gravereaux EC, et al (Mount Sinai School of Medicine, New York)
Ann Vasc Surg 16:24-28, 2002   6–13

Introduction.—The less-invasive nature of thoracic aortic aneurysm (TAA) endovascular grafting potentially enables patients with severe comorbidities that would preclude conventional surgical repair to undergo exclusion of their aneurysm. Many patients, however, have anatomy unsuitable for proximal fixation of the device because of an inadequate segment of normal aorta distal to the last aortic arch vessel origin. The close proximity of the arch vessels to the origin of many TAAs may necessitate placement of

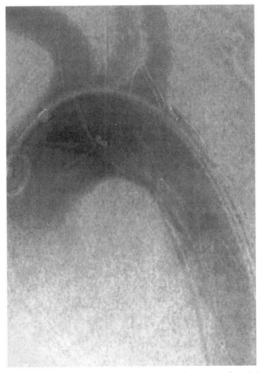

FIGURE 2.—Completion aortogram showing bare stent projection across the origin of the left SCA and left CA. *Abbreviations: SCA*, Subclavian artery; *CA*, carotid artery. (Courtesy of Burks JA Jr, Faries PL, Gravereaux EC, et al: Endovascular repair of thoracic aortic aneurysms: Stent-graft fixation across the aortic arch. *Ann Vasc Surg* 16:24-28, 2002.)

stent struts across the left subclavian or left common carotid ostia. The frequency and impact of deployment of an uncovered stent graft fixation during endovascular repair of TAA were analyzed with regard to proximal endoleaks, the arch vessels crossed, and the subsequent development of important sequelae in that vascular territory.

Methods.—Between May 1997 and July 2000, 51 patients underwent endovascular repair of a TAA by means of an endoluminally placed stent segment (Talent LPS). All patients underwent preoperative and postoperative angiograms and IV contrast-enhanced CT. Patients underwent follow-up contrast CT scans at 1, 3, 6, and 12 months and yearly thereafter.

Results.—Of 20 endografts placed, 9 were positioned without stent strut transversal of any arch vessels, and 11 were fixed across the left subclavian artery (SCA), carotid artery (CA), or both. Two patients had stent strut transversal of both the left SCA and CA orifices (Fig 2), and 2 had transversal of the left CA orifice after undergoing left SCA to CA transposition. No evidence was seen of any of the arch vessel artery orifices being even partially occluded unintentionally by the graft itself. One patient had intentional coverage of the left SCA by the cloth portion of the graft because of an inadequate landing zone distal to the left subclavian origin; the patient was not able to undergo further treatment, yet remained asymptomatic with a patent CA. During a 17-month follow-up, the 11 patients with arch vessel stent transversal had no stenoses, occlusion, or clinically evident upper extremity or cerebral ischemia associated with arch vessel coverage.

Conclusion.—Thoracic aortic endograft fixation across aortic arch vessels is not correlated with early morbidity.

▶ Fixation of stent grafts across the orifice of main vessels seems to be working out in the short run. However, only a few grafts have actually been placed across the origin of the common carotid artery. It seems, however, that fixation of the device in the distal curve of the aortic arch may produce differential stresses on the attachment site. One wonders if this may lead to late development of attachment site problems.

G. L. Moneta, MD

7 Aortic Aneurysm

Immediate Repair Compared With Surveillance of Small Abdominal Aortic Aneurysms

Lederle FA, for the Aneurysm Detection and Management Veterans Affairs Cooperative Study Group (Veterans Affairs Med Ctrs, Minneapolis; et al)

N Engl J Med 346:1437-1444, 2002　　　　　　　　　　　　　　　7–1

Background.—Authorities continue to debate the survival benefit associated with elective surgical repair of small abdominal aortic aneurysms (AAAs). A randomized immediate repair of such aneurysms was compared with surveillance in a randomized trial.

Method.—Patients aged 50 to 76 years with AAAs of 4 to 5.4 cm in diameter and who were not at high surgical risk were enrolled in the study. Five hundred sixty-nine patients were assigned to immediate open surgical repair of the aneurysm; 567 were assigned to surveillance by US or CT every 6 months, with repair reserved for aneurysms that became symptomatic or enlarged to 5.5 cm. Mean follow-up was 4.9 years.

Findings.—By the end of the study, 92.6% of the patients assigned to immediate repair and 61.6% assigned to surveillance had had aneurysm repair. The 2 groups did not significantly differ in rate of death from any cause. Survival trends did not favor immediate repair in subgroups defined by age or aneurysm diameter at study entry. The total operative mortality rate was only 2.7% in the patients having immediate repair. The rates of death related to AAA in the 2 groups were comparable at 3% in the immediate-repair group and 2.6% in the surveillance group. Eleven patients in the surveillance group (0.6%) had AAA rupture, resulting in 7 deaths. The rate of hospitalization associated with AAA was 39% lower in the surveillance group.

Conclusions.—In this study, elective repair of AAAs smaller than 5.5 cm did not improve survival rate. These findings were obtained even though the total operative mortality rate was low.

▶ This is the long-awaited primary article of the Department of Veterans Affairs Aneurysm Detection and Management (ADAM) trial. It has been worth the wait. This is one of the most important articles ever published on the subject of AAAs. The salient points are as follows. (1) The rupture rate of unrepaired AAAs less than 5.5 cm in size is tiny: 0.6% per year. This rate was not reduced by early repair of the aneurysm. (2) Early repair of AAAs less than 5.5 cm in size does not reduce overall mortality rate. (3) By 4 years, 27% of AAAs initially measuring 4 to 4.4 cm had enlarged to greater than 5.5 cm and were therefore repaired; 53% of aneurysms initially measuring 4.5 to 4.9 cm in diameter grew to 5.5 cm over the monitoring period and were repaired. For those aneurysms 5.0 to 5.4 cm in diameter at the time of randomization to surveillance or early repair, 81% in the surveillance group were eventually repaired. Finally, the operative mortality rate in both the immediate-repair group and surveillance group was excellent: 2.7% in the immediate-repair group and 2.1% in the surveillance group. Overall, the results of this study and the United Kingdom Small Aneurysm Trial support a policy in most cases of reserving elective repair of AAAs until they reach at least 5.5 cm in diameter.

G. L. Moneta, MD

Rupture Rate of Large Abdominal Aortic Aneurysms in Patients Refusing or Unfit for Elective Repair
Lederle FA, for the Veterans Affairs Cooperative Study #417 Investigators (Veterans Affairs Med Ctr, Minneapolis; et al)
JAMA 287:2968-2972, 2002   7–2

Background.—In patients with an abdominal aortic aneurysm (AAA) who are at high operative risk, surgical repair is typically delayed until the AAA reaches a diameter at which the risk associated with rupture outweighs that of surgery. However, little is known about the risk of large AAA rupture. The incidence of rupture in patients with large AAAs was reported.

Methods.—Forty-seven Veterans Affairs Medical Centers enrolled a total of 198 patients in the prospective study between 1995 and 2000. All patients had AAAs of 5.5 cm or greater. Elective AAA repair was not scheduled in any of the patients because of medical contraindications or patient refusal. The mean follow-up was 1.52 years.

Findings.—Fifty-seven percent of the patients died during follow-up. Forty-six percent underwent autopsy. Probable AAA rupture was documented in 45 patients. The 1-year incidence of probable rupture was 9.4% for AAAs with initial diameters of 5.5 to 5.9 cm, 10.2% for AAAs with initial diameters of 6 to 6.9 cm, and 32.5% of those with initial diameters of 7 cm or greater. The increased rupture risk among AAAs with diameters of 6.5 to 7.9 cm was largely attributed to the likelihood that these lesions would reach 8 cm in diameter during follow-up, after which 25.7% ruptured within in 6 months.

Conclusions.—Patients with AAAs of 5.5 cm or greater in diameter who are at high operative risk have a substantial risk of AAA rupture. This risk increases with diameter size.

▶ This is an offshoot of the Department of Veterans Affairs Aneurysm Detection and Management Trial (ADAM) (see Abstract 7–1). This study examined the natural history of unrepaired AAAs greater than 5.5 cm in diameter. Aneurysms were not repaired, either because the patient was unfit for surgery or refused operation. Aneurysms greater than 5.5 cm in diameter appeared to have substantial 1-year rupture risk: 9.4% for abdominal aortic aneurysms 5.4 to 5.9 cm, 10.2% for those 6.0 to 6.9 cm, and 32.5% for those greater than 7 cm in diameter. These are reasonably solid data on rupture rates of AAAs, and they support elective repair of aneurysms greater than 5.5 cm in diameter.

G. L. Moneta, MD

Indicators of Infection With *Chlamydia pneumoniae* Are Associated With Expansion of Abdominal Aortic Aneurysms
Lindholt JS, Ashton HA, Scott RAP (Hosp of Viborg, Denmark; St Richard's Hosp, Chichester, England)
J Vasc Surg 34:212-215, 2001   7–3

Background.—Previous research has demonstrated an association between *Chlamydia pneumoniae* and atherosclerosis, myocardial infarction, and abdominal aortic aneurysms (AAAs). The relationship between AAA expansion and *C pneumoniae* infection was assessed.

Methods.—One hundred ten patients with an AAA were considered for surgery, after diagnosis by the Chichester aneurysm screening program in the United Kingdom, as having an initially infrarenal aortic diameter of 3 to 5.9 cm. The patients were monitored by US scanning prospectively for a mean of 4.1 years. Blood samples were obtained from 100 patients (90 men and 10 women) for measurement of immunoglobuli (Ig) G and IgA antibodies against *C pneumoniae*.

Findings.—Forty-four percent of the men with an AAA had an IgA titer of 64 or greater and/or an IgG titer of 128 or greater. After adjustment for initial AAA size and patient age, an IgG titer of 128 or greater correlated significantly with expansion. Both IgA and IgG titers were significantly, positively associated with mean annual expansion. This persisted after adjustment for initial AAA size and patient age. An IgG titer of 128 or greater was present significantly more often in patients with more than 1 cm expansion annually.

Conclusion.—A substantial percentage of men with AAAs had signs of *C pneumoniae* infection. The progression of AAAs was positively associated with *C pneumoniae* infection indicators.

▶ In this article, IgG and IgA antibodies against *C pneumoniae* were measured in patients considered for AAA repair. Evidence of *C pneumoniae* was found in approximately 50% of males with AAA. In addition, there was a positive correlation between both IgG and IgA titers with expansion rate of AAA. This is one of several articles in this year's YEAR BOOK examining the association between *Chlamydia* and various manifestations of arteriovascular disease. The association between the presence of *Chlamydia* and arterial disease seems strong. It is, of course, unclear whether treatment of subclinical *Chlamydial* infections can have any impact on the course of occlusive atherosclerosis or on the expansion rate of AAAs.

G. L. Moneta, MD

Proteolysis of the Abdominal Aortic Aneurysm Wall and the Association With Rupture

Petersen E, Wågberg F, Ängquist K-A (Umeå Univ, Sweden)
Eur J Vasc Endovasc Surg 23:153-157, 2002   7–4

Background.—One of the most significant factors in the formation of abdominal aortic aneurysms (AAAs) is the degradation of extracellular matrix proteins in the aortic wall, resulting in decreased elastin concentration and increased turnover of collagen. Several studies have shown the involvement of matrix metalloproteinases (MMPs) in AAA disease. MMP-2 and MMP-9 are secreted from cells as proenzymes, and various activators and tissue inhibitors of metalloproteinases (TIMPs) control their activities in the extracellular environment. Four TIMPs have been identified; TIMP-1 and TIMP-2 are secreted from cells in complex with pro-MMP-9 and pro-MMP-2, respectively. There is a delicate balance between MMPs and TIMPs in the metabolism of the extracellular matrix during normal physiologic conditions, and disruption of the balance may cause uncontrolled turnover of the extracellular matrix. In AAA, this may ultimately lead to rupture. Increased elastase activity in the AAA wall in combination with low antiproteinase activity has been shown to be associated with rupture. Proteolysis of the AAA wall and its association with rupture were investigated.

Methods.—Levels of MMP-2 and MMP-9 were measured in the wall of 30 medium-sized ruptured AAAs (5 to 7 cm) and large asymptomatic AAAs ($\geq$ 7 cm).

Results.—Levels of MMP-2 were significantly higher in the walls of large asymptomatic AAAs than in medium-sized ruptured AAAs. Conversely, levels of MMP-9 were significantly higher in the walls of medium-sized ruptured AAAs than in large asymptomatic AAAs. The TIMP-1 and TIMP-2 levels were equivalent. A positive correlation was noted between MMP-2 and the diameter of the asymptomatic AAAs, but there was a negative correlation between MMP-9 levels and asymptomatic AAA size. There were no significant correlations between the diameter of large asymptomatic AAAs and TIMP-1 or TIMP-2.

Conclusions.—Rupture of AAA is associated with higher levels of MMP-9 but not with TIMP-1 or TIMP-2. MMP-2 levels are positively correlated with the size of asymptomatic AAAs, while MMP-9 levels are negatively correlated with the size of asymptomatic AAAs. MMP-9 may have a role in the progression of AAAs toward rupture, while MMP-2 may be a factor in the expansion of the aneurysm.

▶ There obviously must be something that leads to expansion and rupture of AAAs. In recent years, the role of MMPs has been examined. In this article, the level of MMP-2 correlated with diameter of AAA, while the level of MMP-9 did not. MMP-9 levels did, however, correlate with AAA rupture. It is postulated that expansion and rupture of AAAs are different biochemical processes. MMP-2 is released by mesenchymal cells and is located preferentially in the media. MMP-2, therefore, may contribute to destruction of medial layers, but preservation of adventitial layers, and may therefore be correlated with aneurysm expansion, but not necessarily rupture. MMP-9 is released from primarily monoclonal cells that are principally located in the adventitial layer. By interfering with collagen deposition in the adventitia, MMP-9 may therefore serve as a permissive factor for rupture. It appears that finally progress is being made in elucidating the clinically relevant biochemistry of AAA. Perhaps someday circulating MMP levels will identify patients at risk for aneurysm rupture and/or expansion.

G. L. Moneta, MD

Plasma Levels of Metalloproteinases-3 and -9 as Markers of Successful Abdominal Aortic Aneurysm Exclusion After Endovascular Graft Treatment
Sangiorgi G, D'Averio R, Mauriello A, et al (Univ of Milan, Italy; San Raffaele Hosp, Milan, Italy; Univ of Rome Tor Vergata)
Circulation 104[suppl I]:I-288-I-295, 2001   7–5

Background.—Histologically, specimens of abdominal aortic aneurysms (AAAs) show evidence of degradation of matrix proteins caused by production of matrix metalloproteinases (MMPs). The effects of AAA repair on plasma MMP levels are unknown. Circulating levels of MMP-3 and MMP-9 in patients undergoing endovascular graft exclusion were compared with those in patients undergoing open repair of AAA.

Methods.—The study included 30 patients undergoing endovascular repair, 15 patients undergoing open surgical repair of AAA, and 10 healthy control subjects. Patients underwent measurement of plasma MMP-3 and MMP-9 levels before AAA repair and at 1-, 3-, and 6-months' follow-up. For patients undergoing open surgery, aneurysmal tissue samples were analyzed for MMP-3 and MMP-9 by immunohistochemical staining.

Results.—As measured by the enzyme-linked immunosorbent assay (ELISA) sandwich technique, baseline MMP levels were higher in the AAA groups than in the control group. The mean MMP-9 values were 32.3 ng/mL in the endovascular group and 28.0 ng/mL in the open surgery group, compared with 8.9 ng/mL in the control group; MMP-3 values for the 3 groups for the same variables were 18.3, 26.7, and 8.2 ng/mL, respectively. Six months after open surgery, MMP-9 decreased to 14.7 ng/mL and MMP-3 to 12.0 ng/mL. In the endovascular group, these values were significantly higher for patients with imaging evidence of endoleak at 6 months' follow-up: MMP-9 was 44.3 ng/mL in patients with endoleak compared with 14.6 ng/mL in those without. Values for MMP-3 were 25.0 versus 10.3 ng/mL, respectively (Fig 2).

Conclusions.—For patients with AAA, open surgical repair leads to significant reductions in plasma MMP-9 and MMP-3 levels. The same is true for patients with successful endovascular graft exclusion; however, MMP levels remain elevated for patients with endoleak. Monitoring of plasma

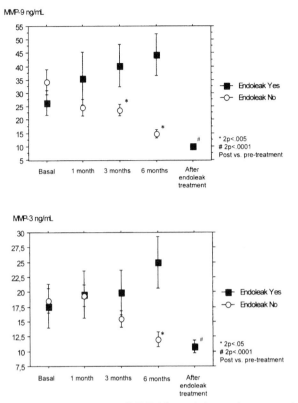

FIGURE 2.—Mean (±SEM) MMP-9 (**top**) and MMP-3 (**bottom**) plasma value concentrations before and during follow-up after stent graft placement. Plasma levels of both MMP-9 and MMP-3 decreased in patients showing no endoleak (n = 23), whereas increase was observed in patients with endoleakage (n = 7). In those who were treated for endoleak presence (n = 5), significant decrease in MMP-9 and MMP-3 plasma levels compared with pretreatment values was observed 6 months after treatment. (Courtesy of Sangiorgi G, D'Averio R, Mauriello A, et al: Plasma levels of metalloproteinases-3 and -9 as markers of successful abdominal aortic aneurysm exclusion after endovascular graft treatment. *Circulation* 104 (suppl I):I-288-I-295, 2001.)

MMP levels after endovascular AAA repair may help in identifying patients with endoleak.

▶ In this study, the reduction of plasma levels of MMP-3 and MMP-9 in patients with AAAs, repaired by open or endovascular techniques, fell with successful exclusion of the aneurysm. Interestingly, aneurysms repaired with endovascular techniques and which manifested persistent endoleak, had an increase in MMP levels. There is, therefore, the intriguing possibility that MMP-9 and MMP-3 levels can be used as biomarkers for successful exclusion of AAAs by endovascular repair. If this hypothesis is confirmed by larger prospective studies, it may be that our endovascular aneurysm patients will be followed with MMP levels rather than serial CT scans.

G. L. Moneta, MD

Arterial Dimensions in the Lower Extremities of Patients With Abdominal Aortic Aneurysms—No Indications of a Generalized Dilating Diathesis

Sandgren T, Sonesson B, Ryden-Ahlgren Å, et al (Univ of Lund, Malmö, Sweden; Univ of Linköping, Jönköping, Sweden)
J Vasc Surg 34:1079-1084, 2001   7–6

Background.—The examination of abdominal aortic aneurysms (AAAs) reveals degradation of the extracellular matrix with disruption of elastic fibers. Both anatomical and mechanical factors are important in this degenerative process. Recent studies that demonstrated defects in mechanical properties in the vascular wall of distant arteries not prone to dilation have led to speculation that AAAs result not only from a local process in the abdominal aorta but indicate a generalized arterial abnormality. The regulation of blood flow has also been shown to be disturbed. Earlier studies have indicated a tendency toward general dilatation of the peripheral arteries in patients with AAAs. One problem with these studies, however, is that the normal diameters of the arteries under study were not known. It has recently been reported that the diameters of peripheral arteries increase about 20% to 25% between 20 and 70 years and that the size of an artery is dependent on both sex and body habitus. Whether a dilating diathesis is present in peripheral arteries of patients with AAAs was investigated.

Methods.—The anteroposterior diameters of the common femoral artery (CFA) and popliteal artery (PA) were measured in a series of 183 patients with an AAA. The group consisted of 158 men and 25 women ages 57 to 78 years. Measurements of the CFA and PA were obtained before elective surgery on the patients with AAA and compared with the same measurements in healthy age-matched control subjects.

Results.—Among male patients, 8 CFA aneurysms and 4 PA aneurysms were found. Of these patients, 46% of patients with aneurysms of the CFA and 49% of patients with aneurysms of the PA were affected by peripheral vascular occlusive disease (PVOD). The CFA diameters of the patients with AAAs were 97.8% of those in healthy control subjects. Exclusion of the CFA aneurysms yielded CFA diameters that were 92.7% of those in control subjects. Similar findings were reported for the PA diameters in patients with AAAs versus those in control subjects.

Conclusions.—Excluding the few patients with AAAs who had peripheral aneurysmal disease and those with PVOD, no dilating diathesis was found in CFAs and PAs. This result is supportive of the hypothesis that specific genetic factors or other factors not present in the majority of AAAs are responsible for the development of concomitant peripheral aneurysms.

▶ The results of this study are somewhat surprising. Many of us feel that patients with AAAs have overall larger arteries than those patients who do not have AAAs. The results of this study clearly indicate that, at least with respect to the common femoral and popliteal arteries, there is no real difference between the size of these vessels in normal patients versus those with AAAs.

The results imply that specific factors leading to the development of AAAs are different than those leading to the development of peripheral artery aneurysms. However, there must be some overlap. It is well known AAAs are more common in patients with peripheral artery aneurysms than in the general population.

G. L. Moneta, MD

Hospital Costs and Benefits of Screening for Abdominal Aortic Aneurysms: Results From a Randomised Population Screening Trial

Lindholt JS, Juul S, Fasting H, et al (Viborg Hosp, Denmark; Univ of Aarhus, Denmark)

Eur J Vasc Endovasc Surg 23:55-60, 2002   7–7

Background.—Whether screening for abdominal aortic aneurysm (AAA) is a cost-effective strategy remains controversial. The hospital costs and benefits of AAA screening in older men were analyzed in a population-based study.

Methods.—Contact information for 12,658 men (ages 65-73 years) living in 1 county in Denmark was obtained in 1994. Subjects were randomly assigned to a control group (n = 6319) or to a group that was offered free hospital-based screening for AAA (n = 6339). Subjects whose AAA was more than 5 cm in diameter were referred for surgery; other subjects with AAA were offered annual scans. In addition, subjects with aortic ectasia were offered screening every 5 years. Patients were followed up through March 2001 (mean follow-up, 5.13 years) to identify operations for AAA and hospital deaths caused by AAA. Cost data (including screening, surveillance, and treatment) were obtained for both groups.

Results.—Of the 6339 subjects invited to undergo AAA screening, 4843 (76%) accepted. Screening identified an AAA in 191 subjects (4%), and in 24 subjects (12.5%), the AAA was more than 5 cm. Another 51 subjects were referred for surgery during follow-up. Overall, of the 75 subjects referred for surgery, 60 either chose to or were able to undergo surgery. This number was not significantly higher than in the control group (41 control subjects underwent surgery), but the number of emergent operations was significantly less in the screened group (7 vs 27 cases). The number of hospital deaths resulting from AAA was also significantly lower in the screened group (6 vs 19 deaths). The costs were 83.50 DKK (approximately $10.50 US) per scan, 81,400 DKK (approximately $10,175 US) per elective operation in the control group, 71,485 DKK (approximately $8935 US) per elective operation in the screened group, and 117,000 DKK (approximately $14,625 US) per emergency operation. The cost of preventing each hospital death caused by AAA (including indirect costs) was 67,855 DKK (approximately $8480 US), and the cost per life-year saved was about 7540 DKK (approximately $945 US).

Conclusions.—AAA screening among elderly men proved to be cost effective by significantly reducing by 74% the number of emergent operations for

AAA and by reducing by 68% the number of hospital deaths caused by AAA. The costs associated with preventing hospital deaths and with each life-year saved are reasonable compared with the costs of other interventions that are also considered to be cost effective.

▶ It is always so very difficult to interpret the cost-effectiveness of screening for treatable diseases. In this study, even given the costs of the screening procedures and the costs of emergency and elective operations, screening for AAAs appeared to be cost-effective and successful in reducing hospital-associated AAA mortality. This study likely was successful in establishing cost-effectiveness for screening because the authors restricted the screening to older males (older than 65 years), the group most likely to have an AAA. In addition, the screening study itself was very inexpensive. At one time in our practice, we routinely screened patients for AAAs. In recent years, we have stopped screening, but perhaps it should be reconsidered in the older male.

G. L. Moneta, MD

Randomized Clinical Trial of Screening for Abdominal Aortic Aneurysm in Women

Scott RAP, Bridgewater SG, Ashton HA (St Richard's Hosp, Chichester, England)
Br J Surg 89:283-285, 2002
7–8

Background.—Most studies of the effectiveness of screening for abdominal aortic aneurysm (AAA) have involved men older than 60 years. One factor in defining a population to screen is the prevalence of AAA. However, the incidence of rupture also is an important consideration, since the aim of screening is not only to detect AAA but also to prevent rupture. Recent studies have suggested that the mortality rate associated with ruptured AAA in women is increasing and that the rate of rupture of AAA is higher in women than in men. To assess the value of screening women for AAA, a screening program was implemented in the United Kingdom as part of a randomized controlled trial. Results after 10 years are reported.

Methods.—The trial, in which 9342 women and 6433 men were screened for AAA, began in Chichester in 1988. Subjects' ages ranged from 65 to 80 years. The women were randomly divided into age-matched screening (4682 women) and control (4660 women) groups. Women in the screening group were invited to undergo US measurement of the abdominal aorta. Those in whom an AAA was detected (aortic diameter 3 cm or greater) were followed up with repeat US at intervals determined by the diameter of the aneurysm. Surgical repair was considered in AAAs in which the aortic diameter measured 6 cm or larger, the diameter increased by at least 1 cm in a year, or the aneurysm became symptomatic.

Results.—The prevalence of AAA was 1.3% in women and 7.6% in men. The incidence of rupture at 5 and 10 years was the same for the screened and control groups of women.

Conclusions.—It would appear from these findings that screening for AAA in women is not indicated and is not cost effective.

▶ Screening for AAAs under appropriate circumstances (older males older than 65 years with an inexpensive US scan) appears cost-effective in identifying AAAs and reducing AAA mortality (see Abstract 7–7). Based on the data in this article, screening should not be extended to women. It appears the incidence of AAA in women is sufficiently low, so screening is neither clinically indicated nor economically cost-effective.

G. L. Moneta, MD

Propranolol for Small Abdominal Aortic Aneurysms: Results of a Randomized Trial

Laupacis A, for the Propranolol Aneurysm Trial Investigators (Inst for Clinical Evaluative Sciences, Toronto)

J Vasc Surg 35:72-79, 2002   7–9

Background.—The observation of patients with a small, asymptomatic abdominal aortic aneurysm (AAA) with regular US scanning until the aneurysm reaches a size where elective resection is considered is widely practiced. A medication to delay the growth rate of AAAs probably would be used by patients and clinicians. Randomized trials have shown that propranolol decreases aneurysm growth and the risk of rupture in animals that spontaneously develop aortic aneurysms. Whether it has the same effect in human patients with small AAAs was investigated.

Methods.—Patients with an asymptomatic AAA of 3 to 5 cm were randomly selected to receive either propranolol (276 patients) or placebo (272 patients) in a double-blind study. They were observed for a mean of 2.5 years. The study's primary end point was the mean annual growth rate of the aneurysm as determined by US scanning every 6 months. Secondary outcomes were death, surgery, withdrawal from study medication, and quality of life as measured by the Short-Form Health Survey (SF-36). Analyses were by intention-to-treat.

Results.—The groups were similar at baseline. Fewer patients in the placebo group stopped their medication (26.8% vs 42.4%) (Fig 2). Both groups had similar growth rates, but there was a trend toward more elective surgery in the placebo group (26.5% vs 20.3%). However, there was no significant difference in the death rate (placebo, 9%; propranolol, 12%). Patients in the propranolol group had a significantly poorer quality of life in the SF-36 areas of physical functioning, physical role, and vitality.

Conclusions.—Propranolol is not well tolerated by patients with AAAs, and it had no significant effect on the growth rate of small AAAs.

FIGURE 2

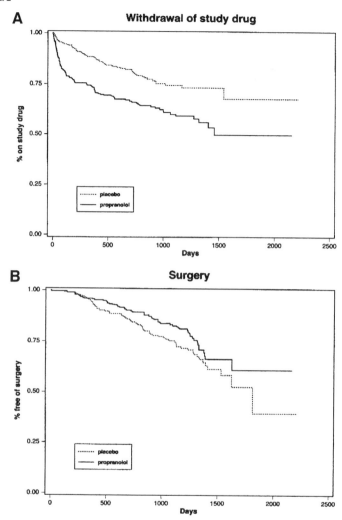

A **Withdrawal of study drug**

% on study drug vs *Days*

placebo
propranolol

B **Surgery**

% free of surgery vs *Days*

placebo
propranolol

(Continued)

▶ In past years, nonrandomized trials have found that the growth rate of AAA in patients receiving a β-blocker was less than in patients not receiving a β-blocker. This study examined the role of β-blockers in preventing aneurysm expansion in a prospective fashion. The results of the study are disappointing for those interested in medical management of AAAs. The results do not sup-

FIGURE 2 (cont.)

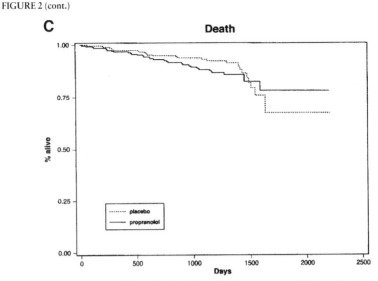

FIGURE 2.—A, Time to withdrawal of study drug. B, Time to surgery. C, Time to death. (Courtesy of Laupacis A, for the Propranolol Aneurysm Trial Investigators: Propranolol for small abdominal aortic aneurysms: Results of a randomized trial. *J Vasc Surg* 35:72-79, 2002.)

port the hypothesis that propranolol reduces expansion rates of AAAs. In addition, patients tolerated propranolol relatively poorly, and the drug did not reduce time to surgery or time to death in patients with AAAs. Propranolol does not appear to affect AAAs.

G. L. Moneta, MD

Prognosis of Patients Turned Down for Conventional Abdominal Aortic Aneurysm Repair in the Endovascular and Sonographic Era: Szilagyi Revisited?
Conway KP, Byrne J, Townsend M, et al (Univ Hosp of Wales, Heath Park, Cardiff)
J Vasc Surg 33:752-757, 2001   7–10

Background.—In 1998, the United Kingdom Small Aneurysm study found a low risk of rupture in abdominal aortic aneurysms (AAAs) less than 5.5 cm in diameter. Autopsy studies based on the clinical and radiographic assessment of aneurysm size have also suggested a correlation between size and risk of rupture. These studies were performed before the availability of current imaging technologies, however, and did not allow risk stratification on the basis of size at presentation.

The UK aneurysm trial is not likely to be repeated for larger AAAs; thus, evidence supporting nonintervention for AAAs larger than 5.5 cm must come from indirect sources. With the development of endoluminal tech-

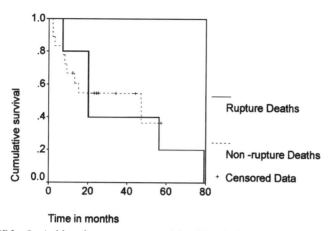

FIGURE 2.—Survival free of rupture, anuerysyms 5.5 to 5.9 cm in diameter. (Courtesy of Conway KP, Byrne J, Townsend M, et al: Prognosis of patients turned down for conventional abdominal aortic aneurysm repair in the endovascular and sonographic era: Szilagyi revisited? *J Vasc Surg* 33:752-757, 2001.)

niques, patients who are not candidates for laparotomy are now considered for endovascular repair. However, the natural history of larger aneurysms is uncertain, particularly in the presence of severe comorbidity. The outcome of patients referred with AAAs larger than 5.5 cm in diameter who were turned down for elective open repair were studied. The cause of death and risk of rupture were determined in all patients.

Methods.—A prospective log was maintained for all patients with AAAs for 10 years, and demographic details on all patients with AAAs larger than 5.5 cm were collected. Copies of death certificates were obtained as well as local in-hospital patient records and general practitioner records. The results of postmortem examinations were also obtained. AAAs were stratified

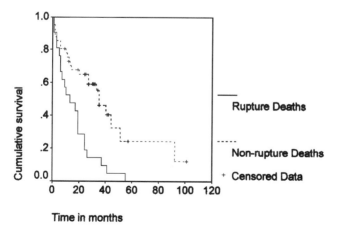

FIGURE 4.—Survival free of rupture, anuerysyms 6.0 to 7.0 cm in diameter. (Courtesy of Conway KP, Byrne J, Townsend M, et al: Prognosis of patients turned down for conventional abdominal aortic aneurysm repair in the endovascular and sonographic era: Szilagyi revisited? *J Vasc Surg* 33:752-757, 2001.)

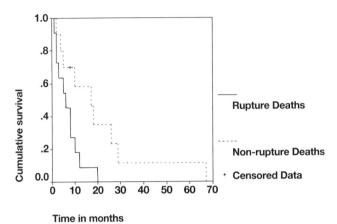

Time in months

FIGURE 6.—Survival free of rupture, anuerysms larger than 7.0 cm in diameter. (Courtesy of Conway KP, Byrne J, Townsend M, et al: Prognosis of patients turned down for conventional abdominal aortic aneurysm repair in the endovascular and sonographic era: Szilagyi revisited? *J Vasc Surg* 33:752-757, 2001.)

on the basis of their size at presentation (5.5-5.9 cm; 6.0-7.0 cm; and >7.0 cm) and reasons for nonintervention were documented.

Results.—Requests for elective repair of AAA were turned down for 106 patients during a 10-year period. The mean age of these patients was 78.4 years, and 76 of the 106 patients had died at the end of the study. The overall 3-year survival rate was 17%. Patients with aneurysms larger than 7.0 cm survived for a median of 9 months. Rupture of AAA was certified as the cause of death in 36% of patients with aneurysms of 5.5 to 5.9 cm (Fig 2), in 50% of patients with aneurysms of 6.0 to 7.0 cm (Fig 4), and in 55% of patients with aneurysms larger than 7.0 cm (Fig 6). The most common reason for not intervening was patient refusal (31 patients), followed by "unfit for surgery" (18 patients), advanced age (18 patients), cardiac disease (9 patients), cancer (9 patients), and respiratory disease (6 patients). Fifteen patients were turned down for AAA repair for other causes.

Conclusions.—Rupture was a significant cause of death in patients with untreated AAAs larger than 5.5 cm. The prognosis appeared to be much worse for patients with AAAs larger than 7.0 cm.

▶ Results of this study should be compared with the Department of Veterans Affairs (ADAM) Trial of untreated large AAAs (Abstract 7–2), as well as Szilagyi's 1972 article[1] examining the fate of patients with asymptomatic AAAs who were judged unfit for surgical treatment. Although the numbers vary among the reports, in essence they indicate a very small rupture risk for small AAAs (<5.5 cm in diameter), a significant risk of rupture for aneurysms greater than 5.5 cm in diameter, and a very high risk of rupture once the aneurysm reaches 7 cm. I believe the data currently available justify withholding elective repair of AAAs until the aneurysm reaches 5.5 cm. In addition, unless the operative risk is prohibitive, or the chance of meaningful recovery truly unlikely, aneurysms greater than 7 cm in diameter need to be repaired.

G. L. Moneta, MD

Reference

1. Szilagyi DE, Elliot JP, Smith RF: Clinical fate of the patient with asymptomatic abdominal aortic aneurysm and unfit for surgical treatment. *Arch Surg* 104:600-606, 1972.

Durability of Open Repair of Infrarenal Abdominal Aortic Aneurysm: A 15-Year Follow-up Study
Biancari F, Ylönen K, Anttila V, et al (Oulu Univ, Finland; Kainuu Central Hosp, Kajaani, Finland)
J Vasc Surg 35:87-93, 2002   7–11

Background.—Only a few studies have evaluated the fate of infrarenal aortic grafts. Anecdotal reports on the complications associated with endovascular repair of abdominal aortic aneurysms (AAAs) have become more frequent as endovascular repair has become more common, and recent studies have questioned the technique's clinical and economic benefits. Of most concern are early and midterm technical failures of endovascular grafting for AAA. The long-term outcome of patients who underwent open repair of infrarenal AAAs was reviewed retrospectively.

Methods.—All 208 patients studied (188 men; mean age, 65.6 years) had survived elective or emergency open repair of infrarenal AAA at a university referral hospital. The main outcome measures were late graft-related complications, survival free from any reintervention, survival free from vascular reintervention, and overall survival rates.

Results.—Thirty-two patients (15.4%) experienced graft-related complications. Six patients (2.9%) experienced a proximal para-anastomotic pseudoaneurysm, and a distal pseudoaneurysm developed in 18 patients (8.7%). Eleven patients (5.3%) developed a graft limb occlusion. These complications required 37 surgical or otherwise-invasive procedures in 27 patients (13%). The rates of survival free from any reintervention were 91.5% at 5 years, 86.2% at 10 years, and 72% at 15 years, and overall survival rates were 66.8%, 39.4%, and 18%, respectively (Fig 3). Age and chronic obstructive pulmonary disease were found to predict poor survival outcome, and chronic obstructive pulmonary disease and lower limb ischemia were found to be associated with an increased need for vascular reintervention to treat graft-related complications.

Conclusions.—Open repair of infrarenal AAAs can provide satisfactory 15-year follow-up rates of survival free from reintervention for graft-related

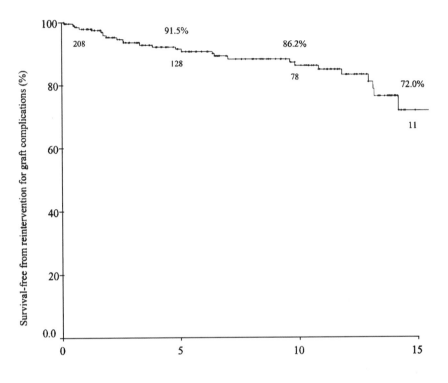

Years

FIGURE 3.—Kaplan–Meier estimates for survival free from any reintervention for graft-related complications (SE < 6.4%). Numbers of patients at risk entering each 5-year interval are given. (Courtesy of Biancari F, Ylönen K, Anttila V, et al: Durability of open repair of infrarenal abdominal aortic aneurysm: A 15-year follow-up study. *J Vasc Surg* 35:87-93, 2002.)

complications. Surgery should be considered the procedure of choice to repair infrarenal AAAs in patients who are suitable candidates.

▶ This study documents the durability of open repair of infrarenal AAAs. With a median follow-up period of 8 years in 208 patients treated with open repair of infrarenal AAA, graft-related complications occurred in 15.4%, and graft-related deaths in 1.9%. The 15-year survival free from any vascular intervention was 74%. These results suggest that if one considers primarily late graft-related complications and late graft-related deaths, open surgery should still be the procedure of choice for infrarenal AAAs. Of course, patient recovery times and the allure of something new cannot be ignored. Endovascular aneurysm repair will not go away just because open repair appears superior in the long run.

G. L. Moneta, MD

Minimal Incision Aortic Surgery

Turnipseed WD, Carr SC, Tefera G, et al (Univ of Wisconsin, Madison)

J Vasc Surg 34:47-53, 2001   7–12

Background.—Clinical trials have shown that endograft repair of aneurysms is feasible and safe. However, durability and performance in the long term have not been established. In addition, no one has proved that such treatment reduces morbidity and mortality rates in high-risk patients or the intensity, duration, and cost of care in less critically ill patients with aortic disease. The clinical outcome and cost of a less invasive method of aortic exposure for routine treatment of abdominal aortic aneurysms (AAAs) and aortoiliac occlusive disease (AIOD) were investigated.

Methods.—Thirty-four patients with AAAs and 16 with AIOD were prospectively treated with minimal incision aortic surgery (MIAS). This group was compared with 50 patients, including 40 with AAAs and 10 with AIOD, treated in the same period with long midline incision and extracavitary small bowel retraction. In addition, a cohort of 32 patients with AAAs treated by endoaortic stent grafts was studied for comparison.

Findings.—Patients with no perioperative complications after MIAS or endovascular repair had briefer hospital stays than patients with uncomplicated aortic repairs done with a traditional long midline abdominal incision. The mean hospital stays for these 3 groups were 3 days, 3 days, and 7.2 days, respectively. Patients undergoing less invasive procedures even had a significantly shorter length of hospitalization when perioperative complications were included. Patients undergoing MIAS and endovascular aortic repair had a briefer stay in the ICU and a faster return to general dietary feeding compared with those undergoing standard open repair. Overall morbidity was 14% for MIAS, 21% for the endovascular technique, and 24% for standard open repair. These rates were not significantly different. Mortality rate was 2%, 3%, and 2%, respectively—also not significantly different. MIAS was more cost effective than either the standard open repair or the endoaortic repair.

Conclusions.—MIAS is as safe as the standard open or endovascular procedure in patients with AAA and AIOD. This less invasive technique is less costly than the other procedures because of shorter ICU and hospital stays and lower direct intraoperative costs, respectively.

▶ Readers of the YEAR BOOK OF VASCULAR SURGERY are encouraged to carefully review the surgical technique of MIAS presented in this article. I have watched Dr Turnipseed perform this operation. To me, it seems a bit of a "goat rope." Nonetheless, if one is willing to struggle a little more than usual, it appears with this procedure that one can reduce hospital stays and costs associated with open abdominal aortic surgery.

G. L. Moneta, MD

Factors Affecting Outcome in Proximal Abdominal Aortic Aneurysm Repair

Anagnostopoulos PV, Shepard AD, Pipinos II, et al (Henry Ford Hosp, Detroit)
Ann Vasc Surg 15:511-519, 2001   7–13

Background.—Repair of abdominal aortic aneurysms (AAAs) involving the proximal abdominal aorta (above the origins of the renal or visceral arteries) is a challenging procedure. These patients are prone to certain cardiac complications, leading to an increased mortality rate. The results of surgery to repair proximal AAA in 65 patients were reviewed, and the factors influencing patient outcomes were analyzed.

Methods.—The study included 65 patients (43 men and 22 women; mean age, 68 years) who underwent nonemergent surgery for repair of a proximal AAA between January 1986 and June 1999. The mean aneurysm diameter was 6.7 cm. In most patients, the repair was done through an extended left flank retroperitoneal exposure. Variables influencing postoperative mortality were assessed by multivariate analysis.

Results.—No perioperative deaths occurred, and no postoperative cases of paraparesis/paraplegia, or symptomatic visceral ischemia were noted. Forty-two percent of patients had postoperative renal dysfunction, and 9% required dialysis, but the permanent dialysis rate was only 2%. Postoperative pulmonary dysfunction developed in 34% of patients, with 6 patients requiring reintubation. On multivariate analysis, the factor most strongly associated with pulmonary dysfunction was radial diaphragm division, followed by operative time and estimated blood loss (Table 5).

Conclusions.—The experience supports the safety of elective repair of proximal AAAs, with acceptable morbidity and mortality rates. Careful surgical planning is essential, particularly concerning the exposure technique and the level of proximal aortic control. For patients undergoing renal artery bypass or reimplantation, the risk of renal dysfunction may be reduced by cold renal perfusion. Radial division of the diaphragm is the main risk factor for pulmonary dysfunction.

▶ In the era of endovascular AAA repair, we, and others, have noted that more and more of our open AAA repairs involve AAAs arising above the visceral and/ or renal arteries. This paper offers a number of technical hints that may help in

TABLE 5.—Multivariate Analysis of Pulmonary Dysfunction

Variable	Odds Ratio	P
Radial diaphragm division	6.65	.003
Operative time (increments of 1 hr)	1.65	.023
Estimated blood loss (increments of 100 mL)	1.03	.019

(Courtesy of Anagnostopoulos PV, Shepard AD, Pipinos II, et al: Factors affecting outcome in proximal abdominal aortic aneurysm repair. *Ann Vasc Surg* 15:511-519, 2001.)

minimizing morbidity and mortality in the repair of such aneurysms. The authors emphasize the use of an extended left flank approach through the 9th or 10th intercostal space, supraceliac clamping of the aorta, avoiding radial division of the diaphragm, and the use of long beveled proximal anastomoses with prosthetic grafting of the left renal artery.

G. L. Moneta, MD

Suprarenal or Supraceliac Aortic Clamping During Repair of Infrarenal Abdominal Aortic Aneurysms
El-Sabrout RA, Reul GJ (Texas Heart Inst, Houston)
Tex Heart Inst J 28:254-264, 2001   7–14

Background.—The majority of infrarenal (IR) abdominal aortic aneurysms (AAAs) can be safely repaired with IR aortic cross-clamping. In some patients, IR clamping can be difficult or impossible because of the presence of unusual lesions or other patient-related factors. Several technical variations can be used to control the IR aorta in these situations, including clamping of the suprarenal (SR), visceral, or supraceliac (SC) aortic segments. The optimal level of proximal aortic control in the treatment of aortic aneurysmal disease has been controversial. Suprarenal or supraceliac aortic clamping during repair of IR AAAs can be complicated by renal, hepatic, and intestinal ischemia. Whether morbidity and mortality in patients with IR AAAs are increased by suprarenal or supraceliac clamping was studied.

Methods.—The authors' experience was retrospectively reviewed in this nonrandomized study. A total of 716 patients underwent elective (682 patients) or urgent (34 patients) IR AAA repair from January 1993 to December 1998.

Results.—IR clamping was used in 516 patients (72.1%) and suprarenal or supraceliac clamping was used in 200 patients (27.9%). The suprarenal/supraceliac group had significantly more patients age 70 years or older (65.5% vs 47.7%) and a higher incidence of preoperative renal insufficiency (7.5% vs 5.5%) compared with the IR clamping group. Suprarenal/supraceliac clamping was used more often than IR clamping in the treatment of ruptured aneurysms (12.5% vs 1.74%). Both groups had similar operative times, but transfusion requirements and length of hospital stay were slightly greater in the suprarenal/supraceliac group. The overall perioperative mortality was 3.1%, but perioperative mortality was higher in the suprarenal/supraceliac group (7.5% vs 1.4%). Postoperative complications developed in 13% of patients in the suprarenal/supraceliac clamping group. Nine other patients in this group required abdominal reexploration.

Conclusions.—Elective suprarenal/supraceliac clamping during repair of IR abdominal aortic aneurysm does not significantly increase mortality. It is a safe technique that facilitates repair, despite associated comorbidities.

▶ The authors in this study were bound and determined to justify a liberal use of supraceliac clamping during repair of infrarenal AAAs. In 200 of 750 patients undergoing infrarenal abdominal aortic aneurysm repair, a supraceliac clamp was used. The mortality in the supraceliac patients was 7.5% versus 1.4% in the infrarenally clamped patients. In more than half the patients in which the supraceliac clamp was utilized, the clamp was used at the discretion of the operating surgeon, and there was no specific indication such as ruptured aneurysm or juxtarenal aneurysm, or need for renal or visceral repair. Perioperative mortality was higher in the supraceliac group (7.5%) than in the infrarenal group (1.4%). Despite this, the authors conclude that suprarenal/supraceliac clamping during infrarenal AAA repair does not significantly increase mortality. I don't see how the authors can make this statement based on the data presented in their report. The ability to accurately and rapidly place a supraceliac aortic clamp should be part of the skills of any vascular surgeon. When it is needed, a supraceliac clamp is clearly preferable to trying to force an infrarenal clamp. However, if the infrarenal aorta can be safely clamped, it seems prudent to utilize this approach rather than a supraceliac clamp.

G. L. Moneta, MD

Risk Factors and Operative Results of Patients Aged Less Than 66 Years Operated on for Asymptomatic Abdominal Aortic Aneurysm
Aune S (Haukeland Univ, Bergen, Norway)
Eur J Vasc Endovasc Surg 22:240-243, 2001   7–15

Background.—Most patients with abominal aortic aneurysm (AAA) are in their seventh or eighth decade of life, and their risk factors, surgical complications, and survival have been well characterized. One author's experience with the risk factors, complications, and survival of patients less than 66 years of age with AAA were described.

Methods.—The subjects were 118 patients (107 men and 11 women) 40 to 65 years of age (mean age, 60.5 years) who underwent surgery for AAA. The preoperative risk factors, early complications, 30-day mortality rates, and survival of these younger patients were compared with those of 333 older patients who underwent surgery during the same period. The mean follow-up of the younger patients was 72 months.

Results.—Preoperative risk factors for the younger patients were similar to those of the older group and included hypertension in 41% of patients, cardiac disease in 27%, pulmonary disease in 14%, and diabetes mellitus in 9%. Coronary artery disease was prevalent in both groups; 22% of the younger patients had had a previous myocardial infarction, 15% had angina pectoris, 2% had atrial fibrillation, 2% had heart failure, and 11% had had previous coronary artery bypass grafting. Thirty-day mortality rates between the younger and older groups did not differ significantly (1.7% and 6%, respectively), nor did the incidence of major surgical complications (9% and 11%, respectively). However, younger patients tended to have more medical complaints (9% vs 4%; $P = .06$).

Observed survival at 8 years was 69% in the younger patients, which is significantly worse than that of a demographically matched population

(83%). Observed survival at 8 years was 47% in the older group, which is significantly worse than that in the younger group but not significantly different than that of a demographically matched population.

Conclusion.—Preoperative risk factors and 30-day complication rates were similar in younger and older patients undergoing surgery for AAA. The younger patients had slightly better operative survival, but their long-term survival was worse relative to that of a demographically matched population. Nonetheless, these results do not suggest that a more aggressive approach to AAA repair is needed for patients less than 66 years of age.

▶ This article emphasizes the fact that young patients with AAAs do not have decreased risk of aneurysm repair simply because of their younger age. The patients were not healthier than older patients, and complications were equally common, and long-term survival was actually poorer than that of the older patient. Therefore, just because the patient is younger and has an AAA, one should not repair an AAA that is smaller than one would normally repair in an older patient. Repair aneurysms based on the presence of symptoms and aneurysm diameter but do not use young patient age as a justification for repairing a small AAA.

G. L. Moneta, MD

A Randomized Study to Evaluate the Effect of a Perioperative Infusion of Dopexamine on Colonic Mucosal Ischemia After Aortic Surgery

Baguneid MS, Welch M, Bukhari M, et al (Manchester Royal Infirmary, England; Univ of Manchester, England)
J Vasc Surg 33:758-763, 2001   7–16

Background.—Colonic ischemia is a well-characterized complication of abdominal aortic surgery, with high morbidity and mortality. The synthetic catecholamine dopexamine hydrochloride was studied for its ability to prevent colonic mucosal ischemia in patients undergoing aortic surgery.

Methods.—The study included 30 patients (mean age, 65 years) who were undergoing elective infrarenal aortic surgery. After optimization of hemodynamic and respiratory variables, patients were randomly assigned to receive perioperative dopexamine in a 2 μg/kg/min infusion or a 0.9% saline solution infusion. Before and 1 week after aortic surgery, colonoscopy with biopsy was performed to assess the presence of mucosal ischemia and selected inflammatory markers.

Results.—Dopexamine made no difference in fluid or blood requirements or hemodynamic/respiratory variables. Mucosal ischemic changes were detected in just 1 of the 12 patients receiving dopexamine versus 8 of the 18 receiving placebo. On comparison of preoperative and postoperative biopsy specimens, 17% of the patients in the dopexamine group had worsening scores compared with 50% in the placebo group. Inflammatory markers were not significantly different between the 2 treatment groups, although patients with evidence of ischemia showed increased expression of mast cell tryptase and myeloperoxidase and increased inducible nitric oxide synthase staining within the vascular and lamina propria compartments of the mucosa.

Conclusions.—In patients undergoing infrarenal aortic surgery, giving dopexamine hydrochloride infusion during the perioperative period may help to prevent colonic mucosal ischemia. In this situation, dopexamine appears to have a significant anti-inflammatory effect in addition to its hemodynamic effect.

▶ It has long been known that the incidence of subclinical colonic ischemia after an aortic operation is much higher than that of clinically evident colonic ischemia. In this study, the use of dopexamine hydrochloride, a synthetic catecholamine, with dopenergic receptor agonist properties for both dopamine-1 and -2 receptors, was associated with significant histologic protection of colonic mucosa after aortic surgery. The drug was given as a 24-hour infusion beginning after induction of anesthesia. It was not associated with any increased complications. Based on this study, dopexamine may be a promising adjunct in reducing colonic ischemic complications after aortic surgery.

G. L. Moneta, MD

8 Aortoiliac Disease

Distal Aortic Diameter and Peripheral Arterial Occlusive Disease
van der Graaf Y, for the SMART Study Group (Univ Med Ctr, Utrecht, The Netherlands)
J Vasc Surg 34:1085-1089, 2001   8–1

Background.—Previous studies have suggested that distal aortic diameter is a factor in the development of peripheral arterial occlusive disease (PAOD). As many as 40% of patients with abdominal aortic aneurysms (AAAs) have PAOD. An association of PAOD with peripheral aortic occlusive disease has also been reported in studies of hypoplasia of the distal aorta. However, no precise estimates have been reported of the relationship between aortic hypoplasia and PAOD. The relationship between abdominal aortic diameter and PAOD was investigated.

Methods.—This cross-sectional study included 1572 patients (ages 18-79 years) who were newly referred to 1 institution's vascular center. All of the patients were referred for either clinically evident atherosclerotic arterial disease or treatment of cardiovascular risk factors. Diameters of AAAs were measured, and results were used to subdivide patients on the basis of tertiles of these measurements. PAOD was assessed by the adjusted Rose questionnaire, ankle-brachial pressure index, and the presence of gangrene or leg ulcers.

Results.—In comparison with patients with a normal aortic diameter, the prevalence of PAOD was twice as high for patients at both ends of the aortic diameter range. A comparison of the lowest tertile with the middle tertile in the male patients yielded an adjusted odds ratio of 1.7. A comparison of the highest tertile with the middle tertile yielded an adjusted odds ratio of 2.1.

Conclusions.—The risk of PAOD was increased at both the lower and the upper distributions of abdominal aortic diameter. This study is the first large-scale investigation to report the association of a small aortic diameter with PAOD.

▶ Well, small aortas appear to be associated with arterial occlusive disease in patients referred to a vascular center with either peripheral arterial disease or risk factors for peripheral arterial disease. I accept the association but don't know what to do with it. If the patient has peripheral arterial disease, it should be managed; if the patient has only risk factors, they should be managed as well. I don't see how to incorporate aortic diameter into the management algorithm.

G. L. Moneta, MD

Femorofemoral Bypass Grafts: Factors Influencing Long-term Patency Rate and Outcome

Mingoli A, Sapienza P, Feldhaus RJ, et al (Univ of Rome La Sapienza; Creighton Univ, Omaha, Neb)
Surgery 129:451-458, 2001   8–2

Background.—Crossover femorofemoral bypass grafting (CFFBG) has been considered a last-resort technique for patients with critical limb ischemia, to be used only in patients with unilateral iliac artery lesions who were considered at high surgical risk. The effects of selected variables on the short-term and long-term outcomes of CFFBG for critical limb ischemia were assessed in a 20-year experience.

Patients.—The retrospective analysis included 228 patients undergoing CFFBG at a university hospital from 1973 to 1993. Sixty-eight percent of the patients were considered to be at high surgical risk, whereas 82% had limb-threatening ischemia as their indication for surgery. One hundred fifty patients underwent CFFBG as their primary procedure, whereas 78 underwent CFFBG after failure or infection of a previous vascular graft. The bypass was preceded by percutaneous transluminal angioplasty in the donor iliac artery in one fourth of the patients. Fifty-six percent underwent an additional vascular procedure aimed at improving outflow.

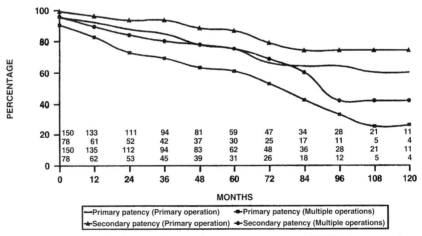

FIGURE 2.—Comparison between primary and secondary patency rates of CFFBG performed as primary operation or for technical reasons and procedures performed after previous graft failures. Graph was tabulated according to the life-table method. (Numbers in the graph represent grafts at risk entering each interval.) (Courtesy of Mingoli A, Sapienza P, Feldhaus RJ, et al: Femorofemoral bypass grafts: Factors influencing long-term patency rate and outcome. *Surgery* 129:451-458, 2001.)

Outcomes.—The postoperative mortality rate was 5.7%. Both morbidity and mortality were significantly elevated in patients older than 65 years. Primary and secondary patency rates were 70.2% and 82.8% at 5 years and 48.1% and 63.2% at 10 years. Limb salvage rates were 85.5% at 5 years and 80.1% at 10 years; survival was 63.3% and 31.0%, respectively.

Long-term patency and limb salvage rates were significantly reduced when CFFBG was performed after a previous graft failure (Fig 2). Graft patency rates were significantly lower when autogenous vein was used rather than synthetic graft materials (ie, expanded polytetrafluoroethylene or polyester). Patency rates were also better with the use of externally supported grafts as opposed to grafts without external support. On multivariate analysis, CFFBG performed after previous graft failure was the only independent predictor of poor primary and secondary patency and limb salvage rates.

Discussion.—Under certain conditions, CFFBG provides good long-term outcomes, comparable to those achieved with reconstructions coming from the aorta. The best results are achieved when CFFBG is performed as a primary procedure, when adequate outflow is present, and when an externally supported graft is used.

▶ We seldom get to do primary femorofemoral bypasses anymore. Most patients with unilateral aortoiliac occlusive disease are treated with percutaneous techniques even when the diseased iliac artery is occluded. By and large, the percutaneous techniques work well for iliac disease, and they avoid groin incisions and a vexing infection rate for prosthetic femorofemoral grafts.

G. L. Moneta, MD

Nerve-Preserving Aortoiliac Reconstruction Surgery: Anatomical Study and Surgical Approach
van Schaik J, van Baalen JM, Visser MJT, et al (Leiden Univ, The Netherlands)
J Vasc Surg 33:983-989, 2001   8–3

Background.—For 49% to 63% of men undergoing aortoiliac vascular reconstruction, dysfunctional ejaculation develops, probably caused by disruption of the efferent sympathetic pathways that supply the bladder neck, vas deferens, and prostate (Fig 1). Dysfunctional erection may also be noted, usually resulting from either proximal disruption of the efferent autonomic pathways or hemodynamic disturbances. Efforts to preserve ejaculation have focused on saving the main trunk of the superior hypogastric plexus (SHP). To provide anatomical evidence-based motivation for preserving functional ejaculation when aortoiliac reconstruction surgery is performed, surgery was performed on human cadavers, and the feasibility of limiting the damage to the lumbar splanchnic nerves (LSN) was assessed.

Methods.—The preaortic and para-aortic retroperitoneal regions were assessed by anatomical and microscopic methods in human cadavers. Two aortoiliac reconstruction operations were performed, 1 of which used a

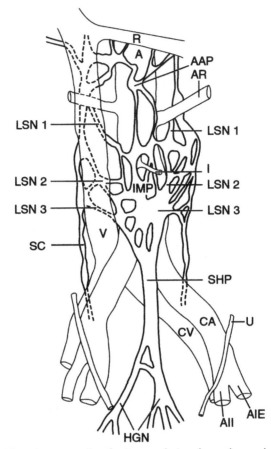

FIGURE 1.—Schematic representation of main sympathetic pathways that supply intrapelvic organs, based on dissection specimen. *Abbreviations: A*, Abdominal aorta; *AAP*, abdominal aortic plexus; *AIE*, external iliac artery; *AII*, internal iliac artery; *AR*, renal artery; *CA*, common iliac artery; *CV*, common iliac vein; *I*, inferior mesenteric artery; *LSN 1, 2, 3*, lumbar splanchnic nerves from lumbar level 1, 2, 3; *R*, left renal vein; *SC*, sympathetic chain; *U*, ureter; *V*, inferior vena cava. (Courtesy of van Schaik J, van Baalen JM, Visser MJT, et al: Nerve-preserving aortoiliac reconstructive surgery: Anatomical study and surgical approach. *J Vasc Surg* 33:983-989, 2001.)

single-blind procedure and the other a modified procedure, and these were then evaluated anatomically.

Results.—On anatomical dissection, the inferior mesenteric plexus (IMP) was a dense mass at the base of the inferior mesenteric artery. The presence of numerous interconnections between the IMP and SHP made it difficult to differentiate between the 2 plexuses. The LSNs fused and redivided, complicating the process of linking those lateral to the aorta to a specific lumbar level. The SHP divided into 2 hypogastric nerves running bilaterally into the small pelvis along the subperitoneal layer between the peritoneum and the endopelvic fascia. The retroperitoneal structures were separated from the overlying fatty mass by a loose connective tissue plane that created distinct compartments. This plane covered the abdominal aorta, common iliac arteries, para-aortic fat compartments, and inferior vena cava. With this plane as a natural plane of cleavage, the abdominal aorta could be exposed. This plane was seen as a thin, dark blue line microscopically, suggesting the presence of collagen fibers. With the single-blind procedure, the SHP and IMP were extensively damaged. When special care was taken to cause only unilateral LSN disruption, generally on the right side, damage to the inferior mesenteric region was avoided. A separate incision of the peritoneum and retroperitoneal tissue layer was performed and the left leg of the bifurcation graft tunneled under the tissue layer, then anastomosed to the left common iliac artery. A cross-stitch closed the orifice on the inside and prevented damage to the inferior mesenteric plexus. The right LSNs that were connected to the SHP were totally disrupted, but the left LSNs, the SHP, and the IMP were intact and undamaged.

Conclusions.—The location and extent of nerve disruption was clearly different between the 2 techniques. The nerve-sparing technique was able to avoid injury on 1 side without sacrificing the usefulness of the procedure. Knowing the anatomical motivation behind the technique should facilitate its incorporation into clinical practice.

▶ This article deserves careful study. Based on precise anatomic dissections, this article offers a technical approach to the infrarenal aorta that should aid in preserving ejaculatory function. Based on these dissections, dissection along the right side of the aorta is to be preferred rather than along the midline of the aorta, or the left side of the aorta. Most of the important nerves are on the left side. Therefore, it would appear a left-sided retroperitoneal approach would also have a greater risk of impairing ejaculatory function. This fact may be an indication for a midline transabdominal approach in some patients requiring open aortic operations.

G. L. Moneta, MD

Incidence of Major Venous and Renal Anomalies Relevant to Aortoiliac Surgery as Demonstrated by Computed Tomography
Aljabri B, MacDonald PS, Satin R, et al (McGill Univ, Montreal)
Ann Vasc Surg 15:615-618, 2001   8–4

Background.—Knowing that major venous anomalies are present facilitates safe aortic surgery. The incidence of major venous and renal anomalies associated with the abdominal aorta in an adult population was estimated.

Methods and Findings.—A total of 1822 IV contrast-enhanced abdominal and pelvic CT scans obtained at 2 centers were selected randomly for prospective review. A staff radiologist indicated the presence or absence of retroaortic left renal vein, circumaortic left venal vein, left-sided inferior vena cava (IVC) without situs inversus, left-sided IVC with situs inversus, duplicate IVC, preaortic confluence of the iliac veins, and horseshoe kidney. The scans had been obtained for a variety of indications. Thirty-four scans

TABLE 1.—Retroperitoneal Venous Anomalies Identified on
Prospective Review of 1788 Contrast-enhanced
Abdominal and Pelvic CT Scans

Anomaly	Total [n (%)]	Male (n)	Female (n)
Retroaortic left renal vein	57 (3.18)	29	28*
Circumaortic left renal vein	29 (1.62)	16	13
Left-sided IVC (without situs inversus	3 (0.17)	0	3†
Left-sided IVC (with situs inversus	0	0	0
Duplicate IVC	7 (0.39)	3	4†
Preaortic confluence of iliac veins	0	0	0
Horseshoe kidney	7 (0.39)	3	4*
Total	103	51	52

*One patient had retroaortic left renal vein and horseshoe kidney.
†One patient had a left-sided inferior vena cava below the left renal vein and a duplicate inferior vena cava above the left renal vein. *Abbreviation:* IVC, Inferior vena cava.
(Courtesy of Aljabri B, MacDonald PS, Satin R, et al: Incidence of major venous and renal anomalies relevant to aortoiliac surgery as demonstrated by computed tomography. *Ann Vasc Surg* 15(6):615-618, 2001.)

were excluded from the analysis for various reasons. The prevalence of major venous and renal anomalies associated with the abdominal aorta and iliac arteries, detected by CT, was 5.65% (Table 1).

Conclusion.—Knowledge of the presence of anomalies before aortic surgery is helpful in operative planning. Such knowledge may decrease the risk of major venous bleeding related to these anomalies.

▶ Stumbling into a venous anomaly during an open aortic procedure guarantees extra blood loss, rousing of the anesthesiologist from the sports page, and an irritated surgeon, not to mention a potentially dead patient. We need to remind ourselves these anomalies are out there; in fact, they are out there about 6% of the time. Unfortunately, the most frequent ones—retroaortic renal vein and renal vein collar—are the least obvious at the time of dissection.

G. L. Moneta, MD

Infrainguinal Arterial Reconstructions in Patients With Aortoiliac Occlusive Disease: The Influence of Iliac Stenting

Timaran CH, Stevens SL, Freeman MB, et al (Univ of Tennessee, Knoxville)
J Vasc Surg 34:971-978, 2001   8–5

Background.—Some patients with multisegment arterial occlusive disease of the lower extremities require infrainguinal arterial reconstruction (IAR) in addition to iliac artery angioplasty (IAA). The outcomes of iliac artery stenting (IAS) for patients undergoing distal bypass procedures are unknown. The outcomes of patients undergoing IAS before IAR were assessed by a retrospective cohort study, and the results were compared with those of patients undergoing IAA alone or aortofemoral bypass grafting before IAR.

Methods.—The study included 105 patients with a history of previous intervention for iliac occlusive disease who underwent IAR. A total of 120 IARs were performed between 1995 and 2000. Risk factors, complications, and outcome variables were defined according to the criteria of the Ad Hoc Committee on Reporting Standards of the Society for Vascular Surgery/International Society for Cardiovascular Surgery. Iliac lesions were classified by TransAtlantic Inter-Society Consensus classification criteria. The effects of perioperative variables on patency rates were assessed by univariate and multivariate analyses.

Results.—The analysis included 45 IARs for patients with a history of IAS placement, 33 for patients with a previous IAA repair, and 42 for patients with previous bypass surgery. Forty percent of patients in the IAS group had polytetrafluoroethylene grafts used for IAR, compared with 15% in the IAA group; otherwise, the 2 groups had similar characteristics. After 5 years, the primary patency rate was 68% for patients with previous IAS, 46% with IAA, and 61% with bypass surgery. On univariate analysis, the primary pa-

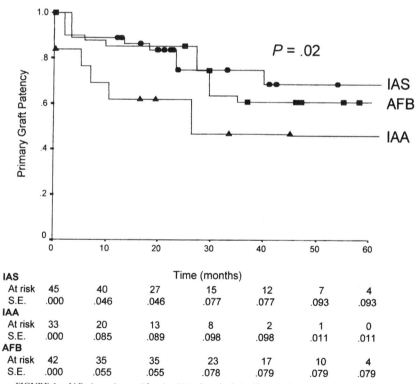

IAS						
At risk	45	40	27	15	12	7	4
S.E.	.000	.046	.046	.077	.077	.093	.093
IAA							
At risk	33	20	13	8	2	1	0
S.E.	.000	.085	.089	.098	.098	.011	.011
AFB							
At risk	42	35	35	23	17	10	4
S.E.	.000	.055	.055	.078	.079	.079	.079

FIGURE 1.—IARs in patients with prior IAA alone had significantly decreased primary graft patency rates with respect to those with previous IAS and AFB (Kaplan-Meier, log-rank test, $P = .02$). (Courtesy of Timaran CH, Stevens SL, Freeman MB, et al: Infrainguinal arterial reconstructions in patients with aortoiliac occlusive disease: The influence of iliac stenting. *J Vasc Surg* 34:971-978, 2001.)

tency rate was significantly higher in the IAS group than in the IAA group (Fig 1). The risk of failure in the new IAR graft was twice as high for patients with previous IAA: (relative risk, 2.2, 95% confidence interval, 1.1-4.8).

Conclusions.—For patients undergoing IAR for aortoiliac occlusive disease, graft patency rate is significantly higher for those with a history of IAS, compared with those with previous IAA alone. Patients with previous IAS have outcomes comparable to those of patients undergoing aortofemoral bypass grafting.

▶ The data suggest that if an infrainguinal bypass is to be performed below an iliac angioplasty, primary stenting of the lesion should be performed.

G. L. Moneta, MD

Outcome of Iliac Kissing Stents
Brittenden J, Beattie G, Bradbury AW (Royal Infirmary, Edinburgh, Scotland)
Eur J Vasc Endovasc Surg 22:466-468, 2001   8–6

Background.—Kissing stents are bilateral common iliac stents that extend into the aorta and allow the 2 adjacent stent walls to appose each other along at least 1 cm in the aorta. The purpose is to reduce the incidence of complications accompanying the "kissing balloon" technique that is used to address intermittent claudication or critical limb ischemia, caused by unilateral or bilateral common iliac artery origin stenosis and/or occlusion. Procedure-related morbidity rates and medium-term hemodynamic and clinical patency were evaluated.

Methods.—The study included 5 men and 7 women (age, 43-73 years; median age, 62 years) who had a planned insertion of kissing stents during elective surgery for proximal common iliac lesions. Six patients had bilateral claudication; 3, unilateral claudication; and 1, claudication and contralateral rest pain and tissue loss. In the 16 limbs with claudication and 4 with critical limb ischemia, only 1 had more than 1 stent inserted. Ten patients received aspirin after the procedure, and 2 received warfarin. During follow-up, stents were classified as normal, stenosed, or occluded.

Results.—One patient had unilateral distal embolization, requiring aspiration and thrombolysis plus surgical repair of a common femoral pseudoaneurysm. Another patient had bilateral stent stenoses, which eventually required bilateral limb amputation, an event considered as a failed reconstruction (Fig 1). Another patient's discharge from the hospital was delayed because of bilateral iliac dissections that responded to heparin. An immediate improvement in symptoms of +2 or +3 on the Rutherford scale was reported by all patients. Symptoms deteriorated to a Rutherford −2 or −3 in 2 to 70 months (median, 27 months) in 13 limbs, with 6 occluded stents and 3 stents with significant stenoses. Aortobifemoral bypass grafting was required for 4 patients. No correlation was noted between type of stent and specific complications.

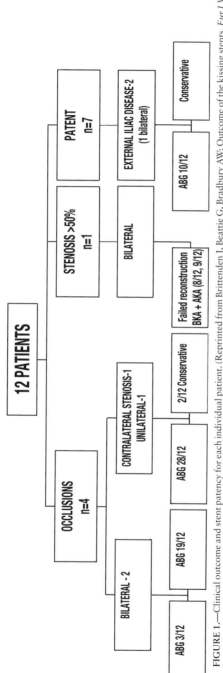
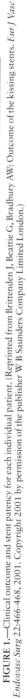

FIGURE 1.—Clinical outcome and stent patency for each individual patient. (Reprinted from Brittenden J, Beattie G, Bradbury AW: Outcome of the kissing stents. *Eur J Vasc Endovasc Surg* 22:466-468, 2001. Copyright 2001 by permission of the publisher W B Saunders Company Limited London.)

Conclusions.—The immediate technical success rate for this series was 100%, and clinical and hemodynamic outcome was excellent after 30 days. However, procedure-related complications developed in 3 of the 12 patients and more than half of the limbs had significant symptomatic deterioration during the course of follow-up, with 6 occluded and 3 stenosed stents. These poor medium-term results may reflect the unfavorable flow dynamics created when the stents appose each other in the midline rather than the vessel wall. Thus, the fault is attributable to the method itself rather than poor technique, suggesting that, at present, it be used only selectively.

▶ This is a chink in the armor of iliac angioplasty. "Kissing stents" did not do well in this small series despite good initial hemodynamic and angiographic success. In 12 patients, 6 stents occluded and 3 stenosed at a median follow-up of 27 months. Two late emergency aortofemoral bypass grafts were required, and another patient required bilateral major lower extremity amputations from late distal embolization associated with the stents. Whereas I generally treat iliac lesions with percutaneous techniques when reasonably possible, I suppose I should give stronger consideration to an aortic graft in patients suitable for both an open procedure and kissing stents.

G. L. Moneta, MD

Sonodynamic Therapy Decreased Neointimal Hyperplasia After Stenting in the Rabbit Iliac Artery

Arakawa K, Hagisawa K, Kusano H, et al (Natl Defense Med College, Saitama, Japan; Photochemical Co Ltd, Okayama, Japan; Hitachi Research Ctr, Tokyo)
Circulation 105:149-151, 2002   8–7

Introduction.—In-stent restenosis continues to be an important problem in patients who have undergone coronary and peripheral stenting. Sonodynamic therapy restricts tumor growth by means of cytotoxic effects after activation of sonochemical sensitizers by US. A water-soluble chlorine derivative, 13,17-bis[1-carboxypropionyl] carbamoylethyl-3-ethenyl-8-ethoxyiminoethylidene-7-hydroxy-2,7,12,18-tetramethyl porphyrin sodium (PAD- S31), the analogue of a new photosensitizer (ATX-S10), has the same biological effect as that of ATX-S10 for tumor treatment and is also considered a sonochemical sensitizer. The efficacy of sonodynamic therapy using PAD-S31 on neointimal hyperplasia was examined in a rabbit stent model.

Methods.—Stents were implanted in the iliac crests of 16 Japanese White rabbits. Thirty-two stented arteries were randomly assigned to either sonodynamic therapy, control, US exposure, or PAD-S31 groups. One hour after the IV administration of PAD-S31 (25 mg/kg body weight), US energy (1 MHz, 0.3 W/cm²) was delivered transdermally to animals in the sonodynamic group. On day 28, all stent sites underwent morphometric evaluation.

Results.—The size of the intimal cross-sectional area was smaller in the sonodynamic therapy group versus the control, US, and PAD-S31 groups (means, 0.31 vs 1.38, 1.66, and 1.61 mm², respectively; $P < .05$). The ratio of the intimal and medial cross-sectional area was smaller in the sonodynamic therapy group versus the control, US, and PAD-S31 groups (means, 0.71 vs 2.53, 2.48, and 3.45 mm^2; $P < .05$).

Conclusion.—Sonodynamic therapy with PAD-S31 may be a feasible treatment approach for noninvasively inhibiting neointimal hyperplasia in a rabbit iliac stent model.

▶ There are several methods under evaluation for prevention of in-stent restenosis. These include various dosages of different drugs attached to the stents, as well as various dosages and delivery methods of applying radiation to the area of stenting. We can now add one more method to those under evaluation.

G. L. Moneta, MD

Diagnosing External Iliac Endofibrosis by Postexercise Ankle to Arm Index in Cyclists
Fernández-García B, Alverez Fernández J, Vega García F, et al (Oviedo Univ, Spain; Central Hosp of Asturias, Oviedo; Central Hosp of Oviedo; et al)
Med Sci Sports Exerc 34:222-227, 2002   8–8

Background.—Arterial problems in cyclists have been described since 1979, including several cases of external iliac endofibrosis. The overall incidence of this condition is unknown as symptoms are generated only during intense exercise. In symptomatic external iliac endofibrosis affecting cyclists, there is a narrowing in the arterial lumen that evolves to decrease muscle perfusion during high-intensity exercise. There are no symptoms at rest, but the condition causes pain and a deterioration in performance during intense cycling, such as climbing hills and time-trial competition. These symptoms predominantly affect the left leg, although 18% are bilateral. The most common symptom is thigh pain. Over the past 5 years, the incidence of confirmed external iliac endofibrosis has been determined to be 0.66 cases per 100 professional cyclists per year. A noninvasive method of evaluating this disorder in cyclists was sought.

Methods.—Eighteen highly trained male cyclists were divided into a pathology group and a control group. Humeral and tibial posterior pressure were measured with Doppler US and the ankle-to-arm index (AAI) before and after an incremental exercise test that was performed to exhaustion on a bike-ergometer.

Results.—The minimal AAI for the pathology group postexercise was 0.76 ± 0.13 for the normal leg and 0.35 ± 0.04 for the ailing leg. There were significant differences between the normal leg and the ailing leg from the first to the fourth minutes after exercise in the pathology group, and from the first to tenth minutes after exercise between the ailing leg in the pathology group and in the control group. Significant differences were observed in leg pressures between the normal and ailing legs in the pathology group from the first to the fourth minutes after exercise, and between the ailing leg in the pathology group versus the control group from the first to the tenth minutes. Discriminant analysis provided a classification of legs as ailing or normal by use of a mathematical function at each recovery time studied.

Conclusions.—External iliac endofibrosis can be noninvasively evaluated with AAI and leg pressure response to maximal exercise.

▶ Cycling fanatics are not just in Europe anymore. We have seen several cyclists who complain of what appears to be claudication with high levels of exertion. These are people who cycle hundreds of miles a week. The authors describe a technique to identify and quantify arterial insufficiency in these high-level athletes. Identification of these lesions is important, as acute limb-threatening iliac artery thrombosis has been reported in these patients.

G. L. Moneta, MD

9 Visceral Renal Artery Disease

Renal Artery End-Diastolic Velocity and Renal Artery Resistance Index as Predictors of Outcome After Renal Stenting
Mukherjee D, Bhatt DL, Robbins M, et al (Univ of Michigan, Ann Arbor; Cleveland Clinic Found, Ohio)
Am J Cardiol 88:1064-1066, 2001   9-1

Background.—Outcome after renal stenting has varied considerably, but patients with increased microvascular resistance are unlikely to benefit clinically from treatment of the renal artery. A review of patients who received treatment for renal artery stenosis sought to determine whether renal artery peak systolic velocity (PSV) and end-diastolic velocity (EDV), and renal artery resistance index (RI) can be used to predict outcome.

Methods.—Between August 2000 and February 2001, 17 patients with renal artery stenosis underwent renal artery stenting at the Cleveland Clinic Foundation, with a 100% procedural success rate. The indication for renal artery stenting was hypertension that was medically refractory or difficult to treat. Renal US was performed before the procedure, with B-mode US guidance and a C5-2 curved array transducer. Measurements of PSV and EDV were obtained, and RI calculated as $[1 - (EDV/PSV)] \times 100$.

Results.—The patients' mean age was 71 years; 58% were men, and 65% had coronary artery disease. Hypercholesterolemia was present in 71%, renal insufficiency in 23%, and diabetes in 23%. The mean US characteristics of the entire cohort included PSV, 366; EDV, 119; and RI, 71. There was a significant correlation between preprocedural EDV and RI in predicting clinical improvement. No clinical benefit was achieved with stenting in patients with RI more than 75 and EDV less than 90. In patients with RI less than 75, the mean blood pressure was reduced by 5 mm Hg; in those with RI more than 75, the mean blood pressure increased by 3 mm Hg. Patients with RI less than 75 showed a minor trend toward reduction in antihypertensive medication use.

Conclusions.—High renal artery EDV and low RI can be used to identify patients who are likely to benefit from renal artery stenting. Despite correction of renal artery stenosis, high RI and low EDV are markers of increased microvascular resistance and poor outcome. Renal revascularization should be reserved for patients in whom improvement in creatinine concentration or reduction in blood pressure is likely.

▶ This is a smaller version of an article in the 2002 YEAR BOOK OF VASCULAR SURGERY[1] indicating that the evaluation of renal parenchymal resistance with US techniques helps predict the result of renal revascularization. The evidence is accumulating that indiscriminate treatment of renal artery stenosis is not indicated, even if you have a catheter and a stent and the skills to use them.

G. L. Moneta, MD

Reference

1. Radermacher J, Chavan A, Bleck J, et al: Use of Doppler ultrasonography to predict the outcome of therapy for renal-artery stenosis. *N Engl J Med* 344:410-417, 2001. (2002 YEAR BOOK OF VASCULAR SURGERY, p 190.)

Long-term Effects of Arterial Stenting on Kidney Function for Patients With Ostial Atherosclerotic Renal Artery Stenosis and Renal Insufficiency
Beutler JJ, van Ampting JMA, van de Ven PJG, et al (Univ Med Ctr, Utrecht, The Netherlands; Twenteborg Hosp, Almelo, The Netherlands)
J Am Soc Nephrol 12:1475-1481, 2001   9–2

Background.—For patients with atherosclerotic renal artery stenosis, the effects of stent placement on subsequent loss of renal function are unknown.

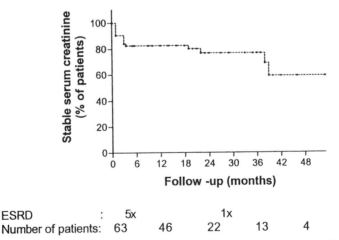

FIGURE 2.—Kaplan-Meier curves for maintained renal function in all patients with atherosclerotic ostial renal artery stenosis and renal dysfunction who were treated with stent placement. Maintained renal function was defined as serum creatinine concentrations that did not increase above 120% of the serum creatinine levels at the time of stent placement. *Abbreviation: ESRD,* Number of patients who developed end-stage renal disease. (Courtesy of Beutler JJ, van Ampting JMA, van de Ven PJG, et al: Long-term effects of arterial stenting on kidney function for patients with ostial atherosclerotic renal artery stenosis and renal insufficiency. *J Am Soc Nephrol* 12:1475-1481, 2001.)

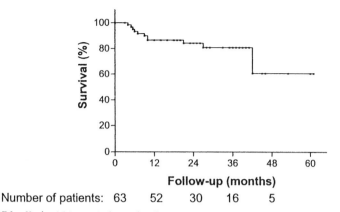

FIGURE 3.—Kaplan-Meier survival curve for all patients with atherosclerotic ostial renal artery stenosis and renal dysfunction who were treated with stent placement. (Courtesy of Beutler JJ, van Ampting JMA, van de Ven PJG, et al: Long-term effects of arterial stenting on kidney function for patients with ostial atherosclerotic renal artery stenosis and renal insufficiency. *J Am Soc Nephrol* 12:1475-1481, 2001.)

The long-term effects of renal artery stenting on renal function outcomes were assessed, with the focus on patients who already had progressive renal dysfunction.

Methods.—The prospective study included 63 patients with ostial atherosclerotic renal artery stenosis plus compromised renal function. All patients had a serum creatinine concentration of more than 120 μmol/L (median value, 171 μmol/L). Before stent placement, 28 patients had stable renal function, and 35 had progressive decline, defined as at least a 20% decline in serum creatinine during 12 months. Angiographic patency and renal function were assessed during a median follow-up of 23 months.

Results.—Twelve patients required angioplasty to treat restenosis. End-stage renal failure occurred within 6 months in 5 patients, 2 of them as a result of stent placement. Also within 6 months, 2 patients died or were lost to follow-up, having stable renal function at the time. In the remaining 56 patients, stent placement did not influence serum creatinine levels if the patient had previously had stable renal function (Fig 2). For those whose renal function had been declining, median serum creatinine levels decreased from 182 to 157 μmol/L in the first year, remaining stable thereafter (Fig 3).

Conclusions.—For patients with ostial atherosclerotic renal artery stenosis and renal dysfunction, renal artery stenting can prevent further loss of renal function. The value of stenting for patients with renal artery stenosis but preserved renal function is unclear.

▶ Some patients with ostial renal artery stenosis benefited in terms of renal function with renal stenting, and others did not. Parenchymal resistance does not appear to have been studied in this investigation, as suggested by Mukherjee et al (Abstract 9–1), and Radermacher et al.[1] Again, as emphasized in the comment on Abstract 9–1, I believe we should be moving away from indiscriminate renal artery stenosis treatment. Some mechanism of trying to predict benefit from treatment of renal artery stenosis should be used in any study evaluating the effects of renal artery angioplasty, stenting, or the effects of renal artery surgery.

G. L. Moneta, MD

Reference

1. Radermacher J, Chavan A, Bleck J, et al: Use of Doppler ultrasonography to predict the outcome of therapy for renal-artery stenosis. *N Engl J Med* 344:410-417, 2001. (2002 YEAR BOOK OF VASCULAR SURGERY, p 190.)

Renal Artery Stenting for Renal Insufficiency in Solitary Kidney in 26 Patients
Chatziioannou A, Mourikis D, Agroyannis B, et al (Univ of Athens, Greece; Baylor College of Medicine, Houston)
Eur J Vasc Endovasc Surg 23:49-54, 2002   9–3

Introduction.—Renal insufficiency combined with renal artery stenosis may result in progressive deterioration of renal function. The role of renal artery stenting in preserving renal function in these patients remains unclear. The experience with Palmaz stents in the treatment of patients with ischemic nephropathy and solitary kidney is discussed.

Methods.—The medical records of 26 patients (mean age, 63 years) who underwent placement of 28 balloon-expandable Palmaz stents during a 5-year period were reviewed. Of the 26 patients, 21 had solitary kidneys resulting from a nonfunctioning contralateral kidney secondary to atherosclerotic renal artery occlusion. The other 5 patients had a solitary kidney owing to other causes (trauma, 2; tumor, 3). All patients had renal insufficiency (serum creatinine > 0.144 mmol/L) and underwent placement of a stent in the remaining stenosed renal artery. Clinical outcome was based on the level of creatinine at 3 months after procedure. Patients were considered to have clinically benefited when a reduction of more than 20% of creatinine compared with baseline creatinine level was observed, or when there was stabilization of the serum creatinine (±20% of the baseline value).

Results.—Sixteen patients (62%) achieved clinical benefit (improvement 35%, stabilization 27%) (Fig 1). Ten (38%) continued to experience deteriorating renal function. The baseline creatinine value was the most important predictor for achievement of clinical benefit (odds ratio: 13; 95% confidence interval, 1.6-107; $P = .01$).

Conclusion.—Improved or stabilized renal function was observed in most patients with solitary kidney and renal artery stenosis with renal insufficiency who undergo renal stenting. High serum creatinine values predict failure of stenting to improve renal function.

▶ The authors contend 62% of patients with solitary kidneys, renal insufficiency, and renal artery stenosis were "improved" with renal artery stenting. The authors improved their odds of achieving success by patient selection (excluding kidneys less than 8 cm in length and with evidence of parenchymal ar-

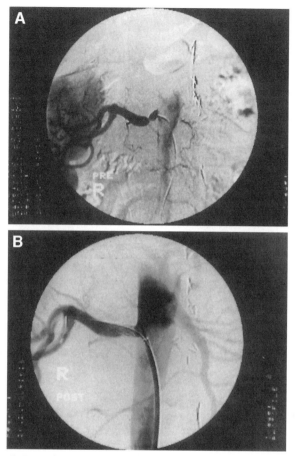

FIGURE 1.—(A) Pre- and (B) post-Palmaz stent (6 mm × 15 mm) placement in a severe stenosis of the renal artery in a solitary kidney. Patient had left nephrectomy due to trauma. Intraparenchymal vascular disease was insignificant. Pretreatment creatinine was 0.2 mmol/L. Patient's renal function status was improved significantly after the intervention (0.138 mmol/L). (Reprinted from Chatziioannou A, Mourikis D, Agoryannis B, et al: Renal artery stenting for renal insufficiency in solitary kidney in 26 patients. *Eur J Vasc Endovasc Surg* 23:49-54, 2002. Copyright 2002, by permission of the publisher W B Saunders Company Limited London.)

terial disease), and by their definition of success (stabilization of renal function decline was considered a success). Thirty-eight percent of kidneys treated with renal stenting were judged as failures. I am not sure "stabilization" should be regarded as a success. Many patients with renal artery stenosis have normal renal function. Perhaps the decline in renal function leading to stenting was secondary to loss of the contralateral kidney. Future studies of this sort need to utilize parenchymal resistance values (see Abstract 9–1) so that success can be further improved by even better patient selection for stenting.

G. L. Moneta, MD

Long-term Follow Up of Renal Transplant Artery Stenosis by Doppler

Buturović-Ponikvar J, Župunski A, Urbančič A, et al (Univ Med Ctr, Ljubljana, Slovenija)
Transplant Proc 33:3390-3391, 2001   9–4

Background.— The rate of progression of renal transplant artery stenosis was assessed in the long term with the use of regular Doppler examination, and the influence of stenosis on renal function and hypertension was determined.

Methods.—Twenty-seven kidney recipients (mean age, 42 years) were studied. All had at least 50% stenosis of the transplanted renal artery. Stenoses were diagnosed and followed up regularly by duplex Doppler US.

Findings.—Overall, there was a tendency toward reduced peak systolic velocity and a corresponding increase in the resistance index. Serum creatinine gradually declined, and hemoglobin levels remained stable. Average blood pressure decreased with an increasing number of antihypertensive medications. There was a trend toward improving stenosis in patients revascularized as well as in patients treated conservatively. Compared with the nonrevascularized patients, the revascularized group had a greater peak systolic velocity and a lower resistance index in the beginning, indicating a greater degree of stenosis at diagnosis.

Conclusion.—Renal transplant artery stenosis can be monitored by Doppler US. In this study, the stenosis tended to be stable over time. Spontaneous regression of stenosis may have occurred, at least in some patients.

▶ In this study, transplant renal artery stenosis was associated with a basically benign prognosis. About 20% of transplant renal artery stenoses actually appear to regress. Based on these data, treatment of transplant renal artery stenosis should be restricted to those kidneys with declining renal function and stenoses greater than 75%.

G. L. Moneta, MD

Isolated Spontaneous Dissection of the Renal Artery

Lacombe M (Hôpital Beaujon, Clichy, France)
J Vasc Surg 33:385-391, 2001   9–5

Background.—The diagnosis of isolated spontaneous dissection of the renal artery (ISRA) is increasingly made in living patients. There is continued debate over the appropriate management of this rare cause of renovascular hypertension. A surgical experience in 22 patients with ISRA is reported.

Patients.—The patients (17 men, 5 women; mean age, 41 years) were treated from 1978 to 1998. All patients were hospitalized and investigated for uncontrolled arterial hypertension. Imaging studies included abdominal aortography in the early part of the series and, more recently, intra-arterial digital angiography (Fig 2A). Three patients had bilateral lesions. Operative

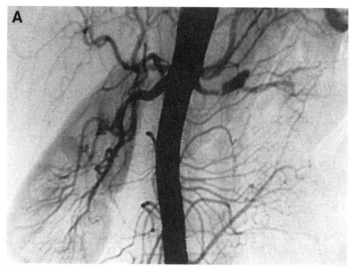

FIGURE 2.—**A,** Preoperative angiography of 49-year-old woman with hypertension: spontaneous dissection of left renal artery. (Courtesy of Lacombe M: Isolated spontaneous dissection of the renal artery. *J Vasc Surg* 33:385-391, 2001.)

treatment included 6 total and 2 partial nephrectomies and 17 arterial repairs—16 performed in situ and 11 extracorporeally.

Outcomes.—There were no postoperative deaths or complications. After surgery, arterial hypertension was cured in 41% of the patients, improved in 50%, and unchanged in 9%. The anatomic results were rated excellent in 81% of the cases and incomplete in the remaining 19%. Two events occurred during long-term follow-up: 1 patient had late thrombosis of a repaired polar artery, and 1 had spontaneous dissection of the contralateral renal artery. Long-term follow-up angiography performed in 8 patients showed that the reconstructions remained stable over time.

Conclusions.—The experience supports the need for surgical treatment in patients with uncontrollable arterial hypertension caused by ISDRA. Arterial repair is the preferred option and can be carried out even in patients with complex lesions. In selected cases, ex vivo surgery is a safe option.

▶ This is a very informative report. Take-home points are that isolated spontaneous dissection of the renal artery is associated with a variety of etiologies (not just fibromuscular disease). Surgical repair is highly successful, but often involves ex vivo (bench) surgery, and the dissecting channels are complex, suggesting endovascular repair may not be feasible in most cases.

G. L. Moneta, MD

Simultaneous Aortic Replacement and Renal Artery Revascularization: The Influence of Preoperative Renal Function on Early Risk and Late Outcome

Tsoukas AI, Hertzer NR, Mascha EJ, et al (Cleveland Clinic Found, Ohio)

J Vasc Surg 34:1041-1049, 2001   9–6

Background.—In a previous report of 89 patients undergoing simultaneous aortic reconstruction and renal artery (RA) revascularization, the authors noted a high rate of operative mortality and an elevated risk of postoperative renal dysfunction among patients with severe bilateral RA disease. In this condition, bilateral RA disease appears to reflect increased serum creatinine levels. The outcomes of patients who had simultaneous infrarenal aortic replacement and RA revascularization were analyzed for serum creatinine levels and other preoperative risk factors.

Methods.—The analysis included 73 consecutive patients (mean age, 69 years) undergoing aortic operatives combined with repair of RA stenosis from 1989 to 1997. The patients were followed up for a mean of 44 months. Patients were divided into 2 risk groups on the basis of their preoperative serum creatinine levels. Group 1 consisted of 45 patients with a serum creatinine of 2 mg/dL or less (median, 1.5 g/dL), and group 2 was 28 patients with a serum creatinine higher than 2 mg/dL (median, 2.5 mg/dL). Surgical indications for aortic procedures were aortic aneurysms in 45 patients, aortoiliac occlusive disease in 15, and both types of lesions in 11 patients.

Results.—In group 1, 15% of patients needed bilateral RA revascularization, compared with 29% of patients in group 2. The rate of medically resistant hypertension was 29% in group 1 versus 57% in group 2. Thirty-day mortality rates were not significantly different between groups (group 1, 2.2%; group 2, 11%). In-hospital mortality rates, however, were much higher for patients undergoing bilateral RA revascularization than for those undergoing unilateral revascularization (13% vs 6.9%). Postoperative dialysis rate was 7% for group 1 versus 36% for group 2; median hospital stay was 9 days for group 1 versus 14 days for group 2. The Kaplan-Meier 5-year survival rate was 85% for group 1 versus 53% for group 2. Still, 88% of patients in group 2 had improvement or resolution in their medically resistant hypertension, and a reduction in serum creatinine with time.

Conclusions.—For patients undergoing aortic surgery with simultaneous RA reconstruction, postoperative risks are higher for those with elevated serum creatinine levels or bilateral RA disease. These patients also appear to have lower long-term survival rates. For this group, endovascular approaches might help to reduce the planned extent of surgery, thus promoting better overall outcomes.

▶ These Cleveland Clinic surgeons performed slightly less than 10 combined aortic/renal procedures per year for 9 years. The overall results of surgery were good, and those patients operated on for hypertension seemed to improve. Like everyone else, they found that the surgical risk was highest when the creatinine was highest, and the operations were bigger (read bilateral). I wish I knew if renal artery surgery for hypertension really does any good. I am deeply suspicious that it does not. Ditto for renal revascularization by angioplasty.

L. M. Taylor, Jr, MD

The Outcome in the United States After Thoracoabdominal Aortic Aneurysm Repair, Renal Artery Bypass, and Mesenteric Revascularization
Derrow AE, Seeger JM, Dame DA, et al (Univ of Florida, Gainesville; Shands HealthCare Inc, Gainesville, Fla; Malcom Randall VA Med Ctr, Gainesville, Fla)
J Vasc Surg 34:54-61, 2001   9–7

Background.—For certain rare, complex vascular surgical procedures, sufficient data are not available on the treatment outcomes. Information from a nationwide data base was used to assess the outcomes of 3 such procedures: repair of thoracoabdominal aneurysm (TAA), renal artery bypass (RAB), and revascularization for chronic mesenteric ischemia (CMI).

Methods.—The retrospective study included data from 1993 to 1997 from the Nationwide Inpatient Sample (INS) on 540 patients undergoing TAA repair, 2058 undergoing RAB, and 336 undergoing CMI. The mean age of the patients was between 66 and 69 years in all 3 groups. Patients undergoing TAA and RAB were more likely to be male (53%, TAA group; 55%, RAB group) compared with only 24% male in the CMI group. Complication and death rates were assessed, along with length of hospital stay, charges, and patient disposition. Risk factors for death were assessed in a multivariate analysis.

Results.—Mortality rates for the TAA, RAB, and CMI groups were 20%, 7%, and 15%, respectively. Complication rates for the TAA, RAB, and CMI groups were 62%, 37%, and 45%, respectively. Proportions of patients discharged to another facility were 21% with TAA, 9% with RAB, and 12% with CMI. For patients undergoing RAB, mortality was significantly increased when another procedure was performed concomitantly: 8% versus 4%. The median length of stay for the TAA, RAB, and CMI groups was 14 days, 9 days, and 14 days, respectively. The median hospital charges for the TAA, RAB, and CMI groups were $64,493, $36,830, and $47,390, respectively. Multivariate analysis identified significant risk factors for the predicted mortality rates for all 3 groups (TAA, 14%-76%; RAB, <1%-46%; CMI, <2%-87%).

Conclusions.—The study provides an overview of the outcomes of TAA repair, RAB, and revascularization for CMI in the United States. All 3 are resource-intensive procedures with high complication and mortality rates. The authors call for a re-evaluation of current treatment approaches to these complex vascular surgical problems.

▶ There are really a lot of problems with studies based on surveys of computerized diagnosis and procedure coding. Most careful reviews, as the authors readily admit, show error rates in diagnosis and procedure codes as high as

25%. Acknowledging this, there is still considerable food for thought in this article, and the thoughts are sobering indeed. Bad outcomes, defined by the authors as death or discharge to someplace besides home, occurred after 41.5% of TAA repairs, 16.4% of RAB operations, and 26.7% of operations for CMI. In reviewing our own experience, I have to say that, thankfully, the mortality rates are lower than found in this study, but a surprisingly similar number of patients who survive require nursing home placement after discharge (thankfully, most often temporary). There are going to be more articles like this, and funding agencies are going to study them carefully. We are going to have to think seriously about whether a 14-day hospitalization followed by nursing home placement is a reasonable outcome for a prophylactic procedure. My bias is that TAA surgery is mostly about the surgeons, not about the patients. And you already know that I think RAB is a bunch of baloney. As my late partner said frequently, "We have spent the last several decades figuring out what we can do in vascular surgery; perhaps it is now time to concentrate upon figuring out what we should do."

L. M. Taylor, Jr, MD

Presentation and Revascularization Outcomes in Patients With Radiation-Induced Renal Artery Stenosis

Fakhouri F, Alanore ALB, Rérolle J-P, et al (Hôpital Européen Georges Pompidou, Paris)
Am J Kidney Dis 38:302-309, 2001   9–8

Background.—Radiation-induced arterial stenosis has been reported primarily in the carotid arteries. However, it can also affect other sites, including the renal arteries. The cases of 7 patients with radiation-induced renal artery stenosis are discussed, including their long-term outcomes after revascularization.

Methods.—The 7 men were identified from a series of 11 who developed renal artery stenosis after abdominal radiation therapy. All had normal blood pressure before irradiation (a radiation dose of greater than 35 Gy to the renal arteries). All had perirenal radiation-induced lesions, with no evidence of arterial disease outside the radiation field. The patients' history, clinical and radiologic findings, and revascularization outcomes were analyzed.

Findings.—At the time of radiation therapy, the patients' median age was 30 years, and they received a median dose of 40 Gy. Patients were referred for evaluation a median of 13 years after irradiation. At that time, their median blood pressure was 171/102 mm Hg, and their median treatment score was 2. The patients had a median glomerular filtration rate of 67 L/min. Six patients had proximal stenoses, 1 had truncal stenoses, and 2 patients had bilateral stenoses. Five patients underwent successful percutaneous transluminal renal artery angioplasty, requiring multiple insufflations. Angioplasty failed in 1 patient, who proceeded to bypass surgery. At a median 36 months' follow-up, 2 patients had died of noncardiovascular causes. Four patients had continued high blood pressure (median, 136/85 mm Hg). No patients had renal artery restenosis, although 1 patient developed aneurysms at the angioplasty site.

Conclusions.—Radiation-induced renal artery stenosis is a rare condition associated with radiation nephritis, ischemic hypertension, and renal failure. This possibility should be considered, however, for any patient who develops hypertension after abdominal radiation, even decades afterward.

▶ Radiation injury to the renal artery is about the same as radiation injury to any other artery. The clinical manifestations may occur years after the radiation dose, and the lesions are difficult to treat. Results of treatment with percutaneous techniques are not great, but they are also not so bad as to preclude an initial endovascular approach.

G. L. Moneta, MD

Percutaneous Transluminal Angioplasty and Stenting in the Treatment of Chronic Mesenteric Ischemia: Results and Longterm Followup
Matsumoto AH, Angle JF, Spinosa DJ, et al (Univ of Virginia, Charlottesville)
J Am Coll Surg 194:S22-S31, 2002   9–9

Background.—Mesenteric ischemia occurs when intestinal blood flow is unable to support the physiologic demands of the gastrointestinal tract. Weight loss and postprandial pain result. The results of percutaneous transluminal angioplasty (PTA), stenting, or both in the treatment of patients who present with symptoms and angiographic findings consistent with chronic mesenteric ischemia were reviewed.

Methods.—A retrospective analysis was conducted for 33 consecutive patients from a single institution who underwent PTA, stenting, or both for treatment of symptoms of chronic mesenteric ischemia. The study group comprised 12 men and 21 women with a mean age of 63 years.

Results.—The median weight loss was 28 pounds. Postprandial pain was evident in 88% of the patients, and all lesions treated were stenoses. Twenty-one patients (32 vessels) underwent PTA alone, and PTA and stenting were performed in 12 patients (15 vessels). PTA was technically successful in 26 of 32 vessels (81.3%), whereas PTA plus stenting was technically successful in 15 of 15 vessels (100%). Twenty-seven patients experienced complete alleviation of symptoms, and 2 patients had improvement in their symptoms. There were 4 immediate clinical failures. Angiographic follow-up was available in 52% of the patients at a mean of 20 months. Primary long-term clinical success was 83.3%. Of the 5 patients with recurrent symptoms, 4 were successfully treated with endovascular therapy. Assisted primary clinical success was 96.6%. Major complications occurred in 13% of the procedures, and the 5-year survival was 76.1% (Fig 7). The 30-day mortality rate was 0%.

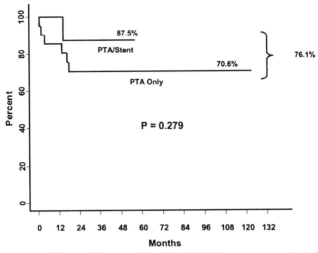

FIGURE 7.—Survival by procedure type. *Abbreviation: PTA*, Percutaneous transluminal angioplasty. (Courtesy of Matsumoto AH, Angle JF, Spinosa DJ, et al: Percutaneous transluminal angioplasty and stenting in the treatment of chronic mesenteric ischemia: Results and longterm followup. *J Am Coll Surg* 194:S22-S31, 2002. By permission of the American College of Surgeons.)

Conclusions.—These findings demonstrate the effectiveness of endovascular therapy for the treatment of mesenteric arterial stenosis in patients with chronic mesenteric ischemia.

▶ Despite my fondness for mesenteric artery bypass surgery (we know the natural history—death is inevitable and the surgery is effective), we too are discovering an increasing number of patients can be treated by angioplasty and stenting. There is no question that the recurrence rate is higher, but many times the recurrences can also be managed by endovascular means. This is a careful review of one of the largest experiences reported that has any follow-up. I recommend it to you.

L. M. Taylor, Jr, MD

Early and Long-term Results of Surgical Treatment of Splenic Artery Aneurysms

Pulli R, Innocenti AA, Barbanti E, et al (Univ of Florence, Italy)
Am J Surg 182:520-523, 2001   9–10

Background.—Splenic artery aneurysm is an uncommon clinical entity but the most frequent aneurysmal disease of visceral arteries and the third most frequent aneurysmal disease among abdominal vessels. The primary focus of this article is on the avoidance of splenectomy in the surgical treatment of splenic artery aneurysms and the feasibility of splenic artery reconstruction and preservation of the spleen as an alternative to aneurysmectomy and splenectomy. The presentation, surgical treatment, and follow-up of patients with splenic artery aneurysms are described.

Methods.—A total of 1952 patients with abdominal aneurysms were referred to a single institution from 1982 to 2000. Of these patients, 15 had splenic artery aneurysms. There were no ruptures. Duplex ultrasonography, CT, MRI, and digital subtraction angiography were performed to evaluate the characteristics of the aneurysm and its relationship with surrounding structures.

Results.—In 14 patients, the aneurysm was resected completely and in 1 case, partial aneurysmectomy was performed. Arterial continuity was restored with end-to-end anastomosis and splenic preservation in 10 patients. Four patients underwent splenectomy primarily because of distal location of the aneurysm. In 1 patient, the spleen was preserved without arterial reconstruction. Follow-up was available for 11 of the 15 patients for a mean of 19.7 months. No deaths or major complications were recorded. In all patients, the reconstructed splenic arteries were patent, without splenic atrophy. One patient had asymptomatic partial splenic infarction.

Conclusions.—These findings support the efficacy and safety of elective surgery for the treatment of splenic artery aneurysms. Arterial reconstruction allows good early and long-term results with preservation of the spleen. Splenectomy may be unavoidable in some patients.

▶ The article emphasizes preservation of the spleen in treatment of splenic artery aneurysms. Splenectomy or splenic artery occlusion by endovascular techniques is commonly performed for splenic artery aneurysms, but the authors note that when the splenic artery aneurysms are located away from the hilum, resection of the aneurysm with end-to-end anastomosis of the splenic artery is usually possible. In addition, late formation of recurrent splenic artery aneurysms does not appear to occur. I think the authors have a good point. Why remove or destroy an organ when it can be preserved?

G. L. Moneta, MD

Visceral Artery Aneurysm Rupture
Carr SC, Mahvi DM, Hoch JR, et al (Univ of Wisconsin, Madison)
J Vasc Surg 33:806-811, 2001   9–11

Background.—Visceral artery aneurysms (VAAs) are rare, and in the past were typically identified only after they ruptured. With the widespread use of CT and angiography, however, many VAAs are being found incidentally. To better characterize the impact of these lesions, a single institution's 10-year experience with the presentation, management, and outcomes of patients with VAA was reviewed.

Methods.—The subjects were 26 patients (15 males and 11 females, 2-86 years of age) with 34 VAAs. In 15 patients (58%), the VAAs were diagnosed before rupture as the result of imaging studies or abdominal symptoms. In 11 patients (42%), the diagnosis was made after rupture.

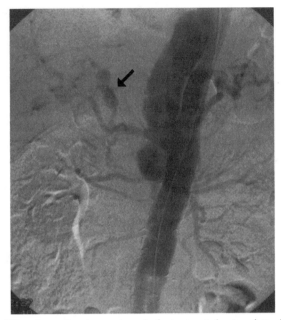

FIGURE 1.—This patient undergoing arteriography for treatment planning of an enlarged thoracoabdominal aneurysm was found to have multiple hepatic artery aneurysms (*arrow*) as well. (Courtesy of Carr SC, Mahvi DM, Hoch JR, et al: Visceral artery aneurysm rupture. *J Vasc Surg* 33:806-811, 2001.)

Results.—Four patients had multiple VAAs: One patient had 3 hepatic artery aneurysms (HAAs), 1 patient had 2 splenic artery aneurysms (SAAs), 1 patient had 3 SAAs, and 1 patient had 3 SAAs and a celiac artery aneurysm. Eight patients (31%) also had associated aneurysms of the abdominal aorta (4 patients), thoracic aorta (3 patients), iliac artery (3 patients), renal arteries (2 patients), lower extremity (1 patient), or intracranium (1 patient). In 4 patients (15%), associated lesions were present in more than 1 location (Fig 1).

The 15 patients in whom a VAA was diagnosed before rupture included 13 SAAs, 3 celiac artery aneurysms, 2 superior mesenteric artery aneurysms, 1 HAA, and 1 gastroduodenal artery aneurysm. Seven of these patients were treated with observation for 2 to 60 months (mean, 15 months). Six of these 7 patients experienced no complications related to their VAAs, but the seventh patient died of a ruptured SAA 6 months after liver transplantation. The remaining 8 patients in whom a VAA was found incidentally underwent elective surgery. Six of these 8 patients had no complications and are doing well. One patient (with an HAA) had postoperative pancreatitis and, later, had an incisional ventral hernia. The last patient (with an SAA) underwent surgery at the time of liver transplantation and subsequently had a nonfatal myocardial infarction and pancreatic duct leak.

The 11 patients first seen with rupture included 4 SSAs, 3 HHAs, 1 right gastric artery aneurysm, 1 gastroduodenal artery aneurysm, 1 pancreaticoduodenal artery aneurysm, and 1 ileal artery aneurysm. All patients promptly underwent surgery; 2 patients died postoperatively. Additionally,

1 patient experienced pneumonia and stroke, 1 patient experienced pneumonia and cardiac arrest, and 1 patient experienced a splenic abscess and prolonged ileus. Overall, then, 12 of these 26 patients (46%) had a ruptured VAA, and 3 of them died, for a mortality rate of 25%.

Conclusion.—VAAs are rare. Rupture is a significant cause of mortality in these patients. Many patients with VAAs have more than 1 VAA, and many have associated aneurysms as well. Given that 25% of patients with a ruptured VAA died, patients with VAAs should be treated aggressively, even those in whom the disease is found incidentally.

▶ VAAs are a hodgepodge of etiologies, associated conditions, and presentations. Some rupture, and the mortality is high, while elective treatment is associated with minimal morbidity and mortality. I agree with the Wisconsin surgeons that treatment of these lesions is indicated when feasible. Who can argue with that?

G. L. Moneta, MD

Is Prosthetic Renal Artery Reconstruction a Durable Procedure? An Analysis of 489 Bypass Grafts
Paty PSK, Darling RC III, Lee D, et al (Albany Med College, NY)
J Vasc Surg 34:127-132, 2001   9–12

Background.—Traditionally, surgical management of renal artery stenosis has consisted of saphenous vein bypass or transaortic endarterectomy, on their own or combined with an aortic procedure. The use of prosthetic grafts in this situation, however, has been questioned. The outcomes of a large series of patients undergoing renal artery reconstruction using prosthetic conduit are discussed.

Methods.—The study included 414 patients who had 489 renal artery bypass procedures performed using prosthetic conduit from 1987 to 1999. Indications for surgery included high-grade renal artery stenosis with concomitant abdominal aortic aneurysm repair or aortoiliac occlusive disease in 63% of patients, renovascular disease in 24%, and renal salvage in 4%. The aorta or aortic graft for inflow was used for 95% of the procedures; iliac or visceral vessels were used for the remainder. A retroperitoneal approach was used for 98% of the operations. Outcome evaluation included postoperative duplex scanning and US follow-up every 6 months.

Results.—The overall rate of nonfatal complications was 11.4%, including early occlusion for 1.4% of cases and late occlusion for 97.8%. Only 3.1% of patients had a worsening of renal function. Patency was well maintained, with secondary patency rates of 98% at 1 year and 96% at 5 years.

Conclusions.—This study demonstrates good and long-lasting results with the use of prosthetic conduit for renal artery reconstruction. Good patency rates and renal function were achieved in both primary reconstructions and reconstructions combined with aortic procedures.

▶ I have always preferred prosthetic for renal artery grafts, and so, to the extent that this article confirms my prejudice, it pleases me. But in classic Albany fashion, the authors have reported excellent patency results in a very large number of cases and completely avoided the issue of whether any of the operations were indicated, and whether they achieved the desired result. Does renal artery revascularization for hypertension or for preservation/restoration of renal function work? You won't find out from this article.

L. M. Taylor, Jr, MD

10 Leg Ischemia

Relationship Between Site of Initial Symptoms and Subsequent Progression of Disease in a Prospective Study of Atherosclerosis Progression in Patients Receiving Long-term Treatment for Symptomatic Peripheral Arterial Disease

Nicoloff AD, and The Homocysteine and Progression of Atherosclerosis Study Investigators (Oregon Health and Science Univ, Portland)

J Vasc Surg 35:38-47, 2002   10–1

Background.—The presence of symptoms distinguishes atherosclerotic disease from atherosclerotic change that is a normal consequence of aging. It may be possible to identify individuals at increased risk for progressive symptoms by examining the relationship between the site of initial symptoms of peripheral artery disease and the incidence of subsequent symptomatic progression. Patients with symptomatic lower extremity disease (LED), cerebrovascular disease (CVD), or both, were followed up prospectively for disease progression.

Methods.—The study included 397 patients with a mean age of 66 years; 38% were women. All underwent comprehensive risk factor assessment and serial noninvasive lower extremity vascular and carotid artery testing. Follow-up examinations were conducted every 6 months for a mean of 48.5 months. Variables considered in the analyses were age, diabetes mellitus, hypertension, smoking, cholesterol level, homocysteine level, lowest initial ankle/brachial index (ABI), worst carotid stenosis, ABI progression, and carotid stenosis progression.

Results.—At study entry, LED was present in 88% of patients, CVD in 37%, and both LED and CVD in 25%. Forty-seven (60%) of 78 deaths during follow-up were due to cardiovascular disease. Disease progression as documented by vascular laboratory findings occurred in 90% of patients by means of life table analysis after 5 years. Rates of progression were 31% for ABI and 40% for carotid stenosis (Fig 5). Symptomatic clinical disease progression occurred in 52% by means of life table analysis after 5 years: LED progression, 22%; CVD progression, 23%; and coronary heart disease progression, 31%. No significant relationship was found between the site of initial peripheral artery disease symptoms and the site or sites of subsequent symptomatic clinical progression.

Conclusion.—Patients with symptomatic peripheral artery disease are at increased risk for death, but symptoms of ongoing LED, CVD, and coronary

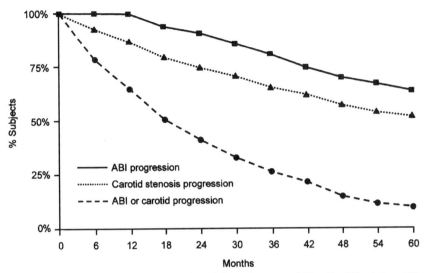

FIGURE 5.—Vascular laboratory progression of disease by means of life table. *Abbreviation: ABI,* Ankle/brachial index. (Courtesy of Nicoloff AD, and The Homocysteine and Progression of Atherosclerosis Study Investigators: Relationship between site of initial symptoms and subsequent progression of disease in a prospective study of atherosclerosis progression in patients receiving long-term treatment for symptomatic peripheral arterial disease. *J Vasc Surg* 35:38-47, 2002.)

heart disease occur with a frequency that is not influenced by the site of the initial symptoms.

▶ This study basically provides a quantitative analysis of what is apparent to all who treat patients with atherosclerosis: once the disease is established, it appears to progress in virtually everyone, although at varying rates. In this study, multiple risk factors were shown to be associated with disease progression. One wonders, given the virtual universal presence of some sort of progression in these patients, if modification of atherosclerotic risk factors really helps these patients all that much. Perhaps once atherosclerosis has progressed to the point of leg ischemia or cerebrovascular disease further progression is the rule, and there may be little to do to change things. We all certainly hope that is not the case, but one really has to wonder.

G. L. Moneta, MD

Peripheral Arterial Disease in Diabetic and Nondiabetic Patients: A Comparison of Severity and Outcome

Jude EB, Chalmers N, Oyibo SO, et al (Manchester Royal Infirmary, England)
Diabetes Care 24:1433-1437, 2001   10–2

Background.—Diabetes mellitus increases one's risk of peripheral arterial disease (PAD), and PAD is itself an important risk factor for amputation in diabetic patients with chronic foot ulcers. However, few studies have examined whether the distribution or severity of PAD differs in diabetic versus nondiabetic patients. The distribution of PAD and its severity and outcomes were compared among patients with PAD who had diabetes and those who did not.

Methods.—The medical records of 136 randomly selected patients with PAD (81 men and 55 women; mean age, 64.7 years) who underwent peripheral angiography were examined. Demographics and clinical characteristics were examined to compare PAD distribution, severity, and outcomes between the 58 diabetic patients (43%) and the 78 nondiabetic patients (57%). A scoring system (0 = normal segment, 15 = total occlusion of more than half the segment) was used to assess the severity of PAD in arterial segments. Outcomes included the need for subsequent revascularization, the need for lower-extremity amputation, and mortality during the year after angiography.

Results.—The diabetic and nondiabetic groups were similar in age (mean ages, 63.9 and 65.3 years, respectively), sex (60% and 62% male), smoking status (81% and 77% current or ex-smokers), and the proportion of patients with ischemic heart disease (41% and 37%) and hypercholesterolemia (24% and 31%). However, diabetic patients were significantly more likely to be hypertensive (74% vs 40%). Compared with nondiabetic patients, diabetic patients had significantly more severe PAD in the profunda femoris artery (median score, 3 vs 0), popliteal artery (median score, 7 vs 3), anterior tibial artery (median score, 13 vs 3), peroneal artery (median score, 5 vs 0), and posterior tibial artery (median score, 15 vs 4). Revascularization rates did not differ significantly between the diabetic and nondiabetic patients (60% and 62%, respectively), nor did the proportion of patients requiring 2 or more revascularization procedures (21% and 22%).

Amputation was required in 33 patients, and the risk of amputation was significantly higher in diabetic patients (41% vs 12%; odds ratio, 5.4). Mortality rates at 1 year after angiography were also significantly higher among diabetic patients (52% vs 26%; odds ratio, 3.1), and diabetic patients who died were significantly younger when they underwent angiography than were nondiabetic patients who died (64.7 vs 71.1 years).

Conclusion.—Among patients with PAD, those with diabetes have more severe PAD in the profundus femoris artery and in arterial segments below the knee. Patients with PAD who are diabetic are also more likely to require amputation than are patients with PAD who are not diabetic. Patients with PAD and diabetes are also more likely to die and to die at an earlier age.

▶ This retrospective review attempts to evaluate the influence of diabetes on the clinical patterns and long-term outcomes of peripheral arterial disease. A cohort of 150 patients who underwent angiography at their institution were randomly selected; a case-control design was not used. Critical ischemia was present in 57% of diabetics (53% with tissue loss) versus 23% of non-diabetics. Consistent with a large body of literature, patients with diabetes had a higher incidence of disease in the profunda and tibioperoneal arteries, a 4-fold increased risk of amputation, and a doubling of mortality over the 4.5 years of follow-up. These are not new findings. However, the authors go on to argue that they found no evidence that revascularization prevented amputation, a conclusion that is far-fetched for their study. Of particular note, despite the high proportion of diabetics with severe tibioperoneal disease and tissue loss, not a single patient with diabetes received a distal revascularization (tibial or pedal) procedure. It's not surprising that the Manchester group is unable to define a role for limb salvage interventions, when severe distal tibial disease is being left untreated in critically ischemic limbs!

M. S. Conte, MD

Natural History of Claudication: Long-term Serial Follow-up Study of 1244 Claudicants
Aquino R, Johnnides C, Makaroun M, et al (Univ of Pittsburgh, Pa; VA Med Ctr, Pittsburgh, Pa)
J Vasc Surg 34:962-970, 2001   10–3

Background.—Relatively little is known about the natural history of intermittent claudication. A long-term follow-up study for a large group of patients with this common lower-extremity vascular disease is discussed, including risk factors for ischemic rest pain (IRP) and ischemic ulcers (IU).

Methods.—The analysis included follow-up data on 1244 patients, all men, with intermittent claudication. Baseline data were collected, with follow-up information including serial assessment of ankle-brachial index (ABI), self-reported walking disease, and development of IRP and IU. The mean follow-up was 45 months, and some patients were followed up for as long as 12 years.

Results.—On average, the patients' ABI decreased by 0.014 per year, and their walking distance by 9.2 yards/y. The cumulative 10-year risk of IU was 23%, with a 30% risk of IRP. On multivariate analysis including various clinical risk factors, the only independent predictors of IRP were diabetes re-

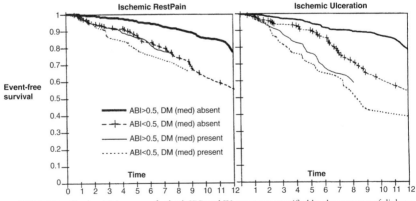

FIGURE 2.—Kaplan-Meier curves for both IRP and IU outcomes stratified by the presence of diabetes requiring medication (DM) and baseline ABI. (Courtesy of Aquino R, Johnnides C, Makaroun M, et al: Natural history of claudication: Long-term serial follow-up study of 1244 claudicants. *J Vasc Surg* 34:962-970, 2001.)

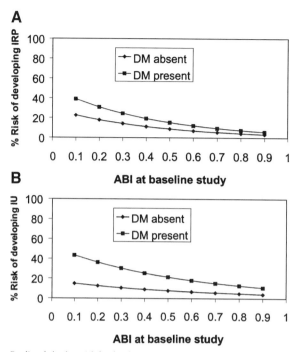

FIGURE 3.—Predicted absolute risk for development of IRP (A) and IU (B). *Abbreviation: DM,* Diabetes requiring medication. (Courtesy of Aquino R, Johnnides C, Makaroun M, et al: Natural history of claudication: Long-term serial follow-up study of 1244 claudicants. *J Vasc Surg* 34:962-970, 2001.)

quiring medication (relative risk, 1.8); and ABI (relative risk, 2.2) for each 0.1 decrease. The same 2 factors were also independent predictors of IU: (relative risk, 3.0 and 1.9, respectively) (Figs 2 and 3).

Conclusions.—The findings lend new insight into the long-term clinical outcomes of intermittent claudication. For patients with this condition, the presence of diabetes mellitus and the baseline ABI are key risk factors for IRP and IU.

▶ The authors have a reasonably conducted prospective study of male veteran cigarette smoking claudicants from which we have already had several reports. This reasonably thick salami slice addresses the issue of occurrence of IRP and IU in this cohort, none of whom had these symptoms/findings at the time of study entry. The incidence was higher than you might expect, establishing that this is a cohort with advanced disease compared with some other studies. Lower ABI and diabetes were associated with more likelihood of progression—exactly as predicted by multiple other studies. There was no association with smoking, but then there couldn't be. They had almost no nonsmokers. Prospectively collected data are precious—this article is worth your time to read.

L. M. Taylor, Jr, MD

Developing the Vascular Quality of Life Questionnaire: A New Disease-Specific Quality of Life Measure for Use in Lower Limb Ischemia

Morgan MBF, Crayford T, Murrin B, et al (King's College Hosp, London)
J Vasc Surg 33:679-687, 2001   10–4

Background.—Quality of life (QOL) is an important outcome measure for assessing patients with chronic lower limb ischemia. However, current tools for measuring QOL in this population are either not disease specific or are limited to patients with claudication. The development and testing of a disease-specific QOL instrument that can be used for all patients with chronic lower limb ischemia were described.

Methods.—During the first phase, a panel of physicians, nurses, and patients developed 89 items they believed were most important to patients with lower limb ischemia. Then 137 patients rated the importance of these 89 factors on a 5-point scale. The questions with the highest scores that were important to 40% of the patients or more were selected for pretesting by 20 additional patients. The final 25-item King's College Hospital VascuQol questionnaire included 5 domains: pain, symptoms, activities, social, and emotional.

During the second phase, 39 patients (24 men and 15 women; median age, 67 years) completed the questionnaire and the Short-Form 36 (SF- 36), a general measure of health, at baseline and again 4 weeks later. Treadmill walking distance and ankle/brachial pressure indexes were also recorded at these times. Test-retest scores of patients whose symptoms and objective measurements had not changed were compared to determine the questionnaire's reliability. The responsiveness of the questionnaire was determined by comparing changes in a patient's score with changes in other indexes. Scores on the questionnaire were correlated with those on the SF-36 and with treadmill walking distance results to determine the questionnaire's validity.

Results.—Among 17 patients whose condition remained unchanged between weeks 0 and 4, the test-retest scores had an intraclass (reliability) coefficient of 0.94 ($P < .001$). Item-total score Cronbach α values were greater than 0.90, and all item-domain α scores were between 0.7 and 0.8. The questionnaire was responsive to changes, and correlated significantly with both global (SF-36) and clinical indicators of change. Finally, the questionnaire was valid: the total score correlated significantly with disease severity and treadmill walking distance, and domain scores correlated significantly with those on the SF-36.

Conclusion.—The 25-item King's College Hospital VascuQol questionnaire is a reliable, responsive, and valid tool for assessing outcomes in patients with chronic lower limb ischemia.

▶ This article is recommended as a brief synopsis on developing a disease-specific questionnaire. Patency results remain important in vascular surgery, but assessment of quality of life issues is rapidly emerging, along with endografting, as a fertile area of clinical research. We have waited too long to properly assess the impact of vascular disease on the patients' quality of life.

G. L. Moneta, MD

Peripheral Artery Disease, Diabetes, and Reduced Lower Extremity Functioning
Dolan NC, Chan C, Liu K, et al (Northwestern Univ, Chicago; Univ of California at San Diego; Natl Inst on Aging, Bethesda, Md; et al)
Diabetes Care 25:113-120, 2002   10–5

Background.—In the general population, patients with diabetes mellitus have a greater risk of disability than patients without this disease. Whether this is also true in the population of patients with peripheral artery disease (PAD) was examined, with particular emphasis on lower extremity function.

Methods.—The subjects were 460 adults 55 years of age and older with PAD (ankle/brachial index [ABI] less than 0.90). All subjects completed questionnaires to determine their leg symptoms (San Diego Claudication Questionnaire) and to assess their difficulty with walking (Walking Impairment Questionnaire). They also underwent lower extremity functional measurements, including the 6-minute walk (to assess endurance), the usual and fast-pace 4-m walking velocity test (to measure speed), and tandem stand and repeated chair rises (to measure balance and strength). A summary performance score (SPS) was calculated by assigning scores of 0-4 to results of each of the 3 lower extremity functional tests based on cut points derived from normative data (maximum SPS, 12). Results of these assessments were compared between the 147 patients with diabetes (32%; 63% men) and the 313 patients without diabetes (68%; 58% men).

Results.—The mean ABI was similar in the patients with and without diabetes (0.64 and 0.65, respectively). Patients with diabetes were significantly younger (mean, 69.2 vs 73.1 years) and more likely to be black (24% vs 13%). After data adjustment for age, patients with diabetes were significantly more likely to have comorbidities (mean, 2.4 vs 2.0), especially cardiovascular disease (68% vs 56%); to have neuropathic pain (mean scores on a 22-point scale, 5.6 vs 3.5); and to report leg pain with exertion and rest (29% vs 14%). However, they were significantly less likely than nondiabetic patients to report intermittent claudication (25% vs 36%).

Patients with diabetes had significantly worse scores on the Walking Impairment Questionnaire (both shorter distances and lower speeds), and their performance on the lower extremity functional tests was significantly poorer. Specifically, their 6-minute walking distance was shorter (1040 vs 1168 feet), their fast-pace 4-m walking velocity was slower (0.83 vs 0.90 m/s), and they were less likely to complete a full tandem stand (42% vs 62%). Their SPS was also significantly lower than for patients without diabetes (mean, 7.3 vs 8.6). The differences between diabetics and nondiabetics in fast-pace 4-m walking velocity and SPS remained significant after stepwise multiple linear analyses that adjusted for type of exertional leg pain, neuropathy score, and number of cardiovascular comorbidities.

The severity of diabetes also influenced leg function: After data adjustment for age, sex, race, and body mass index, performance on all 3 lower extremity function tests was significantly worse among patients whose diabetes was controlled by medication compared with diabetics whose disease was controlled by diet.

Conclusion.—Patients with PAD who also have diabetes have significantly worse lower extremity function than patients with PAD who are not diabetic. Furthermore, those with more severe diabetes (ie, requiring medication) have significantly worse lower leg function than those with less severe disease (ie, controlled by diet). Much of the difference in lower leg function between patients with PAD and diabetes and patients with PAD without diabetes can be explained by differences in exertional leg symptoms, cardiovascular disease, and diabetes-associated neuropathy.

▶ While it is fun to poke fun at the vascular medicine specialists when they appear to rediscover the wheel, in some aspects of vascular disease vascular medicine has made significant contributions. Assessment of quality of life issues is one of these areas. In this study, comorbidities associated with diabetes combine to apparently adversely impact lower extremity function, more than function is improved in patients with PAD and without diabetes. This occurs in spite of the fact there are similar ABIs in both groups. The authors correctly acknowledge that patients with diabetes may have had falsely elevated ABIs and therefore actually worse PAD than the controls. However, it is interesting to note symptoms of lower extremity leg pain in diabetic patients do not always seem to be those of classic claudication. I think we should keep this in mind when assessing the outcomes of revascularization in patients with diabetes. The underlying comorbidities may make such patients comparatively worse candidates for a procedure for claudication. Residual symptoms will be adversely impacted by neuropathy, atypical angina, and perhaps altered foot bone structure.

G. L. Moneta, MD

A New Device for the Measurement of Disease Severity in Patients With Intermittent Claudication
Coughlin PA, Kent PJ, Turton EP, et al (St James's Univ, Leeds, England)
Eur J Vasc Endovasc Surg 22:516-522, 2001   10–6

Background.—For patients with peripheral vascular disease, the most common symptom is intermittent claudication. Its severity is assessed by using measures of walking distance, usually treadmill tests, but these have limitations. To allow physicians to gain a better understanding of the functional impairments from intermittent claudication, the Peripheral Arterial Disease Holter Control Device (PADHOC) was developed for outpatient use (Fig 1). Comparisons were made of walking distance between the PADHOC and a

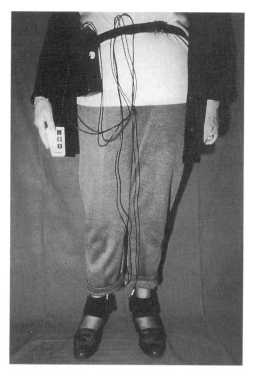

FIGURE 1.—The main unit worn by the patient. (Reprinted from Coughlin PA, Kent PJ, Turton EP, et al: A new device for the measurement of disease severity in patients with intermittent claudication. *Eur J Vasc Endovasc Surg* 22:516-522, 2001. Copyright 2001 by permission of the publisher W B Saunders Company Limited London.)

standard constant load treadmill assessment for patients with intermittent claudication. In addition, patients' self-assessment of walking distance was compared with results of the Double Physiological Walking Test (DPWT), using the PADHOC device. Finally, the characteristics of patients who could and could not perform a treadmill test were evaluated.

Methods.—The study included 36 men and 27 women (age, 48-86 years; median age, 69 years) who underwent DPWT testing and 49 patients who did the standard treadmill test. Patients who did not complete the treadmill test had ischemic heart disease, chronic obstructive pulmonary disease, or osteoarthritis. Measurements obtained were initial claudication distance (ICD), maximum walking distance (MWD), and speed of walking. Patients estimated their own claudication distance and had ankle-brachial pressure indices (ABPIs) determined after resting 45 minutes.

Results.—The resting ABPIs of patients who could and could not perform the treadmill test showed no significant differences. The postexercise ABPI was significantly lower than the initial resting ABPI in those who completed the treadmill test. Of those completing the treadmill test, claudication was mild in 6 patients, moderate in 25, and severe in 18. Lower estimated claudication distances were reported by those who could not complete the treadmill test than those who could. No significant differences were found between estimated claudication distances and actual claudication distances measured by the DPWT. A strong correlation was found between estimated claudication distance, treadmill initial claudicating distance (ICD), and initial PADHOC ICD among those completing the treadmill test. Maximal treadmill walking distance and MWD on both parts of the DPWT showed a strong correlation. The ICD obtained on the first part of the DPWT and the treadmill ICD were also strongly correlated, although no significant correlation was shown with the ICDs posted on the DPWT's second part. Disease severity as determined by DPWT correlated significantly with disease severity by the treadmill test. Resting ABPIs and walking ratios showed no correlation. Significant differences occurred in walking speeds, MWDs, and ICDs of the first walking test between those patients who could complete the treadmill test and those who could not. For the second part of the DPWT, no significant differences were seen in ICD, nor were there significant differences between the ratios for ICD or MWD in both groups.

Conclusions.—The PADHOC device and subsequent DPWT provided accurate estimates of patients' functional limitations caused by intermittent claudication. The device is safe and easy to use; its results appear to be free of observer bias. Patients who cannot undergo treadmill testing can be assessed with the use of the PADHOC device, which was also found to be easily transportable for use in various settings.

▶ This device for assessing claudication in patients with peripheral arterial disease looks cumbersome (see Fig 1), but it may serve as an alternative to treadmill walking in patients unable to perform a treadmill test. There is a surprising number of such patients: 22% in this series. I wonder, however, if a patient can't walk on a treadmill for reasons other than obvious severity of disease, why in the world would such a patient be considered for revascularization for any reason other than limb salvage? I see this device as a research tool but doubt it will have utility in clinical practice.

G. L. Moneta, MD

Muscle Fiber Characteristics in Patients With Peripheral Arterial Disease
McGuigan MRM, Bronks R, Newton RU, et al (Univ of Wisconsin, La Crosse; Southern Cross Univ, Lismore, New South Wales, Australia; St Vincents Hosp, Lismore, New South Wales, Australia; et al)
Med Sci Sports Exerc 33:2016-2021, 2001   10–7

Background.—As many as 20% of older persons suffer from atherosclerosis, and symptomatic peripheral arterial disease (PAD) often occurs with this condition, increasing the risk of other cardiovascular diseases. For patients with PAD, muscle fiber type changes as a mechanism for the disorder have been postulated, but findings are as yet equivocal. The gastrocnemius muscle in patients with PAD was evaluated for myosin heavy chain (MHC) expression and potential histochemical changes associated with symptom-

A

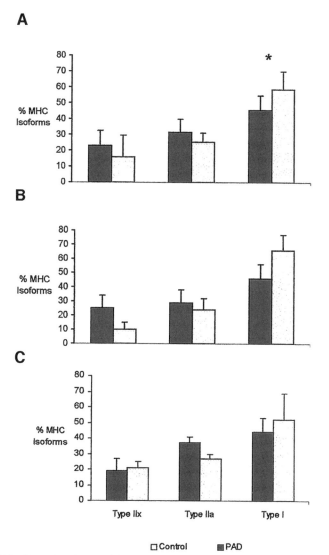

B

C

□ Control　　■ PAD

FIGURE 1.—Expression of MHC isoforms in subjects with PAD and control subjects. $*P < .05$. (**A**), Combined, (**B**), women, and (**C**), men. (Courtesy of McGuigan MRM, Bronks R, Newton RU, et al: Muscle fiber characteristics in patients with peripheral arterial disease. *Med Sci Sports Exerc* 33:2016-2021, 2001.)

atic PAD. The results obtained were compared with those in an activity-matched group of control subjects.

Methods.—The study included 14 patients (8 women, 6 men; mean age, 69.7 years) with PAD and 8 activity-matched control subjects (4 women, 4 men; mean age, 65.1 years). Both groups completed the PAD Physical Activity Recall questionnaire, had treadmill testing to determine maximal walking performance, and submitted to hemodynamic measurements (ankle-brachial index [ABI] using Doppler US). All participants underwent needle biopsy, with the specimens extracted from the medial head of the gastrocnemius muscle. These samples were analyzed for the expression of MHC isoforms.

Results.—Compared with the control group, PAD patients had significantly lower ABI values at rest that decreased still further with exercise. Control subjects were able to walk a significantly longer time than PAD patients on the treadmill test. PAD patients had a significantly smaller proportion of MHC I than control subjects, but no significant differences were noted in MHC IIa or MHC IIx expression (Fig 1). PAD patients had a significantly smaller percentage of type I fibers than control subjects, and these fibers were significantly smaller than those in the control group. No difference was found between the 2 groups in the percentage of type IIA fibers, although these fibers were significantly smaller in the PAD patients compared with those in the control group. Individuals with PAD had a significantly greater percentage of type IIx fibers, which were somewhat reduced. In comparison with control subjects, women with PAD had significantly reduced fiber areas for all 3 fiber types, whereas men with PAD only showed a reduced size in the type I and IIA fibers. A significantly greater capillary density was found in those with PAD, and the capillary/fiber ratio and number of capillaries in contact with each muscle fiber were significantly increased.

Conclusions.—The gastrocnemius muscle of patients with PAD showed significant changes in MHC isoform expression, in fiber types, and in fiber areas when compared with those of the control subjects. For patients with PAD, reductions were found in the MHC 1 isoforms, and percentages of type I fibers, while fiber area and percentages of type IIA fibers were significantly increased. Type I fibers are apparently converted to type IIA fibers, allowing a greater capacity for nonoxidative metabolism in PAD muscles than for oxidative metabolism. Capillary density, number of capillaries in contact with each muscle fiber, and capillary/fiber ratio were also increased in PAD muscles. These changes reflect the effects of ischemia. Muscle performance on the treadmill test was compromised for patients with PAD, illustrating the reduced endurance capacity of the muscles in this disorder.

▶ The purpose of these studies was to determine whether MHC expression (protein) is modulated in patients with PAD. This topic has been studied by others, and these authors hoped to extend our understanding of this issue by increasing the number of patients studied and by ensuring the patients had similar degrees of ischemia. Skeletal muscle biopsies were obtained from age-matched individuals. The authors found that patients with PAD had increased density of capillaries when compared with normal patients. Furthermore, there appears to be evidence of conversion of MHCs to include fibers that have a greater capacity for nonoxidative than oxidative metabolism. Since the arterial diseased tissue appears to have greater capillaries than normal tissue, the authors conclude that the fiber type composition rather than oxygen demand limits the endurance capacity of the muscle. This conclusion is conjectural at best, and it does not appear to be supported by any data to show that oxygen delivery is adequate during exercise in patients with arterial disease and increased capillaries.

M. T. Watkins, MD

Prior Exercise Training Produces NO-Dependent Increases in Collateral Blood Flow After Acute Arterial Occlusion
Yang HT, Ren J, Laughlin MH, et al (Univ of Missouri, Columbia)
Am J Physiol 282:H301-H310, 2002   10–8

Background.—In a previous study, these authors showed that prior exercise training improves collateral blood flow (BF) to the rat calf muscles after acute occlusion of the femoral artery. In this study, they investigated a possible mechanism for this effect.

Methods.—Adult male Sprague-Dawley rats were randomly assigned to either the sedentary group (28 animals) or the exercise group (30 animals). Rats in the exercise group underwent daily treadmill exercises for 6 weeks. After 6 weeks, animals were instrumented for measuring BF to the calf muscles and distal limb arterial pressure. All animals underwent surgical occlusion of the femoral arteries. Additionally, half of each group were injected with either the nitric oxide synthase inhibitor N^G-nitro-L-arginine methyl ester (L-NAME) or saline 30 minutes before BF measurements. BF was measured 4 hours after surgery while animals performed treadmill testing at 2 speeds (20, then 25 m/min, both at a 15% grade). Differences between untreated controls, controls treated with L-NAME, untreated exercise-trained animals, and exercised animals treated with L-NAME were compared.

Results.—BF did not increase during the second treadmill test compared with the first, which indicates that the maximal BF had been achieved. BF to the proximal and distal hindlimb and to the calf muscles was significantly greater in the untreated exercise group than in the untreated controls. This was also true for the treated groups, but the increased collateral BF in the treated exercise group was significantly attenuated compared with that of the untreated exercised animals. Collateral circuit resistance was significantly lower in the exercise groups compared with the control groups, but again, L-NAME treatment attenuated this effect. Collateral circuit conductance was significantly increased in the untreated exercised animals compared with the untreated controls. With L-NAME treatment, collateral circuit conductance in the trained animals did not differ significantly from that in either the untreated or treated controls. Distal tissue resistance was significantly lower only in the untreated exercise group, while distal tissue conductance was significantly higher only in the untreated exercise group.

Conclusion.—In this rat model, exercise training improved collateral-dependent BF to the hindlimb and calf muscles after acute femoral artery occlusion. The primary determinant of this effect is resistance of the upstream collateral circuits. These findings support the hypothesis that training causes enhanced endothelium-mediated dilation that increases collateral BF after acute arterial occlusion.

▶ Patients with acute arterial occlusion are symptomatically worse at the onset of the occlusion. If the leg remains viable, improvement over the subsequent days to weeks is the rule. Where collateral development is often cited as the explanation, one might infer from this study that the "development" of collaterals is really an upregulation of NO production and collateral "dilatation" rather than "development." It is interesting to speculate, therefore, that patients with acute arterial occlusion may someday be candidates for drugs specifically targeting collateral vasodilatation.

G. L. Moneta, MD

Medical Treatment of Peripheral Arterial Disease and Claudication
Hiatt WR (Univ of Colorado, Denver)
N Engl J Med 344:1608-1621, 2001   10–9

Background.—Peripheral arterial disease, an important manifestation of systemic atherosclerosis, results from atherosclerotic occlusion of the arteries to the legs. It is associated with marked impairment of ambulation and quality of life as well as a substantial risk of illness and death. The treatment of peripheral arterial disease and claudication was reviewed.

Discussion.—Risk factor modification, antiplatelet agents, and symptom treatment are underused in patients with peripheral arterial disease. Clinical trials involving patients with peripheral arterial disease are needed to investigate the value of treating hyperlipidemia, diabetes, hyperhomocysteinemia, and other prevalent risk factors. Currently, affected patients should be considered for secondary prevention strategies, as are patients with coronary artery disease. Angiotensin-converting-enzyme inhibitors may reduce the risk of ischemic events in patients with peripheral arterial disease. Antiplatelet drugs successfully decrease the risk of fatal and nonfatal ischemic events in this patient population. Evidence supporting the use of antiplatelet therapy is stronger than that for angiotensin-converting-enzyme inhibitors. In all patients, the use of aspirin should be considered, with clopidogrel as an alternative. Treatment of claudication and limited mobility should begin with a supervised walking-based program. This approach is associated with low risk and the likelihood of marked improvement in functional capacity. In addition, drugs are available to improve functional status. The efficacy of pentoxifylline is limited, but cilostazol has been found to improve pain-free and maximal treadmill walking distance and quality of life. Other compounds, including propionyl levocarnitine, are currently being studied for their utility in claudication and critical leg ischemia treatment.

▶ This review article is succinct, covers all the important points, and is quite readable. I recommend it highly as a compact source of information regarding pharmacotherapy of peripheral arterial disease. I wish Bill Hiatt had included some information about long-term warfarin therapy, but with this exception I agree with everything he says. I pretty much have to because I learned a lot of this stuff from him in the first place.

L. M. Taylor, Jr, MD

Duplex Scanning as the Sole Preoperative Imaging Method for Infrainguinal Arterial Surgery
Boström A, Ljungman C, Hellberg A, et al (Univ Hosp, Uppsala, Sweden)
Eur J Vasc Endovasc Surg 23:140-145, 2002   10–10

Background.—Conventional angiography remains the traditional method for evaluating inflow and outflow arteries before infrainguinal arterial reconstruction, but it is associated with a low but significant rate of local and systemic complications. Recent experience with duplex scanning has suggested that its accuracy approaches that of angiography and provides hemodynamic as well as anatomic information. The use of duplex scanning as the only preoperative diagnostic investigation before lower limb reconstruction was studied.

Methods.—A retrospective evaluation reviewed 329 surgical interventions for chronic infrainguinal arterial occlusive or aneurysmal disease. All patients underwent duplex scanning, and 157 of the 329 interventions were performed without preoperative angiography.

Results.—Among the patients who underwent femoral artery endarterectomy, duplex scanning correctly diagnosed the extent of the stenosis and the status of the distal deep femoral artery in all but 1 patient. Among those undergoing infrainguinal bypass, the duplex scan findings agreed with the findings of on-table angiography in terms of the selection of optimal outflow anastomotic sites in 98% of patients. The status of runoff was correctly evaluated by duplex scanning in 90% of these patients. There were no significant differences in the 30-day occlusion rate and patency at 12 months between reconstructions in patients with or without preoperative angiography.

Conclusions.—Preoperative angiography is not necessary in patients undergoing infrainguinal arterial reconstruction when the duplex scanning findings are conclusive.

▶ Infrainguinal bypass can be performed on the basis of duplex scanning alone with good results. However, it is important to keep in mind that even in centers dedicated to this concept, many scans will be inconclusive. For those contemplating this approach, I suggest beginning with bypasses to the popliteal only when duplex demonstrates at least 1 tibial vessel in continuity with the popliteal, and that tibial vessel to also be in continuity to the level of the ankle. The inflow status also must be normal, either by pulse palpation or normal femoral artery waveform.

G. L. Moneta, MD

Femoropopliteal Bypass Is Not a Generic Procedure: A Survey of the Practice Patterns of the Florida Vascular Society

Samson RH (Mote Vascular Found, Sarasota, Fla)
Ann Vasc Surg 15:544-547, 2001   10–11

Background.—The long-term results for femoropopliteal bypass grafts differ, depending on the type of graft material and the choice of an above-knee or below-knee site for the distal anastomosis. Evaluation of recent literature on femoropopliteal bypass reveals that there may be many other factors affecting the outcome of this procedure. However, there has not been a study of the nuances of surgical technique and intraoperative choices and practice patterns. The surgical techniques used by vascular surgeons in Florida were evaluated, and their practice preferences were analyzed to determine whether there is a standard method for performance of the femoropopliteal bypass. In addition, the long-term patency of the grafts inserted by these surgeons was determined.

Methods.—All 83 members of the Florida Vascular Society received a multiple-choice questionnaire. The questions covered all aspects of the operative and immediate perioperative experience. The questionnaire was not a validated instrument, but 5 questions were specifically duplicated by rephrasing to assess the respondents' understanding of the questions.

Results.—Fifty-three surgeons (64%) responded to the survey. The respondents performed from 10 to 80 femoropopliteal bypasses per year, with a mean of 38 per year. Only 7 surgeons (13%) were aware of their patency rates, and only 4 could provide life tables. Only 2 surgeons were aware of mortality rates. The survey did not question surgeons regarding complications. After adjustment for separate analysis of the most important variables, it was found that no 2 surgeons were in agreement regarding the manner in which the procedure is performed.

Conclusions.—Femoropopliteal bypass has been considered a benchmark procedure that is relatively straightforward and consistently performed by most vascular surgeons. However, these findings contradict this view. The variation in practice identified in this survey may explain the discrepancy in the reported patency rates for femoropopliteal bypass.

▶ The members of the Florida Vascular Society (FVS) have demonstrated that there are many ways to skin a cat. Unfortunately, they are also unaware of exactly how well the cat is skinned, in that only 13% know their patency rates for femoropopliteal bypass. I attended one of the FVS meetings and am convinced the members are both responsible and competent. Being unaware of patency rates, I believe, reflects realties of what there is time to do in vascular practice in the managed care paperwork world we live in.

G. L. Moneta, MD

Usefulness of Autogenous Bypass Grafts Originating Distal to the Groin

Reed AB, Conte MS, Belkin M, et al (Brigham and Women's Hosp, Boston)
J Vasc Surg 35:48-55, 2002   10–12

Background.—When the amount of autogenous vein available for infrainguinal arterial reconstruction is limited, bypass grafts originating distal to the common femoral are useful for certain patients with critical limb ischemia. These distal origin grafts (DOGs) may also reduce the morbidity of surgery and the time required for recovery. The performance of DOGs over the past 20 years was assessed, with special attention to comparisons between patients with and without diabetes mellitus.

Methods.—A computerized registry provided the data for a retrospective review of consecutive autogenous DOG procedures done from 1978 to 2000. None of the procedures was a revision of an earlier infrainguinal bypass grafting procedure or was performed for popliteal aneurysm.

Results.—A total of 249 autogenous DOG procedures (217 patients) were performed, with 159 of them in patients with diabetes mellitus. Patients with diabetes mellitus tended to be significantly older than those without and were more likely to have hypertension, previous coronary artery bypass grafts, congestive heart failure, and chronic renal disease than those without. The most commonly used conduit was the nonreversed greater saphenous vein. Postoperative morbidity occurred in 24% (61 procedures), with major morbid events being myocardial infarction, renal failure, or pulmonary failure (22 procedures). Operative mortality was 2.0%. Complete follow-up was achieved for 92% of patients in a mean of 27 months. The cumulative primary graft patency rate was 62% at 5 years, 73% for those with diabetes and 45% for those without diabetes. Limb salvage rates were 79% overall, 84% for those with diabetes and 69% for those without diabetes. Overall, the patient survival rate was 45% for those both with or without diabetes.

Conclusions.—The use of the DOG procedure is most appropriate among patients with diabetes mellitus, who can expect good long-term results even in the presence of renal failure. Patients without diabetes mellitus undergoing this procedure should be chosen carefully as results are marginal in terms of long-term graft patency.

▶ To me, one of the basic principles of infrainguinal grafting is to use the best vein available and keep the graft as short as possible. In this article examining the fate of grafts originating distal to the femoral artery, only rarely did a significant stenosis in the superficial femoral artery develop above the distal origin grafts. The authors apparently did not use the profunda femoris artery as an inflow source. This is a vessel frequently used on our service. It is often relatively less diseased than either the common femoral or femoral artery, and it often allows proximal anastomosis to be performed to a thin-walled vessel rather than the more thickly walled common femoral or superficial femoral artery.

G. L. Moneta, MD

Long-term Assessment of Cryopreserved Vein Bypass Grafting Success

Harris L, O'Brien-Irr M, Ricotta JJ (State Univ of New York, Buffalo; State Univ of New York, Stony Brook)
J Vasc Surg 33:528-532, 2001   10–13

Purpose.—When autogenous vein is unavailable, cryopreserved veins have been used in patients as a means of attempted limb salvage. We evaluated the long-term patency and limb salvage rates for patients undergoing bypass grafting with cryopreserved veins.

Methods.—Medical records were reviewed for patients undergoing cryovein bypass grafting at 2 hospitals from 1992 to 1997. Follow-up data were obtained from subsequent admissions and office records. Primary outcomes were death, amputation, and primary patency. Skin integrity and additional bypass grafting procedures were assessed when data were available. Analysis was performed by means of life-table and χ^2 analyses with the Statistical Package for Social Sciences (SPSS).

Results.—Seventy-six patients (mean age, 70 ± 11 years) underwent 80 procedures. Indications for surgery were tissue loss (63%), rest pain (24%), acute ischemia (11%), and other (2%). Early complications included 3 deaths (4%), 14 acute thromboses (18%), and 7 major amputations (9%). The mean follow-up period was 17.8 ± 20.89 months (range, 0-77 months). The primary patency rate was determined to be 36.8% at 1 year and 23.6% at 3 years by means of life-table analysis. The limb salvage rate was 65.5% at 1 year and 62.3% at 3 years. Skin integrity was found to be compromised in 17 (55%) of 31 patients who were available to follow-up. Nine patients (11.3%) underwent additional ipsilateral revascularization or revisions, with 1 of 3 of these patients eventually requiring a major amputation.

Conclusion.—Cryopreserved vein may be a reasonable alternative conduit for limb salvage when no autogenous tissue is available; it has an acceptable limb salvage rate (62.3%) at 3 years. Long-term patency remains relatively poor, with only 23.6% of originally placed grafts patent at 3 years. The use of cryopreserved veins should be strictly confined to limb salvage after a thorough search for autogenous tissue has been exhausted.

▶ This article documents the long-term outcomes of infrainguinal grafting with the use of a cryopreserved vein in a series of 67 patients (80 procedures). Not surprisingly, the results remain dismal, with patency rates of 37% at 1 year and 24% at 3 years. Given the improved results that have been recently noted with prosthetic grafts that feature adjunctive cuffs or patches, combined with anticoagulation, it would appear that cryopreserved allograft conduits have little or no role in lower extremity bypass.

M. S. Conte, MD

Optimal Oral Anticoagulant Intensity to Prevent Secondary Ischemic and Hemorrhagic Events in Patients After Infrainguinal Bypass Graft Surgery

Tangelder MJD, for the Dutch BOA Study Group (Univ Hosp Utrecht, The Netherlands; et al)
J Vasc Surg 33:522-527, 2001

10–14

Background.—How intensive should oral anticoagulant therapy be to prevent fatal ischemia and hemorrhage after infrainguinal bypass surgery? Data from the Dutch Bypass Oral Anticoagulants or Aspirin (BOA) Study were used to determine the optimal international normalized ratio (INR) for oral anticoagulants in this population.

Methods.—The subjects were 1326 patients (65% male; mean age, 69 years) who received oral anticoagulant therapy after infrainguinal bypass graft surgery. The target INR was 3.0 to 4.5, and each patient's INR was measured in 0.5-unit increments to determine the time spent in each INR class. These data (41,928 INR measurements) were plotted to determine the total patient-time spent in each class. Then the rates of fatal ischemia and fatal hemorrhage during 1698 patient-years of follow-up were calculated for each INR class, as the number of events that occurred while a patient was in that INR class divided by the total patient-time spent in that INR class.

Results.—Anticoagulant levels were within the target INR range about half the time; about 40% of the time they were below it, and about 10% of the time they were above it. During follow-up, 121 patients died as the result

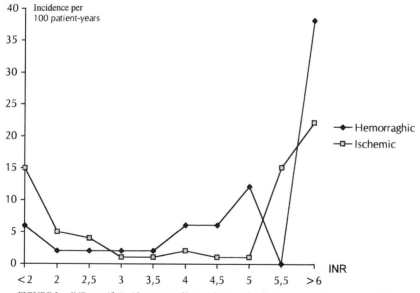

FIGURE 2.—INR-specific incidence rate of hemorrhagic and ischemic events. *Abbreviation: INR*, International normalized ratio. (Courtesy of Tangelder MJD, for the Dutch BOA Study Group. Optimal oral anticoagulant intensity to prevent secondary ischemic and hemorrhagic events in patients after infrainguinal bypass graft surgery. *J Vasc Surg* 33:522-527, 2001.)

of ischemia and 16 died from hemorrhage. The lowest incidence of ischemic and hemorrhagic events occurred at INRs of 3.0 to 4.0 (3.8 events per 100 patient-years) (Fig 2).

Conclusion.—An oral anticoagulant INR of 3.0 to 4.0 is the optimal range for preventing fatal ischemic and hemorrhagic events after infrainguinal bypass graft surgery.

▶ The implication of this study is that the use of warfarin routinely with an INR of 3.0-4.0 is desirable in patients with infrainguinal vein grafts. I disagree. From looking at the figure, one can see that hemorrhagic complications exist at all levels of INR. I would much rather deal with an ischemic leg than an intracranial hemorrhage. I don't think using warfarin routinely provides a favorable risk/benefit ratio for most patients with infrainguinal vein grafts, especially at an INR of greater than 3.0. However, the risk/benefit ratio may shift in patients with multiple failures or identified hypercoagulable states. It is these types of patients in whom we utilize warfarin anticoagulation but generally at an INR of 2.5-3.0.

G. L. Moneta, MD

Reintervention as a Clinical Trial Endpoint After Peripheral Arterial Bypass Surgery

Watson HR, Belcher G, Horrocks M (Univ of Bath, England; Takeda Europe Research and Development Centre, London)
Br J Surg 88:1376-1381, 2001   10–15

Background.—Most studies of peripheral arterial bypass surgery have used graft patency as the main outcome measure. However, the patency rate may not provide a true reflection of clinical outcomes. The 1-year reintervention rate after femorodistal bypass surgery was evaluated in patients from a multicenter trial.

Methods.—The analysis included 517 patients with severe leg ischemia who participated in a prospective study of adjuvant drug therapy in femorodistal bypass surgery. Through 12 months' follow-up, information was collected on symptoms, graft patency, vascular interventions, and clinical outcomes. Follow-up was 96% complete.

Results.—Overall, 239 patients underwent a total of 426 reinterventions within 12 months. In 90% of cases, information on the need for reintervention agreed with the patients' clinical outcome. By comparison, patency rates showed lower rates of agreement with clinical outcomes: 80% with the primary patency rate and 81% with the secondary patency rate. The best overall concordance of end point and clinical outcome was achieved with patients who had no reintervention or were "alive without reintervention" (Fig 3).

Conclusion.—Compared with other technical end points, avoidance of the need for reintervention 12 months after femorodistal bypass for ischemia provides a more accurate picture of the patients' clinical outcomes.

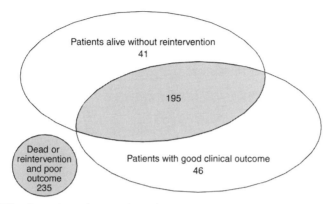

FIGURE 3.—Concordance of "patient alive without reintervention" and clinical outcome at 12 months. *Shading* represents concordance between technical and clinical outcome (517 patients). (Courtesy of Watson HR, Belcher G, Horrocks M: Reintervention as a clinical trial endpoint after peripheral arterial bypass surgery. *Br J Surg* 88:1376-1381, 2001. Reprinted by permission of Blackwell Science, Inc.)

Adding patient survival to this end point further increases its clinical applicability.

▶ If one considers all the undesirable things after bypass surgery (ie, reintervention, need for intervention on the opposite leg, failure of the surgical or pedal wound to heal, failure to regain independent living status, etc), it becomes very clear the current state of the art of bypass surgery, while better than 20 years ago, still has a very long way to go. The large majority of patients never achieve an ideal result of being pain-free, with healed wounds, no amputation, and living and walking independently.

G. L. Moneta, MD

Critical Assessment of the Outcome of Infrainguinal Vein Bypass
Golledge J, Iannos J, Walsh JA, et al (Repatriation Gen Hosp, Daw Park, Adelaide, South Australia)
Ann Surg 234:697-701, 2001   10–16

Background.—Graft patency may provide an unrealistic impression of bypass surgery outcomes. The functional outcome of patients undergoing infrainguinal vein bypass grafting was assessed by documenting freedom from further surgery, hospital admission, and complications.

Methods.—Two hundred thirty-six patients undergoing primary vein grafts during a 6-year period were studied. An ideal outcome was defined as patient survival for 12 months with a patent graft as seen on duplex scanning, no perioperative complications, and no further related open or endovascular surgery or hospital admission.

Findings.—Secondary graft patency at 12 months was 82%. However, only 22% of patients had ideal outcomes. By 1 year, 19% of patients had died, 39% needed further ipsilateral intervention, and 17% needed further

B

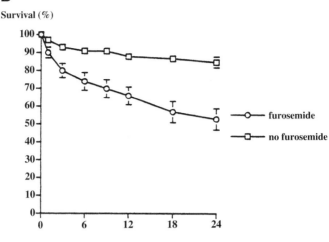

Survival (%)

FIGURE 2.—B, The effect of furosemide on survival rates after infrainguinal vein bypass. *Vertical bars* refer to standard errors. (Courtesy of Golledge J, Iannos J, Walsh JA, et al: Critical assessment of the outcome of infrainguinal vein bypass. *Ann Surg* 234:697-701, 2001.)

contralateral intervention. Forty-six percent of the patients were readmitted to the hospital. Patients receiving calcium channel blockers were more likely to have an ideal outcome, mainly because of improved primary patency. Ideal outcomes were less likely in patients with cardiac failure who needed furosemide, mainly because of these patients' lower survival rate (Fig 2, B).

Conclusions.—Few patients have ideal outcomes after infrainguinal vein bypass. The use of calcium channel blockers may improve outcomes. Clinicians need to carefully consider whether revascularization is appropriate in patients with cardiac failure.

▶ Nearly all vascular surgeons have now done enough lower extremity bypass surgery to understand that patency is not the whole story, nor even the most important part of the story. Patients who need leg bypass for critical limb ischemia are nearing the end of life, and they have all the features of that population. These authors have analyzed the results of 236 bypass grafts and found that ideal and/or good results occurred in half the patients. They looked for factors associated with an ideal result, and their logistic regression spit out only calcium channel blocker use—surely a statistical quirk. I think the central message here is that critical limb ischemia and the need for leg bypass indicate near-term onset of a terminal decline, one which is characterized by multiple hospitalizations, frequent need for repair surgery, and rapidly declining functional status.

L. M. Taylor, Jr, MD

Contemporary Analysis of Outcomes Following Lower Extremity Bypass in Patients With End-Stage Renal Disease

Cox MH, Robison JG, Brothers TE, et al (Med Univ of South Carolina, Charleston)
Ann Vasc Surg 15:374-382, 2001   10–17

Introduction.—The decision on whether to perform infrainguinal bypass or amputation for patients with end-stage renal disease (ESRD) and life-threatening arterial occlusive disease of the lower extremity is difficult, because both options are associated with considerable morbidity and mortality rates. The quality of life for patients with ESRD after infrainguinal bypass was assessed by comparing their outcome with that for patients with normal renal function (NRF) who also underwent infrainguinal bypass.

Methods.—Patients were identified through a computerized registry for the years 1990 through 1999. The study included 63 patients with ESRD who underwent 78 infrainguinal bypasses, and a control group of 132 age-, race-, and sex-matched patients with NRF who underwent 148 bypasses. Primary and secondary patency, limb salvage, and patient survival were calculated using Kaplan-Meier analysis. Markov decision analysis was used to calculate expected quality-adjusted life years (QALY) with intervention.

Results.—The ESRD and NRF groups differed in that diabetes and the presence of tissue necrosis were more prevalent in the ESRD group. The predominant conduit used in both groups was autogenous saphenous vein graft. Primary and cumulative secondary patencies were similar in the 2 groups. Limb salvage at 36 months was 62% for patients with ESRD and 68% for those with NRF, not a statistically significant difference. Five-year survival rate was significantly lower in the ESRD group (55%) than in the NRF group (62%). For all treatment options (nonoperative management, primary amputation, and bypass operation), patients with ESRD had poorer predicted QALY outcomes than patients with NRF. Sensitivity analysis showed, however, that the bypass operation offered greater improvement in QALY than did amputation and nonoperative management. The improvement was over a broad range of operative mortality and limb salvage rates in both ESRD and NRF groups. And in both groups, primary amputation did not appear to be a cost-effective alternative to nonoperative management.

Conclusion.—Results of a Markov decision analysis suggest that bypass is a viable treatment option for patients with ESRD, but the margin of overall benefit may be small, particularly when tissue necrosis is also present. For an individual case, the surgeon's clinical judgment and informed patient choice remain paramount.

▶ This is another article that uses so-called "decision analysis" in an attempt to tell us the consequences of our decisions to proceed with a particular therapeutic option in a particular group of patients. I have never found this type of analysis to be of any use whatsoever when faced with an individual patient. As long as doctors get to be doctors, I find this type of research to be a waste of time. I have a sneaking suspicion the only physicians who read these are people who write these types of papers. They may ultimately prove useful but more properly belong in journals of health care policy or insurance policy. I just don't think practicing physicians find them useful.

G. L. Moneta, MD

Peripheral Artery Occlusion: Treatment With Abciximab Plus Urokinase Versus With Urokinase Alone—A Randomized Pilot Trial (the PROMPT Study)
Duda SH, Tepe G, Luz O, et al (Univ of Tübingen, Germany; Cleveland Clinic Found, Ohio; Eli Lilly and Company, Bad Hamburg, Germany)
Radiology 221:689-696, 2001   10–18

Background.—Previous studies have shown promising results for the glycoprotein IIb/IIIa receptor inhibitor abciximab for the treatment of peripheral arterial occlusion. The Platelet Receptor Antibodies in Order to Manage Peripheral Artery Thrombosis (PROMPT) trial compared the role of abciximab plus urokinase for patients with recent arterial occlusion of the lower extremities.

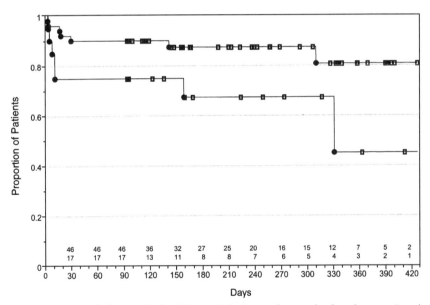

FIGURE 2.—Graph illustrates Kaplan-Meier survival estimates of patients free from the composite end point of surgical revascularization or limb amputation based on treatment with urokinase plus abciximab (*upper line*) or urokinase alone (*lower line*). Circles = time points where clinical events occurred; *squares* = time points where patients were censored. The respective numbers of patients at risk are above the x-axis: the numbers on the top represent the urokinase-plus-abciximab group, and the numbers on the bottom represent the urokinase-alone group. (Courtesy of Duda SH, Tepe G, Luz O, et al: Peripheral artery occlusion: Treatment with abciximab plus urokinase versus with urokinase alone—a randomized pilot trial (the PROMPT Study]. *Radiology* 221:689-696, 2001. Radiological Society of North America.)

Methods.—The randomized pilot trial included 70 patients who had developed occlusion of the arteries of the lower extremity within 6 weeks previously. They were assigned to receive urokinase plus either abciximab (n = 50) or placebo (n = 20). The major complication rate was assessed at 30 days; amputation-free survival was assessed at 90 days. Digital subtraction angiograms were read without knowledge of the patients' assigned treatment group.

Results.—Patients receiving urokinase plus abciximab had a faster thrombolysis time, relative to the length of the treated clot: odds ratio, 0.52; 95% confidence interval, 0.35 to 0.76. None of the patients died of causes related to the procedure or from intracranial hemorrhage. Nonfatal major hemorrhage, however, occurred in 8% of the urokinase plus abciximab group versus none of the urokinase plus placebo group. Ninety-day amputation-free survival rates were significantly better for the combination group: 96% with urokinase plus abciximab versus 80% with urokinase plus placebo (Fig 2). The corresponding hazard ratio was 0.42, 95% confidence interval, 0.16 to 0.96.

Conclusions.—The addition of abciximab to urokinase for thrombolysis appears to improve outcomes for patients with recent lower-extremity arterial occlusion. The combination approach yields shorter thrombus dissolution times and better amputation-free survival rates. The risk of major hemorrhage, however, appears higher than with urokinase alone.

▶ The IIb/IIIa inhibitors are widely used in conjunction with coronary artery angioplasty and stent procedures. In this study, IIb/IIIa inhibitors marginally improved the outcome of patients treated with lytic therapy for acute limb ischemia. Both the IIb/IIIa and placebo groups, however, had a considerable incidence of adjunctive angioplasty and/or surgery in addition to thrombolytic therapy. There are so many confounding variables that the value of adding a IIb/IIIa inhibitor to lytic therapy cannot really be assessed from a study this size. All we can really conclude is it doesn't hurt much.

G. L. Moneta, MD

Value of POSSUM Physiology Scoring to Assess Outcome After Intra-arterial Thrombolysis for Acute Leg Ischaemia (Short Note)
Neary B, Whitman B, Foy C, et al (Gloucestershire Royal Hosp, Gloucester, England)
Br J Surg 88:1344-1345, 2001   10–19

Background.—The Physiological and Operative Severity Score for the enUmeration of Morbidity and mortality (POSSUM) scoring system was developed to predict outcome for surgical patients. The 14-variable physiology component of the POSSUM score was assessed for its ability to predict the outcomes of patients undergoing intra-arterial thrombolysis for acute lower-extremity ischemia.

Methods.—The analysis included 100 patients (53 men, 47 women; median age, 72 years) who underwent 121 attempts at intra-arterial thrombolysis for acute critical leg ischemia. The data were collected prospectively as part of a UK audit of thrombolysis for acute leg ischemia. For each patient, the POSSUM physiology score was calculated retrospectively and correlated with mortality outcomes.

Findings.—The initial results were rated as complete lysis in 40% of cases, partial lysis in 23%, lysis without runoff in 17%, and no lysis in 20%. At 30 days, 70% of patients had successful limb salvage, 7% had undergone amputation, and 22% had died. The POSSUM physiology score significantly predicted each patient's mortality. None of 44 patients in the lowest POSSUM risk category died, compared with 7 of 8 in the highest category.

Conclusions.—The POSSUM physiology score is useful in predicting the risk of death for patients undergoing attempted intra-arterial thrombolysis for acute leg ischemia. This score could provide useful information for pre-treatment counseling of patients being considered for this high-risk, nonsurgical intervention.

▶ The authors have shown that they can use a standardized measure of risk assessment to predict death associated with lytic therapy. The authors indicate the high death rate in their population may have been due to inclusion of high-risk patients. I find the value of risk scoring systems like POSSUM to be primarily in quantitatively comparing patients in different series from different institutions. I think most surgeons are reasonably proficient in recognizing a high-risk patient in their office—even without a risk score stamped on their forehead.

G. L. Moneta, MD

Intermittent Claudication: Cost-Effectiveness of Revascularization Versus Exercise Therapy

de Vries SO, Visser K, de Vries JA, et al (Univ of Groningen, The Netherlands; Tufts Univ, Boston; Harvard Med School, Boston; et al)
Radiology 222:25-36, 2002   10–20

Background.—Exercise is generally considered an inexpensive, effective method of improving claudication symptoms. Many clinicians recommend it as the initial treatment. However, individual responses to exercise vary greatly. Long-term compliance has been reported to be as low as 65%. Furthermore, the time spent exercising represents a cost that has not been previously considered. The costs, efficacy, and cost effectiveness of alternative treatments for intermittent claudication were compared.

Methods.—Data from the literature and original patient data were combined to develop a Markov decision model to assess societal cost effectiveness. Patients had previously untreated intermittent claudication. Treatment options were exercise; percutaneous transluminal angioplasty with stent placement, when necessary; and/or bypass surgery. Treatment strategies were defined as the initial treatment combined with secondary therapeutic options if the initial approach failed.

Findings.—Compared with exercise, revascularization, either with angioplasty or bypass surgery, improved efficacy by 33 to 61 quality-adjusted life days among patients with no history of coronary artery disease. Compared with exercise alone, angioplasty (when feasible) was associated with an incremental cost-efficacy ratio of $38,000 per quality-adjusted life year gained. With additional bypass surgery, this value was $311,000. Incremental cost-effectiveness ratios were sensitive to age, history of coronary artery disease, estimated health values for no or mild claudication compared with severe disease, and the cost of revascularization.

Conclusion.—On average, the expected gain in efficacy obtained with bypass surgery for intermittent claudication appears to be minor compared with the costs. Angioplasty, when feasible, is more effective than exercise alone, with a cost-effectiveness ratio within the accepted range.

▶ I have grown so weary of Markov decision models and QALYs I don't think it is possible for me to be objective anymore. I present this article as it seems well done, and somebody somewhere might be interested.

G. L. Moneta, MD

Comparison of the Long-term Results Between Surgical and Conservative Treatment in Patients With Intermittent Claudication
Mori E, Komori K, Kume M, et al (Kyushu Univ, Fukuoka, Japan)
Surgery 131:S269-S274, 2002
10–21

Background.—Therapy for intermittent claudication is controversial because its natural history is generally benign and it is not a limb-threatening condition. The goal of therapy for claudication is to relieve symptoms and improve the patient's quality of life. The effectiveness of surgical and conservative therapies in attaining these objectives was compared.

Methods.—The study group comprised 427 patients who were admitted with intermittent claudication from January 1984 to December 1999. The patients were separated into 2 groups, with 259 patients (362 legs) treated surgically and 168 patients treated conservatively.

Results.—The surgery group showed a significantly better rate of improvement in the above-the-knee regions compared with the conservative group. However, in the below-the-knee area, there were no significant differences between the 2 groups. For the surgically treated patients, the 3- and 5-year patency rates were satisfactory for arterial reconstruction in the above-the-knee regions, but patency rates were not good below the knee, even when an auto vein was used.

Conclusions.—In patients with intermittent claudication, aggressive surgical management is recommended for those whose distal anastomotic region is above the knee. However, conservative treatment may be as effective as surgery in patients whose distal anastomotic region is below the knee.

▶ More and more, the traditional action that one should, if at all possible, avoid procedures for claudication is being challenged. Treatment for basically a benign disease must, however, have minimal complications. (In recent years, I have taken to offering patients with claudication angioplasty of favorable common iliac artery lesions.) The details of this article are important and I believe suggest that if you choose to perform above-knee popliteal bypass for claudication, an autogenous graft is preferred. The 5-year patency of an autogenous above-knee vein graft in this series was 85.7% versus 64% for an above-the-knee prosthetic graft. When operating for claudication, you certainly want everything to be as optimal as possible. I also suggest prior to performing this operation that the patients undergo preoperative vein mapping and only undergo operation if they have an excellent potential conduit.

G. L. Moneta, MD

Lower Extremity Nontraumatic Amputation Among Veterans With Peripheral Arterial Disease: Is Race an Independent Factor?
Collins TC, Johnson M, Henderson W, et al (Houston VA Med Ctr; Baylor College of Medicine, Houston)
Med Care s40:I106-I116, 2002   10–22

Background.—More black patients undergo amputation than white patients, and more Hispanic patients than black patients have lower-extremity amputations resulting from diabetes, a major risk factor for amputation that can coexist with peripheral arterial disease (PAD). With respect to the patient's race or ethnicity, the number of lower-extremity nontraumatic amputations was compared with the number of lower-extremity bypass revascularizations for patients with PAD.

Methods.—Data were taken from the National VA Surgical Quality Improvement Program (NSQIP) and the Veterans Affairs Patient Treatment File (PTF). Patients were classified into 3 groups: non-Hispanic white, black, and Hispanic. Bivariate analysis was performed, and a multiple logistic regression model was used to assess those factors that independently predicted lower-extremity amputation compared with those predicting lower-extremity bypass.

Results.—Of 11,494 outcome cases identified, 3085 (26.8%) were amputations of the lower extremity and 8409 (73.2%) were bypass revascularizations. Of the patients undergoing revascularization, 3.1% were Hispanic, 28.9% black, and 66.2% non-Hispanic white. Of those having amputations, 48.4% were aged 70 years or more. Patients who had amputations were more likely to present a history of impaired sensorium, previous revascularization or amputation, congestive heart failure, MI, diabetes that required insulin, renal failure requiring dialysis, open wound infection, and rest pain. In addition to 14 preoperative atherosclerotic-related variables that independently predicted amputation versus revascularization, black patients were 1.5 times more likely to have amputation than non-Hispanic white patients, and Hispanic patients were 1.4 times more likely than non-Hispanic white patients to have amputation.

Conclusions.—Within the population of Veterans Administration hospitals, patients who are non-Hispanic whites have a much lower risk for lower-extremity nontraumatic amputation than those who are black or Hispanic. An independent association with lower-extremity nontraumatic amputation was found for both black race and Hispanic ethnic background. The increased rate of atherosclerotic risk factors in black and Hispanic patients does not account for the increased risk faced by these racial or ethnic groups of undergoing amputation rather than bypass revascularization for advanced PAD.

▶ Those who believe risk of amputation is solely tied to definable medical risk factors are living in a dream world. Social factors can play a huge role in treatment outcomes of many conditions, and there is no reason PAD should be any different. Acknowledging there is a problem is the first step to solving it.

G. L. Moneta, MD

Limb Salvage Using High-Pressure Intermittent Compression Arterial Assist Device in Cases Unsuitable for Surgical Revascularization
van Bemmelen PS, Gitlitz DB, Faruqi RM, et al (VA Med Ctr, Northport, NY; State Univ of New York at Stony Brook)
Arch Surg 136:1280-1285, 2001   10–23

Background.—Previous studies have suggested that intermittent compression therapy may be of value for patients with chronic critical ischemia that is not correctable by surgery. An experience with this technique in 14 ischemic lower extremities was reported.

Methods.—The experience included 13 patients treated over a 2½-year period at a Veterans Affairs hospital. All legs had critical ischemia that was not amenable to surgical reconstruction; 14 legs had rest pain and 13 had tissue loss. The patients' mean age was 76 years, and 8 of the 13 were diabetic. Revascularization was considered impossible because of lack of outflow arteries in 7 patients, lack of autogenous vein in 5, and poor medical condition in 3. Patients were provided with an arterial assist device and instructed to use it at home 4 h/d for 3 months. Outcomes included limb salvage rate and calibrated pulse volume amplitude.

Results.—At the end of the 3-month protocol, pulse volume amplitude was significantly increased in 9 of the 14 legs. All 9 legs were salvaged. In contrast, 4 legs required amputation, and none of these showed hemodynamic improvement on compression therapy. Patient compliance had a major impact on the success of therapy. The mean time of compression device use—measured objectively by a built-in counter—was 2.38 h/d in patients with successful limb salvage, compared with 1.14 h/d in those whose limbs were amputated.

Conclusion.—For patients with critical ischemia who are not candidates for surgery, intermittent compression therapy can improve limb hemodynamics and improve the limb salvage rate. The authors call for further studies to evaluate the use of high-pressure intermittent compression for patients with limb-threatening ischemia.

▶ Occasionally, those on the fringes may stumble onto something. There is a body of literature that, taken as a whole, suggests intermittent compression therapy may be useful in patients with lower extremity arterial insufficiency. I would be interested to see if the company that makes this device has the courage to sponsor a randomized trial of this device in a series of patients with chronic limb ischemia. The whole thing looks promising, but I fear it will remain on the fringes until more patients are evaluated in multiple centers by authors lacking financial ties to the company.

G. L. Moneta, MD

Reversal of Angiogenic Growth Factor Upregulation by Revascularization of Lower Limb Ischemia

Porcu P, Emanueli C, Kapatsoris M, et al (Med Univ of Sassari, Italy; Natl Inst of Biostructures and Biosystems, Osilo, Italy; Med Univ of South Carolina, Charleston)
Circulation 105:67-72, 2002   10–24

Background.—Angiogenic molecules have been proposed for the promotion of reparative collateral growth and acceleration of tissue healing in patients with arterial ischemia. Such an approach should overcome the impaired expression of endogenous angiogenic factors that limits spontaneous reparative response to ischemia that is caused by atherosclerosis-induced vascular obstruction. Tissue kallikrein (tK) and vascular endothelial growth factor (VEGF) are potent angiogenic agents, and the upregulation of these agents has been documented in animal models of acute ischemia. However, it is not known whether these angiogenic agents are overexpressed in human beings with chronic peripheral vascular insufficiency. The question of whether circulating levels of tK and VEGF are modulated by chronic limb ischemia and are correlated with the severity of disease was evaluated.

Methods.—The study group comprised 36 patients with symptomatic peripheral vascular disease before and after surgical revascularization. Circulating tK and VEGF were measured in these patients. In 6 patients who had no symptoms at rest, tK was assayed after an exercise stress test.

Results.—In all patients, VEGF levels were within the normal range and were unchanged after revascularization (Table 2). However, tK expression was upregulated in 34 of the 36 patients, and there was no further increase after exercise. A positive correlation was found between tK levels in the venous effluent of ischemic limbs and the number of angiographically recog-

TABLE 2.—Growth Factor Levels Before and After Revascularization

		Before		After	
		tK	VEGF	tK	VEGF
Hypertension	+	856±215	91±19	308±85*	94±31
	−	1278±523	99±22	550±229*	99±21
Diabetes mellitus	+	830±219	96±18	409±133*	93±37
	−	1129±377	97±15	413±167*	98±16
Hypercholesterolemia	+	945±178	76±18	229±48*	81±15
	−	1234±458	109±29	666±201*	118±33

Note: Values are mean ± SEM (pg/mL). Patients were grouped according to presence (+) or absence (−) of each single risk factor indicated in the raw. Hypertension, diabetes, and hypercholesterolemia were diagnosed in 20, 8, and 15 of the 36 patients, respectively.
*$P < .05$ before revascularization.
(Courtesy of Porcu P, Emanueli C, Kapatsoris M, et al: Reversal of angiogenic growth factor upregulation by revascularization of lower limb ischemia. *Circulation* 105:67-72, 2002.)

nizable collateral vessels. Follow-up studies showed a reversal of upregulation of tK after revascularization, whereas no change was observed in venous samples from untouched legs.

Conclusions.—The induction of tK could indicate a compensatory response to chronic arterial insufficiency with the goal of maintaining adequate tissue perfusion. Growth factors may have important roles in reparative and therapeutic angiogenesis associated with chronic lower extremity ischemia.

▶ Tissue kallikrein (tK) is a vasodilator and appears to have a role in angiogenesis. In this study, tK was found to be upregulated in patients with symptomatic peripheral vascular disease, and this upregulation was reversed with revascularization. The implications are that specific growth factors may be able to be targeted for delivery via gene therapy in patients with chronic limb ischemia. Obviously, many details remain to be worked out, such as potential toxicities and appropriate doses and methods of delivery, as well as perhaps identifying additional growth factors that may also be required. In addition, of course, the relative proportions of each and when to deliver them will need to be determined.

G. L. Moneta, MD

Indications for Directed Thrombolysis or New Bypass in Treatment of Occlusion of Lower Extremity Arterial Bypass Reconstruction
Schwierz T, Gschwendtner M, Havlicek W, et al (Elisabethinen Hosp Linz, Austria)
Ann Vasc Surg 15:644-652, 2001   10–25

Introduction.—When broad indications are used to treat bypass graft thromboses with thrombolysis, the long-term outcomes are overall discouraging. The literature does not offer a satisfactory answer regarding the conditions under which directed thrombolysis can be expected to provide good versus poor long-term results. Criteria for determining the indications for bypass thrombolysis or the insertion of a new bypass were presented.

Methods.—Between 1988 and 1997, thrombolysis for bypass graft thrombosis was performed in 82 infrainguinal reconstructions. The secondary cumulative patency was compared retrospectively with that of 143 patients who had occluded infrainguinal bypasses that were replaced by new bypass grafts between 1973 and 1998. Multivariate analysis was used to determine the influence of prognostic factors on secondary long-term patency.

Results.—Complete recanalization of the occluded bypass was accomplished by thrombolysis in 59 patients (72%). In 7 patients (8.5%), residual thrombi remained and were removed by additional thrombectomy after restoration of antegrade flow in the bypass. In 16 patients (19.5%), there was no recanalization or the treatment had to be interrupted early because of complications. Life-table analysis for all 82 patients from the time of thrombolysis on showed a total mean secondary cumulative patency rate of 57.1% after 1 month, 31.6% after 1 year, and 27.2% after 3 years. For the 143 patients who underwent bypass replacement, the total mean secondary cumulative patency rate was 83.9% after 1 month, 69.5% after 1 year, 54.4% after 3 years, and 43.5% after 5 years (Fig 1). There were 2 primary prognostic factors: bypass age of at least 11 months, and duration of occlusion of 3 days or less. If both primary prognostic factors were present, along with the 2 secondary prognostic factors (corrective operation, good runoff), the secondary 3-year patency rate was 77.8%. If the 2 primary prognostic factors were present but only 1 or neither secondary prognostic factor was present, the maximal secondary 3-year patency rate, depending on the factor combination, was 31.8%. When only 1 or neither primary prognostic factor was present, the secondary cumulative 3-year patency rate was 13.2% ($P <$ .004). The 3-year patency rate was 77.7% with autologous (nonreversed) veins, and 65.8% with umbilical veins. The long-term outcomes for polytet-

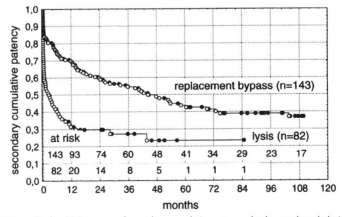

FIGURE 1.—Kaplan-Meier curves of secondary cumulative patency after bypass thrombolysis (n = 82) and replacement bypass (n = 143) in total patient population (broad indications). (Courtesy of Schwierz T, Gschwendtner M, Havlicek W, et al: Indications for directed thrombolysis or new bypass in treatment of occlusion of lower extremity arterial bypass reconstruction. *Ann Vasc Surg* 15:644-652, 2001.)

rafluoroethylene (PTFE) grafts and PTFE-vein composite bypass were significantly poorer.

Conclusion.—Brief graft occlusions (≤3 days) in older bypass grafts (≥11 months) should be treated via thrombolysis. In all other circumstances, the bypass should be replaced with autologous vein. In the absence of autologous vein, umbilical vein is suitable for vessel replacement. With the use of specific indications, the outcome after thrombolytic therapy can be improved, the failure rate can be decreased, and the cost can be reduced.

▶ The authors' conclusion that thrombolysis of an older bypass graft may be amenable to treatment with lytic agents is not new. We prefer to treat vein graft thromboses with a new vein graft, but we will occasionally use lytic therapy in a patient with limited available autogenous conduit to treat thrombosis of a graft placed more than 1 year previously. Thrombolysis and surgical repair of any underlying lesion probably followed by anticoagulation would be our choice, rather than prosthetic grafting, in such patients.

G. L. Moneta, MD

Tibioperoneal (Outflow Lesion) Angioplasty Can Be Used as Primary Treatment in 235 Patients With Critical Limb Ischemia: Five-Year Follow-up
Dorros G, Jaff MR, Dorros AM, et al (William Dorros-Isadore Feuer Interventional Cardiovascular Disease Found Ltd, Grafton, Wis; Heart and Vascular Inst, Morristown, NY; St Luke's Med Ctr, Milwaukee, Wis)
Circulation 104:2057-2062, 2001   10–26

Background.—Because of the need for revascularization of inflow lesions and the questionable success of emergency surgery, angioplasty of the tibioperoneal vessels has generally not been used as a primary revascularization strategy for critical limb ischemia (CLI). However, the need for emergency surgery after tibioperoneal vessel angioplasty (TPVA) seems to be overstated. Data on patients with CLI were analyzed to determine the immediate and longer term outcomes of TPVA.

Methods and Findings.—Two hundred eighty-four consecutively treated critically ischemic limbs were included in the analysis. Clinical success was defined as relief of rest pain or improvement of lower extremity blood flow. TPVA was successful in 95%. One hundred sixty-seven limbs required dilation of 333 ipsilateral inflow obstructions to access and successfully dilate 486 of 529 (92%) tibioperoneal lesions. Two hundred fifteen of the 221 successfully treated patients were followed up clinically for 5 years. Bypass surgery was performed in 8%, and significant amputations were performed in 9% of limbs during follow-up. Ninety-one percent of the limbs were salvaged. Overall, the probability of survival was 56%–58% for Fontaine class III patients and 33% for class IV patients. Compared with class IV patients, those in class III had significantly fewer surgical bypasses and amputations.

Conclusions.—These data show that TPVA, often combined with inflow lesions, is effective in the primary treatment of CLI. The low cumulative survival rate is an indication of severe comorbidities, which may be ameliorated by aggressive cardiovascular diagnostic and treatment strategies.

▶ This article is included as a yardstick of how not to do clinical research. Clearly it is possible to dilate almost anything, and the authors apparently will do just that. No objective measure of ischemia is presented in the data. To not perform ankle-brachial indexes or waveform analysis because the patients have "obvious advanced ischemic disease" is ridiculous. We all know it can be difficult to distinguish ischemia from neuropathy; many ulcerated lesions heal with conservative therapy, and many toe amputations can heal without proximal revascularization. The authors present no data on how the treated sites fared over time. It is reasonable to expect the tibial-treated sides to do worse than superficial femoral artery lesions, which only have a 60% success rate at 2 years, at best. If the tibial arteries fared worse than this, the minimal need for late amputation in these patients in this study suggests many patients probably did not need to be treated in the first place.

G. L. Moneta, MD

11 Upper Extremity Vascular and Hemoaccess

Vascular Access Use in Europe and the United States: Results From the DOPPS

Pisoni RL, Young EW, Dykstra DM, et al (Univ of Michigan, Ann Arbor; Lister Hosp, Stevenage, England; Augusta-Kranken-Anstalt, Bochum, Germany; et al)
Kidney Int 61:305-316, 2002   11–1

Introduction.—Case series reports suggest that vascular access practices vary significantly between Europe and the United States, but a direct broad-based comparison of vascular access use in Europe and the United States has never been made. Data were used from the Dialysis Outcomes and Practice Patterns Study (DOPPS) with the same data collection protocol for more than 6400 patients on hemodialysis (HD) to compare vascular access use at 145 US dialysis units and 101 units in 5 European countries (France, Germany, Italy, Spain, and the United Kingdom).

Methods.—The factors related to the use of native arteriovenous fistula (AVF) versus graft or permanent venous catheters for HD were analyzed. Time to failure for AVF and grafts were evaluated.

Results.—An AVF was used by 80% and 24% of European and US prevalent patients (Fig 1), respectively. The use of an AVF was significantly correlated with younger age, male sex, lower body mass index, nondiabetic status, lack of peripheral vascular disease, and no angina. After adjusting for these factors, the use of AVF versus graft still remained higher in Europe than in the United States ($P < .0001$). The use of AVF ranged within facilities in the United States from 0 to 87% (median, 21%) and in Europe, from 39% to 100% (median, 83%). In patients new to HD, AVF access was 66% in Europe versus 15% in the United States ($P < .0001$), catheter access was 31% in Europe versus 60% in the United States, and graft access was 2% in Europe versus 24% in the United States. Twenty-five percent of European and 46% of US incident patients did not have a permanent access placed before initiation of HD. In Europe, 84% of new patients on HD had seen a nephrologist

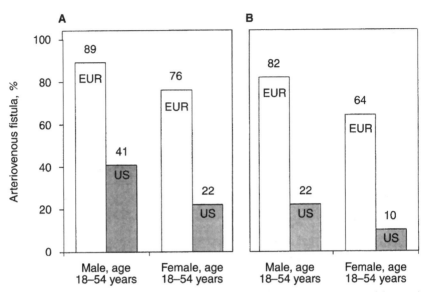

FIGURE 1.—Arteriovenous fistula (AVF) use among prevalent patients in Europe (EUR) and the United States (US) for patient group (A) without diabetes, peripheral vascular disease (PVD), and coronary artery disease (CAD). B, Patients with diabetes, PVD, and/or CAD. The percent of patients using an AVF at the time of study enrollment in a cross-sectional sample of patients was determined for the two subgroups shown. (Courtesy of Pisoni RL, Young EW, Dykstra DM, et al: Vascular access in Europe and the United States: Results from the DOPPS. *Kidney Int* 61:305-316, 2002. Reprinted by permission of Blackwell Science, Inc.)

for more than 30 days before end stage renal disease (ESRD) in contrast to 74% of US patients ($P < .0001$). Pre-ESRD care was correlated with increased odds of AVF versus graft use ($P = .01$). A 1.8-fold greater odds ($P = .002$) was calculated for a patient starting HD with a permanent access if a facility's usual time from referral to access placement was 2 weeks or less. The rate of AVF use was significantly lower ($P = .04$) when surgical trainees assessed or performed access placements. When AVF was the first access, the survival of AVF was superior to grafts in time-to-first failure ($P = .0002$); AVF survival was longer in Europe than in the United States ($P = .0005$). Both AVFs and grafts had better survival if used when initiating HD versus being used after patients began catheter dialysis.

Conclusion.—Large differences were observed in vascular access use between Europe and the United States, even after adjusting for patient characteristics. A facility's preferences and approaches to vascular access practice are important determinants of vascular access use.

▶ The data indicate that US surgeons are behind European colleagues in providing autogenous vascular access for HD. There are no excuses for this. Nephrologists and internists must do a better job in identifying patients for dialysis before actual institution of dialysis and therefore help avoid the temporary use of venous catheters. I wonder how much the commercialization of dialysis in the United States has contributed to our dependence on grafts rather than fistulas? The emphasis on profit in dialysis centers seems to have resulted, in some cases, in less-skilled dialysis technicians, such that many are unable to cannulate anything but enormous autogenous fistulas.

G. L. Moneta, MD

The Transposed Forearm Loop Arteriovenous Fistula: A Valuable Option for Primary Hemodialysis Access in Diabetic Patients
Gefen JY, Fox D, Giangola G, et al (St Luke's-Roosevelt Hosp, New York)
Ann Vasc Surg 16:89-94, 2002   11–2

Introduction.—The Brescia-Cimino fistula has an overall long-term patency rate of nearly 83%; results are lower, however, for patients with diabetes. The early experience with the transposed forearm loop arteriovenous fistula (AVF) (Fig 1), an underused option for autologous hemodialysis access for patients with diabetes is discussed. This approach avoids using forearm arteries, which are often atherosclerotic and inadequate for fistula formation, while still making full use of the forearm veins.

Methods.—Between 1999 and 2001, 16 patients with diabetes and with forearm arteries inadequate for a Brescia-Cimino fistula underwent a transposed forearm loop AVF. All patients underwent preoperative Doppler US vein mapping and examination of the radial and ulnar arteries at the level of the wrist. Nine patients also underwent examination of the brachial artery at the level of the elbow. In all patients, the forearm segment of the basilic or cephalic vein was transposed to create a U-shaped loop and was anastomosed to the brachial, proximal radial, or proximal ulnar artery distal to the antecubital fossa. Functional patency was considered as usability for dialy-

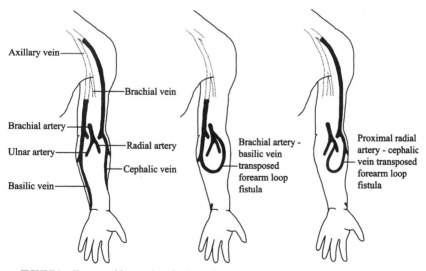

FIGURE 1.—Transposed forearm loop fistula configurations. (Courtesy of Gefen JY, Fox D, Giangola G, et al: The transposed forearm loop arteriovenous fistula: A valuable option for primary hemodialysis access in diabetic patients. *Ann Vasc Surg* 16:89-94, 2002.)

sis. Patency rates were determined by means of Kaplan-Meier survival analysis.

Results.—The median follow-up was 11 months (range, 1-18 months). No perioperative complications or deaths and no ischemic complications or steal syndromes occurred. Six (37%) early failures occurred as a result of thrombosis or failure to mature (2 and 4 patients, respectively). One fistula occluded at 3 months and another at 5 months. The primary patency was 43% at 18 months and overall patency was 62% at 18 months.

Conclusion.—The transposed forearm loop fistula is the primary access procedure of choice for patients with diabetes with significant forearm arterial disease.

▶ This article represents a retrospective analysis of a single hospital group's experience with transposed vein forearm loop fistulae for dialysis access. The article acknowledges the high failure rate of forearm Brescia-Cimino fistulas in patients with diabetes. The authors purport that a transposed forearm loop arteriovenous fistula provides a valuable and durable alternative for dialysis access. The number of patients reported is small and follow-up is limited. The patients who underwent transposed venous fistula were not compared with another age-matched (even retrospectively matched) group of patients undergoing alternative autogenous access procedures. The primary patency reported is comparable to the disappointing patency of prosthetic grafts in the same position, and it is vastly inferior to primary upper arm venous fistulae. I believe there are no data in this article to support its title or conclusions.

M. T. Watkins, MD

Brachial-Jugular Expanded PTFE Grafts for Dialysis

Vega D, Polo JR, Polo J, et al (HGU "Gregorio Marañón", Madrid)
Ann Vasc Surg 15:553-556, 2001   11–3

Introduction.—Only isolated case reports have described the use of jugular veins in vascular access for dialysis. The effectiveness of brachial-jugular grafts for dialysis was analyzed, focusing on the long-term outcome for patients.

Methods.—The study included 51 patients (age, 8 to 72 years; mean, 49 years), 22% of whom had diabetic nephropathy. Expanded, standard-wall polytetrafluoroethylene (ePTFE) grafts were used in all cases, and all surgical procedures were performed under local anesthesia. Data analyzed included patient age, presence of diabetic nephropathy, complications of angioaccess, and therapeutic methods of treating complications. The life-table method was used to analyze primary and secondary patency rates.

Results.—The brachial-jugular anatomical position represented 7% of all grafts during the study period (September 1986 to June 1998). The external jugular vein was used in 21 cases (Fig 3). In the remaining 31 cases, the graft was anastomosed to the internal jugular vein. Thirty-three patients received 6- to 8-mm tapered grafts, and 18 had 6-mm grafts. No early failures oc-

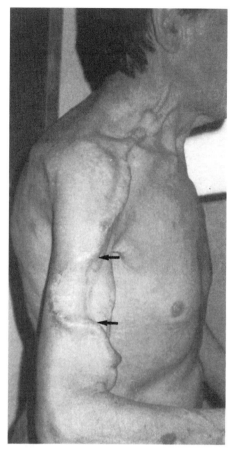

FIGURE 3.—Patient with a brachiojugular graft to the external jugular vein for more than 8 years. A bypass to treat periprostetic infection was performed (*arrows*). (Courtesy of Vega D, Polo JR, Polo J, et al: Brachial-jugular expanded PTFE grafts for dialysis. Ann Vasc Surg 15:553-556, 2001.)

curred. During an overall follow-up time of 1391 graft months, the complication rate was 0.72 episodes per graft year. The most common complication (60 patients) was thrombosis. Primary patency rates (the interval between graft construction and the occurrence of any complication requiring surgical or radiologic therapy) were 57% at 1 year, 43% at 2 years, and 30% at 3 years; secondary patency rates (the interval between graft placement and definitive loss of function because of a nonrecoverable complication) were 74% at 1 year, 63% at 2 years, 59% at 3 years, and 54% at both 4 and 5 years.

Conclusion.—Brachial-jugular grafts can be used as an alternative to other, more complex operations, such as axillofemoral graft or intrathoracic vein bypass for patients with nondilatable axillary or subclavian vein stenosis. Because jugular veins can be the last resort for maintaining an upper-arm graft, dialysis catheters should not be used through the jugular vein route.

▶ I have used this configuration for dialysis access on occasion. These grafts work for awhile but are nothing special.

G. L. Moneta, MD

Prophylaxis of Hemodialysis Graft Thrombosis With Fish Oil: Double-blind, Randomized, Prospective Trial

Schmitz PG, McCloud LK, Reikes ST, et al (St Louis Univ)
J Am Soc Nephrol 13:184-190, 2002   11–4

Background.—Recent studies have indicated that most vascular access grafts in patients with end-stage renal disease (ESRD) experience thrombo-

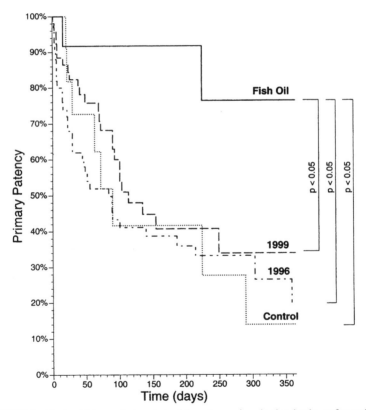

FIGURE 1.—Kaplan–Meier survival analysis of the patency of newly placed polytetrafluoroethylene grafts among cohorts of patients monitored for 1 year before study commencement in 1996 (n = 50) or 1 year after study closure in 1999 (n = 48), compared with control patients (n = 12) and patients who received fish oil (n = 12). (Courtesy of Schmitz PG, McCloud LK, Reikes ST, et al: Prophylaxis of hemodialysis graft thrombosis with fish oil: Double-blind, randomized, prospective trial. *J Am Soc Nephrol* 13:184-190, 2002.)

sis within 1 year of placement, and more than 75% require a salvage procedure to maintain patency. Many strategies have been used to limit the incidence of vascular access thrombosis, including pharmacologic agents, but the relative frequency of side effects and the inconsistent clinical results have dampened enthusiasm for these approaches. In searching for new strategies to prevent dialysis access thrombosis, the need to reduce the cost and morbidity of maintenance dialysis are of paramount concern. The use of diets enriched with omega-3 fatty acids derived from fish oil concentrates represents a novel approach. Such diets might have a beneficial effect on the vascular perturbations that underlie synthetic graft thrombosis. Whether diets enriched with omega-3 fatty acids can decrease the incidence of thrombosis in newly constructed polytetrafluoroethylene grafts was investigated.

Methods.—In a double-blind trial, 24 patients were randomly chosen to receive either 4000 mg of fish oil or 4000 mg of control oil, both enriched with antioxidants and deodorized with peppermint. Patients began therapy within 2 weeks of graft placement and were monitored for 12 months or until thrombosis developed.

Results.—Primary patency at 1 year was 14.9% for the control group and 75.6% for the fish oil–treated group (Fig 1). Survival analysis demonstrated a significant difference between fish oil–treated and untreated patients, with a power of 90%. Analysis of significant covariables confirmed that this effect resulted primarily from the administration of fish oil. This treatment also decreased venous outflow resistance and systemic blood pressure compared with the control group.

Conclusions.—The unique biologic properties of fish oil appear to have a beneficial effect in reducing the incidence of polytetrafluoroethylene graft thrombosis. The use of diets enriched with fish oil is a potential treatment strategy for the prevention of vascular access thrombosis in dialysis patients.

▶ In this small study, the ability of fish oil to prolong patency of hemodialysis grafts was striking. The differences between the treated and untreated patients were perhaps driven as much by the poor patency of the control group at 1 year (15%) versus the excellent patency of the fish oil treated patients (75%) at 1 year. Certainly, however, further investigation should be considered. In the meantime, some consideration should be given to treating your patients on dialysis grafts with fish oil. My partner says fish oil is pretty much good for everything.

G. L. Moneta, MD

Surgical Bypass for Subclavian Vein Occlusion in Hemodialysis Patients
Chandler NM, Mistry BM, Garvin PJ (St Louis Univ)
J Am Coll Surg 194:416-421, 2002   11–5

Introduction.—More than 86% of patients with end-stage renal disease are dependent on hemodialysis. Significant stenosis or occlusion of the subclavian vein occurs in 20% to 50% of patients with central venous catheters in the subclavian or internal jugular veins. An experience with surgical bypass in patients undergoing hemodialysis who also had subclavian vein occlusion was examined retrospectively.

Methods.—All subclavian venous bypass procedures performed between May 1987 and May 2000 were analyzed. Twelve procedures were performed during this period. The mean patient age of 11 males and 1 female was 55.5 years (range, 17-72 years). All patients underwent bilateral venography to assess their central venous systems before undergoing surgical bypass.

Results.—All patients underwent an extra-anatomical surgical bypass procedure. Follow-up was a mean of 16 months (range, 1-79 months). At 1 month, 100% of hemodialysis access sites were functional; at 1 year, 2 years, and 3 years, 80%, 60%, and 25% were functional, respectively. One patient underwent a thrombectomy of the bypass graft at 14 months' follow-up.

Conclusion.—Subclavian vein bypass is an effective and low-risk surgical option with an acceptable patency rate that prolongs the life of a functioning hemodialysis access after complete occlusion or reocclusion.

▶ Many dialysis grafts fail secondary to subclavian vein stenosis or occlusion. When the vein is occluded, subclavian vein bypass appears to significantly extend the life of an ipsilateral hemodialysis access. The procedure is simple but probably best utilized when the subclavian vein is completely occluded. I think most would still prefer an endovascular treatment for a narrow but patent subclavian vein.

G. L. Moneta, MD

Forearm Arteries Entrapment Syndrome: A Rare Cause of Recurrent Angioaccess Thrombosis

Chemla ES, Raynaud A, Mongrédien B, et al (Hôpital Européen Georges Pompidou, Paris; Clinique Labrouste, Paris)
J Vasc Surg 34:743-747, 2001   11–6

Background.—Entrapment syndrome below or just above the elbow is not often reported, and the rare published cases of vascular entrapment syndrome are linked to an anomalous anatomical structure: the ligament of Struthers. The first 2 cases in which entrapment of forearm arteries occurred in patients with angioaccess for hemodialysis are discussed.

> *Case 1.*—Woman, 66, referred for angiography of her vascular access for dialysis, a 9-year-old ulnar-to-basilic artery graft that had required treatment previously (4 times in the past 5 years) for acute thrombosis. Two days before referral, acute thrombosis was successfully treated with local fibrinolysis and manual aspiration thromboembolectomy. Angiography showed the radial artery to be occluded, and the ulnar artery to be occluded in supination, the result of an external compression just below its takeoff. On MRI, the ulnar ar-

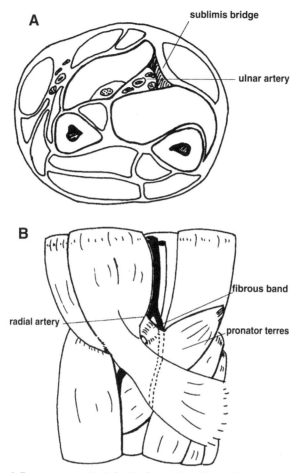

FIGURE 6.—A, Forearm cross section's drawing figuring the sublimis bridge. During supination, the ulnar artery is compressed between both superficialis and profundus flexor digitorum. **B,** Anterior view of forearm, showing fibrosis arcade compressing the radial artery in pronator teres syndrome. (Courtesy of Chemla ES, Raynaud A, Mongrédien B, et al: Forearm arteries entrapment syndrome: A rare cause of recurrent angioaccess thrombosis. *J Vasc Surg* 34:743-747, 2001.)

tery was seen to be compressed in a flexor digitorum fibrosis arcade (a slip connecting the flexor digitorum superficialis and profundus muscles). Because the polytetrafluoroethylene graft had 2 large aneurysms, and no ischemic symptoms were present, angioaccess was ligated, and a new fistula was created at the other forearm.

Case 2.—Man, 69, referred for angiography of his angioaccess for hemodialysis (a 4-year old wrist radio cephalic native fistula) was seen 5 times before for acute thromboses and treated with local fibrinolysis and manual aspiration embolectomy. Previous angiograms could find no causes for occlusion or stenosis. Patient had no ischemic symptoms or pain during dialysis. Angiography with the patient in both the pronated and supinated positions indicated that in the pronated position, the radial and interosseous arteries were normally patent but were occluded in supination by an external compression 2 cm below takeoff of the radial artery. The cause was shown to be pronator teres syndrome (a fibrous band from the pronator teres muscle compressing the radial artery) (Fig 6). After surgery, patency in the supine position was normal, and after a follow-up of 1 year, no new thromboses had occurred.

Discussion.—Upper-limb compression at the thoracic level is often reported, but entrapment at other locations below or just above the elbow is uncommon. Most patients with entrapment syndrome at this level have neurologic symptoms, but in these 2 cases, forearm claudication and neurologic symptoms were absent. Both entrapment syndromes were demonstrated by angioaccess repetitive thromboses. Involvement of an arterial entrapment syndrome should be ruled out in cases of unexplained recurring forearm angioaccess thrombosis.

▶ A decreasing thrill in a forearm angioaccess with supernation of the forearm is a clue to the presence of possible entrapment as a cause of repetitive access failure.

G. L. Moneta, MD

Percutaneous Thrombolysis of Thrombosed Haemodialysis Access Grafts: Comparison of Three Mechanical Devices

Smits HFM, Smits JHM, Wüst AFJ, et al (Univ Med Ctr, Utrecht, The Netherlands)
Nephrol Dial Transplant 17:467-473, 2002   11–7

Background.—Thrombosed hemodialysis access grafts are often treated with mechanical percutaneous thrombolysis. However, few data comparing the effectiveness of different mechanical devices are available. The efficacy of 3 such devices—a rotating brush catheter, a hydrodynamic catheter, and a rotating basket catheter—in removing clots from thrombosed hemodialysis access grafts and in restoring graft patency was examined.

Methods.—The subjects were 55 patients who underwent mechanical thrombolysis for a total of 68 thrombosed hemodialysis access grafts. Patients found to have more than 50% stenosis of the vessel diameter also underwent percutaneous transluminal angioplasty (PTA) immediately after thrombolysis. In 13 cases, the Cragg rotating brush catheter (Cragg Thrombolytic Brush, Micro Therapeutics, San Clemente, Calif) was used, combined with urokinase injection into the thrombosed graft. In 18 cases, the Hydrolyser hydrodynamic catheter (Cordis Europa NV, Roden, The Netherlands) was used. In 37 cases, a rotating basket catheter, the Arrow-Trerotola Percutaneous Thrombolytic Device (PTD) (Arrow International, Reading, Pa.), was used. The efficacy of these 3 devices was evaluated by comparing complete clot removal rates, initial technical success rates, clinical success rates, residual stenosis rates after PTA, complications, and graft patency at 30, 60, and 90 days after the procedure.

Results.—The Cragg brush and the PTD completely or almost completely removed the clot in 92% and 95% of cases, respectively, while complete clot removal was significantly less likely with the Hydrolyser (44% of cases). Otherwise, the Cragg brush, the Hydrolyser, and the PTD did not differ significantly in initial technical success rates (85%, 83%, and 95%, respectively), clinical success rates (62%, 67%, and 86%), or residual stenosis rates after PTA (33%, 46%, and 21%). In the Cragg brush group, there were 1 major complication (8%; the brush broke) and 4 minor complications (31%). In the Hydrolyser group, there were 1 major complication (6%; pulmonary embolism) and 10 minor complications (56%; most commonly hematoma). In the PTD group, there were no major complications but 16 minor complications (43%; most commonly minor bleeding).

The mean graft patency rates with the Cragg brush, the Hydrolyser, and the PTD were similar: 73%, 60%, and 55%, respectively, at 30 days; 61%, 53%, and 49% at 60 days; and 49%, 40%, and 43% at 90 days. Cox's proportional hazards analysis indicated that the only significant determinant of long-term graft patency was residual stenosis after PTA: Each 1% of residual stenosis increased the risk of graft failure by 2.5% per day.

Conclusion.—Clot removal was more complete with the rotation devices than with the hydrodynamic catheter. Clot removal with the PTD was similar to that with the Cragg brush but did not require urokinase injection. Nonetheless, the success of PTA had a greater effect on graft patency than did the type of mechanical thrombolysis device used.

▶ Apparently, it doesn't matter how you get rid of the clot. What matters is improving the venous outflow. This is probably not new news to most of us.

G. L. Moneta, MD

Patency and Life-Spans of Failing Hemodialysis Grafts in Patients Undergoing Repeated Percutaneous De-Clotting

Mansilla AV, Toombs BD, Vaughn WK, et al (Texas Heart Inst, Houston; Univ of Texas, Houston)
Tex Heart Inst J 28:249-253, 2001   11–8

Background.—A steady decline has occurred in the number of hospital admissions related to vascular access for hemodialysis in patients with end-stage renal disease (ESRD), with admissions decreasing 17% from 1994 to 1998. This decline is related in part to the development and improvement of outpatient procedures for the management of hemodialysis access. Many patients with ESRD requiring dialysis are managed with polytetrafluoroethylene arteriovenous (PTFE A-V) grafts. The failure of these grafts as a consequence of thrombosis is a common problem that requires prompt intervention. This retrospective study evaluated the primary and secondary

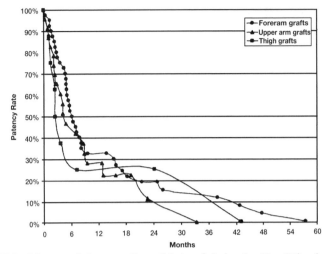

FIGURE 1.—Primary surgical patency of hemodialysis grafts by location. *Note*: SE less than 0.05 at all points. (Courtesy of Mansill AV, Toombs BD, Vaughn WK, et al: Patency and life-spans of failing hemodialysis grafts in patients undergoing repeated percutaneous de-clotting. *Tex Heart Inst J* 28:249-253, 2001.)

patency rates and life spans of failing polytetrafluoroethylene dialysis grafts after repeated percutaneous mechanical declotting.

Methods.—The study group comprised all patients who had undergone percutaneous mechanical declotting, balloon angioplasty, or angiography of their PTFE hemodialysis grafts at a single institution from January 1 through April 30, 1999. Kaplan-Meier analysis was used to calculate the patency of the hemodialysis grafts. There were 161 percutaneous procedures performed on 59 of 71 patients.

Results.—At 1 year, the primary patency rate of the grafts was 29% and the secondary patency rate was 61.4% (Fig 1). The PTFE grafts had lifespans after repeated percutaneous declotting and surgical interventions of 93.5% at 6 months, 78% at 1 year, 58.8% at 2 years, and 35% at 3 years. The patency rates after the first, second, and third declotting procedures were similar (55.9%, 61.9%, and 55.8% at 3 months and 32.2%, 40.8%, and 31.4% at 6 months, respectively) (Fig 4). No statistical difference was noted in the patency rate of grafts after mechanical declotting with use of the Arrow-Trerotola thrombectomy device compared with the crossed angioplasty balloon technique alone. In addition, no difference was noted in the life spans of the grafts whether they were performed in the upper or lower extremity.

Conclusions.—These findings indicate that reocclusion rates are similar after the first, second, and third occlusions, regardless of the percutaneous mechanical declotting technique used. These results indicate that repeated percutaneous management should be used to preserve each graft, regardless of the number of previous declotting procedures.

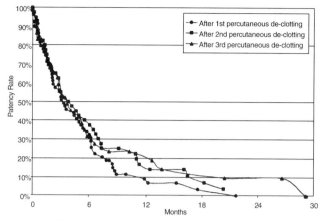

FIGURE 4.—Hemodialysis graft patency following the first, second, and third percutaneous declotting procedures is very similar. Patency was determined for each consecutive declotting procedure and was defined as the period of time the graft remained patent, to the next occlusion event. *Note*: SE less than 0.06, less than 0.07, and less than 0.09 for the first, second, and third declotting procedures, respectively. (Courtesy of Mansill AV, Toombs BD, Vaughn WK, et al: Patency and life-spans of failing hemodialysis grafts in patients undergoing repeated percutaneous de-clotting. *Tex Heart Inst J* 28:249-253, 2001.)

▶ The message here is not to give up when an angioaccess requires multiple percutaneous declottings. Patency rates are similar after 1, 2, or 3 mechanical declottings. (See also Abstract 11–7.)

G. L. Moneta, MD

Impact of Reintervention for Failing Upper-Extremity Arteriovenous Autogenous Access for Hemodialysis
Hingorani A, Ascher E, Kallakuri S, et al (Maimonides Med Ctr, Brooklyn, New York)
J Vasc Surg 34:1004-1009, 2001   11–9

Background.—With the increasing average age of patients requiring hemodialysis for end-stage renal disease, additional upper-arm arteriovenous fistulas (AVFs) will be required, and the number of failing upper-arm AVFs may increase. Few studies, however, have addressed the management of failing AVFs. At the study institution, 75 revisions were performed for 46 patients (49 AVFs). The outcomes of these revisions are discussed.

Methods.—During the period reviewed (between June 1997 and March 2001), 474 AVFs were placed in 380 patients. A standard protocol was used in the original construction of the AVF. The mean age of the patients requiring revision was 68 years; 51% were diabetic and 75% were hypertensive. Twenty of the 46 patients underwent 26 vein patch angioplasties, and 17 underwent 24 balloon angioplasties. Vein interpositions were required in 4 patients, and 12 underwent 12 revisions of the fistula to a more proximal level. When extended salvage procedures were performed, 4 were of turn-downs to the basilic vein for proximal cephalic vein thrombosis or stenosis, and 5

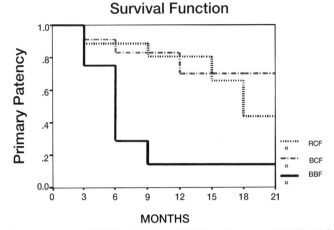

Survival Function

FIGURE 2.—Comparison of RCAVFs, BCAVFs, and BBAVFs. *Abbreviations: RCAVFs,* Radial-cephalic arteriovenous fistulae; *BCAVFs,* brachial-cephalic arteriovenous fistulae; *BBAVFs,* brachial-basilic arteriovenous fistulae. (Courtesy of Hingorani A, Ascher E, Kallakuri S, et al: Impact of reintervention for failing upper-extremity arteriovenous autogenous access for hemodialysis. *J Vasc Surg* 34:1004-1009, 2001.)

were extension bypasses to the axillary or jugular vein for subclavian vein thrombosis. Patients were followed up for patency after revision with duplex US and physical examination.

Results.—After a mean follow-up of 10 months, the patients who had undergone open revision tended to require fewer additional procedures. But by life table analysis, primary patency of the vein patch angioplasty was not significantly better than with balloon angioplasty. No statistically significant difference in patency was noted after revision of a radial cephalic fistula and brachial cephalic fistula (Fig 2). One interposition failed and 1 revision to a more proximal level thrombosed during follow-up. Of the 4 turn-down procedures, 2 thrombosed at 2 and 11 months and 2 were functional at 1 and 24 months. Four of 5 extensions had remained functional at periods ranging from 1 to 8 months, whereas 1 thrombosed at 8 months.

Conclusion.—The cost of maintaining dialysis access in patients with end-stage renal disease is expected to increase significantly in the coming decade. Simple and extended salvage procedures as used in this study may allow maturation and add to the life span of AVFs. Open techniques may have an advantage over percutaneous techniques.

▶ A variety of surgical and percutaneous techniques can be used to salvage an autogenous AVF. Note that this applies only to fistulas that have not thrombosed. While a failing autogenous fistula can be salvaged, the failed fistula is best let go.

G. L. Moneta, MD

Brachial Artery Reconstruction for Occlusive Disease: A 12-Year Experience
Roddy SP, Darling RC III, Chang BB, et al (Albany Med College, NY)
J Vasc Surg 33:802-805, 2001   11–10

Background.—Upper extremity ischemia is rather uncommon, and its pathology differs markedly from that of lower limb ischemia. The clinical characteristics and outcomes of brachial artery reconstruction in patients with symptomatic atherosclerotic occlusive disease of the upper extremity were compared with those of patients undergoing infrainguinal bypass graft surgery during the same 12-year period.

Methods.—From 1986 to 1998, 56 patients with symptomatic atherosclerotic occlusive disease of the upper extremity (group 1) and 3886 patients undergoing infrainguinal bypass graft surgery (group 2) were studied. Exclusion criteria were the presence of embolus, pseudoaneurysm, or trauma at presentation. Patient demographics, clinical characteristics, and outcomes were evaluated.

Results.—The 56 patients in group 1 received 61 bypass grafts; 51 (83%) were performed with autogenous conduit and 10 (17%) were performed with polytetrafluoroethylene. Compared with group 2, patients with upper extremity symptomatic arterial disease were significantly younger (mean age, 58 vs 68 years), significantly more likely to be women (57% vs 36%), and more likely to be smokers (73% vs 36%). Conversely, patients in group 1 were significantly less likely to have diabetes (13% vs 52%). Additionally, 48% of patients in group 1 also had lower extremity occlusive disease; for comparison, only 1.5% of patients in group 2 also required upper extremity revascularization.

Indications for brachial artery bypass graft surgery were arm pain with exertion in 30% of cases, arm pain at rest in 57%, and tissue loss in 13%. There was only 1 postoperative death (of cardiac origin); thus, the 30-day mortality rate was 1.8%. During an average follow-up of 23.3 months, there were 6 early occlusions (10%) and 2 late occlusions (3.3%). All but 1 of these 8 occlusions occurred in women with a smoking history. There were no cases of limb loss. Early and late occlusion rates and 30-day limb loss did not differ significantly between the 2 groups. Life-table analysis indicated a 1-year patency rate of 90.5%. Patency was significantly better for grafts that did not cross a joint (96%) than for grafts that did (80%).

Conclusion.—Revascularization of an occluded brachial artery is safe, with reasonably good 1-year patency rates. Patients who require brachial artery reconstruction for symptomatic atherosclerotic occlusive disease differ significantly from those with ischemia of the lower limbs in that they are more likely to be women, to be smokers, and less likely to have diabetes.

▶ Arm bypass grafts seem to work remarkably well when the indication is a manifestation of atherosclerotic occlusive disease. Based on these data and personal experience, the basic principles are the same as for lower extremity bypass. Use autogenous conduit whenever possible, and keep the grafts as short as possible.

G. L. Moneta, MD

Palmar Hyperhidrosis: Evidence of Genetic Transmission

Ro KM, Cantor RM, Lange KL, et al (Univ of California, Los Angeles)
J Vasc Surg 35:382–386, 2002   11–11

Introduction.—Primary palmar hyperhidrosis is characterized by excessive perspiration. It affects 1% of the Western population. The cause of this condition is unknown, and epidemiologic data are scarce and inadequate. This potentially disabling disorder interferes with social, psychological, and professional activities. Several reports have noted a positive family history for patients with hyperhidrosis. Between September 1993 and July 1999, 58 consecutive patients with palmar, plantar, and axillary hyperhidrosis who were treated with thoracoscopic sympathectomy underwent genetic evaluations in a prospective investigation.

Methods.—Of the 58 probands, 49 volunteered a detailed family history data (response rate, 84%). Study patients and a control group of 20 healthy research subjects completed a standardized questionnaire during the postoperative visit or underwent a telephone interview. The familial aggregation of hyperhidrosis was quantified by an estimate of the recurrence risks to the offspring, parents, siblings, aunts, uncles, and cousins of 49 probands and 20 control subjects. Penetrance was estimated by means of a genetic analysis program.

Results.—Of the 49 probands, 32 (65%) reported a positive family history in the hyperhidrosis group. No family history of hyperhidrosis was reported for anyone in the control group. A recurrence risk of 0.28 in the offspring of probands versus 0.01 in the general population is strong evidence for vertical transmission of this disorder in pedigrees and is further reinforced by the 0.14 risk to the parents of the probands. The disease allele is present in about 5% of the population. One or 2 copies of the allele can result in hyperhidrosis 25% of the time. The normal allele will result in hyperhidrosis less than 1% of the time.

Conclusion.—Primary palmar hyperhidrosis is a hereditary disorder that has variable penetrance and no proof of sex-linked transmission. This does not exclude other possible causes. Genetic verification of this disorder may allow earlier diagnoses and advances in medical and psychosocial interventions.

▶ Treatment of palmar hyperhidrosis is, like neurogenic thoracic outlet syndrome, one of the fringe areas of vascular surgical practice. Most of us know very little about these fringe areas. Because of limitations in data quality and acquisition, which to their credit the authors acknowledged, the exact genetic pattern of this disorder cannot be precisely identified from this study. Nevertheless, it is clear some sort of genetic pattern exists. It appears the disease allele is more common (5%) than I would have thought.

G. L. Moneta, MD

Outcomes After Surgery for Thoracic Outlet Syndrome
Axelrod DA, Proctor MC, Geisser ME, et al (Univ of Michigan, Ann Arbor)
J Vasc Surg 33:1220-1225, 2001   11–12

Background.—Many studies have identified anatomical and physiologic risk factors for disability after surgery for neurogenic thoracic outlet syndrome (N-TOS). The influence of psychological and socioeconomic factors on outcomes after N-TOS surgery was examined.

Methods.—The subjects were 170 patients with N-TOS (40 men and 130 women; mean age, 35.5 years) who underwent thoracic outlet decompression via a supraclavicular approach. Most patients (101, or 59%) underwent preoperative psychological testing, which included an interview by a psychologist experienced in chronic pain evaluation and questionnaires to assess pain and psychological symptoms, including depression and distress. Results of psychological testing, clinical characteristics, and outcome data at a mean of 10.4 months after surgery were extracted from medical records for 98% of the patients. Additionally, 89 patients (52%) completed a questionnaire at an average follow-up of 47 months to assess long-term outcomes, activity level, and overall satisfaction with the surgery.

Results.—No major operative complications occurred, and only 11% of patients experienced minor complications, most commonly the need for chest tube placement as the result of pneumothorax. At short-term follow-up, most patients had improved pain levels (80%), paresthesias (81%), and range of motion (82%). Overall, 67% of the patients were judged to have made good or average progress after surgery. At long-term follow-up, residual symptoms were present in 65% of patients, and 35% took medication for pain. Nonetheless, 64% said they were satisfied with the operation, and 69% said they would undergo the procedure again. Only 18% said they were disabled. Multivariate logistic regression analysis identified 3 preoperative psychosocial variables that were significantly and independently associated with long-term disability: major depression (a Beck Depression Inventory score of more than 21 (odds ratio [OR], 15.7), having a less-than–high school education (OR, 8.1), and not being married (OR, 7.88).

Conclusion.—Brachial plexus decompression improved pain, paresthesias, and range of motion in most of these patients with N-TOS. About two thirds of patients were satisfied with their results at long-term follow-up. Poorer long-term results were significantly associated with preoperative depression, marital status, and education level. Prospective studies are needed to determine whether treatment of depression before thoracic outlet decompression would improve outcomes after T-NOS surgery.

▶ Two questions about neurogenic thoracic outlet syndrome remain unanswered. Is the clinical syndrome (which is very real) caused by compression of the brachial plexus nerves in the thoracic outlet? Is the natural history of the condition altered by surgery? This report in which 170 patients underwent a variety of procedures and were evaluated by a variety of means (some had psychological evaluation, some did not; some had pain/depression scores, some did not; etc) clearly establishes that the authors performed the operations safely. Unfortunately, it answers neither of my 2 questions. Someday, someone is going to figure out a way to prove/disprove the brachial plexus compression theory, and some other day someone else is going to conduct a randomized trial of thoracic outlet surgery. Until then, I will continue to abstain from performing surgery for neurogenic symptoms that can be diagnosed only by subjective means.

L. M. Taylor, Jr, MD

Outcome After Thrombolysis and Selective Thoracic Outlet Decompression for Primary Axillary Vein Thrombosis
Lokanathan R, Salvian AJ, Chen JC, et al (Univ of British Columbia, Vancouver, Canada)
J Vasc Surg 33:783-788, 2001   11–13

Background.—At the authors' center, primary subclavian–axillary vein thrombosis (SAVT) is treated by thrombolysis and anticoagulation for 3 months. A small number of patients have been treated by thoracic outlet decompression. The functional outcomes of this treatment were reviewed.

Methods and Findings.—The medical records of all 28 patients treated for a first episode of SAVT at 1 center in the past 10 years were reviewed. Patients also completed the Disabilities of the Arm, Shoulder, and Hand (DASH) questionnaire developed by the American Academy of Orthopedic Surgeons. The patients were 20 men and 8 women (mean age, 36 years). The median length of time between symptom onset and treatment was 5.5 days. Venography confirmed the diagnosis in all patients. Twenty-five patients

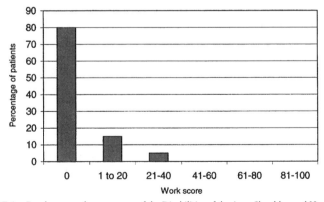

FIGURE 4.—Results on work component of the Disabilities of the Arm, Shoulder, and Hand questionnaire. (Courtesy of Lokanathan R, Salvian AJ, Chen JC, et al: Outcome after thrombolysis and selective thoracic outlet decompression for primary axillary vein thrombosis. *J Vasc Surg* 33:783-788, 2001.)

were treated with catheter-directed urokinase infusions. The vein was chronically occluded in the other 3 patients. In 12 patients with some degree of residual stenosis, percutaneous transluminal angioplasty was performed after thrombolysis. Two patients required decompressive surgery. Of the 21 patients responding to the DASH questionnaire a mean 2.9 years after their SAVT episode, 28% reported being completely symptom free, 62% had DASH scores consistent with mild symptoms, and 2 had more severe symptoms (Fig 4). Twenty percent of the patients reported having some difficulty with work.

Conclusion.—Thrombolysis followed by selective thoracic outlet decompression based on symptom severity can be used to treat SAVT with minimal morbidity. The DASH questionnaire is useful for assessing findings after SAVT treatment.

▶ The results of this series of selected thoracic outlet decompression for axillary-subclavian vein thrombosis from the University of British Columbia, I believe, parallel the clinical experience of most practicing and savvy vascular surgeons who lack an agenda to remove ribs whenever a patient lies still. While I am sure some patients with venous thoracic outlet benefit significantly from first rib removal, I am equally sure most patients will get along fine after thrombolysis with their first rib left in situ.

G. L. Moneta, MD

12 Carotid and Cerebrovascular Disease

Prognosis After Transient Monocular Blindness Associated With Carotid Artery Stenosis
Benavente O, for the North American Symptomatic Carotid Endarterectomy Trial Collaborators (Univ of Texas, San Antonio; et al)
N Engl J Med 345:1084-1090, 2001   12–1

Background.—Transient monocular blindness is a common type of transient ischemic attack and a risk factor for stroke. Endarterectomy has been reported to be beneficial for stroke patients, but its usefulness for patients with transient monocular blindness is less clear. By using data from the North American Symptomatic Endarterectomy Trial, the risk of stroke after transient monocular blindness was compared with that after hemispheric transient ischemic attack. The usefulness of carotid endarterectomy was also examined.

Study Design.—Patients participated in the North American Symptomatic Carotid Endarterectomy Trial if they had transient ischemic attacks or nondisabling strokes associated with carotid artery stenosis. Between December 1987 and December 1996, 2885 patients were randomly assigned to receive optimal medical therapy or optimal medical therapy plus endarterectomy. Patients were followed up through December 1997. All patients underwent a detailed clinical evaluation at baseline and were evaluated every 4 months. The risk of stroke was compared between patients with transient monocular blindness and those with hemispheric transient ischemic attack. Baseline characteristics and risk factors were compared by χ-square test. Data were analyzed by the intention-to-treat principle. Kaplan-Meier survival curves were used to estimate risk.

Findings.—The 198 medically treated patients with transient monocular blindness had a 3-year risk of ipsilateral stroke that was about half of that of the 417 medically treated patients with hemispheric transient ischemic attack (Fig 1). Of the strokes that occurred among the patients with transient monocular blindness, 31% were retinal and the remainder were hemi-

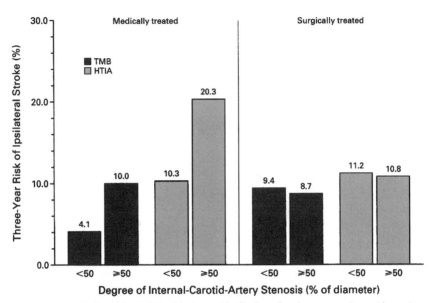

FIGURE 1.—Kaplan-Meier analysis of the 3-year risk of ipsilateral stroke among patients with transient monocular blindness (*TMB*) and hemispheric transient ischemic attack (*HTIA*), according to treatment group and degree of internal carotid artery stenosis. The risk estimates (as percentages) are shown *above the bars*. The numbers of patients represented by the bars are, from left to right, 56, 142, 202, 215, 57, 142, 215 and 197. (Reprinted with permission from Benavente O, for the North American Symptomatic Carotid Endarterectomy Trial Collaborators: Prognosis after transient monocular blindness associated with carotid artery stenosis. *N Engl J Med* 345:1084-1090, 2001. Copyright 2001, Massachusetts Medical Society. All rights reserved.)

spheric. Of the hemispheric strokes, 18% were fatal or disabling. In the patients presenting with monocular blindness, older age; male sex; history of transient ischemic attack, stroke, or intermittent claudication; stenosis; and absence of collateral circulation were associated with increased stroke risk. The 3-year stroke risk with optimal medical treatment for patients with 0 to 1 risk factor was 1.8%; for those with 2 risk factors it was 12.3%, and for those with 3 risk factors it was 24.2%. The 3-year absolute reduction in stroke risk with endarterectomy for patients with 0 to 1 risk factor was −2.2% (an increase); for those with 2 risk factors it was 4.9%, and for those with 3 risk factors it was 14.3%.

Conclusion.—The prognosis was better for patients seen with transient monocular blindness than for those with hemispheric transient ischemic attack. Among patients with transient monocular blindness, carotid endarterectomy appears to be beneficial for patients with other risk factors for stroke.

▶ Although on scientific grounds I object to the NASCET Investigators' extraordinary proclivity to spew forth these post hoc analyses of their data, the secondary papers derived from the NASCET Study have proved to be well-written and usually interesting. Such papers, however, should not, in my opinion, be given the same weight of evidence as the initial reports. I think the reasonable conclusions from this article are that: (1) ocular transient ischemic attacks are not as bad as hemispheric transient ischemic attacks in terms of stroke prognosis, and (2) patient risk factors and very high grade stenosis are what drive the prognosis, not the number and duration of episodes of monocular blindness. I will now think about patients with amaurosis fugax a little differently. Whereas previously I regarded multiple episodes of amaurosis fugax as a stronger indication for surgery than a single episode, I will now regard their prognosis as equal and pay more attention to patient risk factors (see abstract) in deciding which patients with amaurosis fugax to treat surgically.

G. L. Moneta, MD

Recurrent Cerebrovascular Events Associated With Patent Foramen Ovale, Atrial Septal Aneurysm, or Both
Mas J-L, for the Patent Foramen Ovale and Atrial Septal Aneurysm Study Group (Paris V Univ; et al)
N Engl J Med 345:1740-1746, 2001   12–2

Background.—Patent foramen ovale and atrial septal aneurysm are potential risk factors for ischemic stroke, but limited data are available on the effect of these septal abnormalities on the risk for recurrent stroke. In a multicenter follow-up study of patients with ischemic stroke, the risk for recurrent stroke was compared among patients with and without patent foramen ovale or atrial septal aneurysm.

Methods.—The study included 581 patients between the ages of 18 and 55 years. All had had an ischemic stroke of unknown origin within the 3 months preceding enrollment, and no definite cause for the stroke was found after a standardized workup. All patients underwent transthoracic and transesophageal echocardiography, and received aspirin (300 mg/d) for secondary prevention. Outcome events recorded were stroke, transient ischemic attack, systemic embolism, myocardial infarction, and death.

Results.—No atrial septal abnormalities were found in 304 patients; 216 had patent foramen ovale alone, 10 had atrial septal aneurysm alone, and 51 had both abnormalities. Four years after the initial ischemic stroke, risk for recurrent stroke was 4.2% among patients without either cardiac abnormality, 2.3% among those with patent foramen ovale alone, and 15.2% among those with both cardiac abnormalities (Fig 1). The presence of both atrial septal abnormalities was a significant predictor of increased risk for recurrent cerebrovascular events, but the presence of either abnormality alone was not. Risk for recurrent stroke increased with age.

Conclusion.—Preventive strategies other than aspirin should be considered for patients with both patent foramen ovale and atrial septal aneurysm who have had a stroke. The presence of both cardiac abnormalities substantially increases risk for recurrent stroke.

▶ I believe many people consider cryptogenic stroke in a young person with a patent foramen ovale to be an indication for closure of the patent foramen

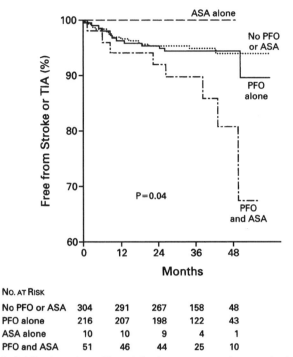

FIGURE 1.—Probability that patients will remain free from recurrent stroke or transient ischemic attack, according to the presence or absence of atrial septal abnormalities. The log-rank test was used to calculate the P value. Abbreviations: TIA, Transient ischemic attack; PFO, patent foramen ovale; ASA, atrial septal aneurysm. (Reprinted by permission of *The New England Journal of Medicine* from Mas J-L, for the Patent Foramen Ovale and Atrial Septal Aneurysm Study Group: Recurrent cerebrovascular events associated with patent foramen ovale, atrial septal aneurysm, or both. *N Engl J Med* 345:1740-1746, 2001. Copyright 2001, Massachusetts Medical Society. All rights reserved.)

ovale. It appears, however, that treatment with aspirin is sufficient in such patients, and that treatment of the foramen ovale is only indicated in patients who also have atrial septal aneurysms. Of course, this study addresses only recurrent stroke and doesn't tell us what to do with asymptomatic patients with patent foramen ovale and no history of stroke. Interestingly, the precise cause of recurrent stroke in these patients remains largely undetermined. It appeared not to be associated with deep venous thrombosis.

G. L. Moneta, MD

Cerebral Atherosclerosis as Predictor of Stroke and Mortality in Representative Elderly Population

Lernfelt B, Forsberg M, Blomstrand C, et al (Sahlgrenska Univ, Gothenburg, Sweden)
Stroke 33:224-229, 2002

12–3

Background.—The association between cardiovascular risk factors and carotid atherosclerosis is less distinct in elderly subjects than in middle-aged subjects. Elderly populations have a high prevalence of carotid atherosclerosis. However, it is not clear to what extent carotid atherosclerosis is associated with different cardiovascular risk factors in patients older than 75 years. The degree of atherosclerotic carotid disease was analyzed with cervical duplex scans and transcranial Doppler US at age 78 in a group of elderly men and women followed up since age 70 with respect to their cardiovascular risk factors. The study assessed the relationship between extracranial carotid artery disease, pulsatility index changes, and cardiovascular risk factors and evaluated the correlation between atherosclerosis in the carotid arteries and the incidence of stroke, cardiac disease, and death in these elderly patients.

Methods.—The study group comprised 142 men and women, who were assessed at the ages of 70 and 76 years before the final evaluation at age 78. Extracranial and intracranial circulation were evaluated by duplex sonography and transcranial Doppler. Mortality rates and hospitalization for stroke were analyzed over 5 years to age 83.

Results.—Carotid plaques were identified in 82% of the men and 79% of the women at age 78. The pulsatility index (PI) was between 1.0 and 1.4 in 63% of the study population and 1.5 or greater in 13% of the subjects. PI correlated with hypertension, stenosis greater than 50%, and presence of carotid plaques. Bilateral plaques occurred in 57% of the men and 46% of the women. Carotid stenosis greater than 75% was observed in 7 patients. The presence of bilateral plaques at age 78 years was correlated with increased systolic blood pressure and the presence of ischemic heart disease at age 70 years. Unilateral plaques at age 78 years were not associated with atherosclerotic risk factors or cardiovascular disease at age 70 years. Men with bilateral carotid plaques at age 78 were at increased risk of stroke or death during the 5-year follow-up period (74% vs 21% for patients with unilateral or no plaques) (Fig 2). However, this increased risk was not seen among the women.

Conclusions.—Carotid atherosclerosis is prevalent in the elderly population. Bilateral plaques were correlated with systolic blood pressure and ischemic heart disease in patients aged 70 years and were predictive of the risk of stroke and death in men but not in women.

▶ This study once again confirms that while some degree of atherosclerosis is common in elderly patients with severe carotid stenosis, in unselected patients severe carotid stenosis is very uncommon (0.5% of patients). I include this article in the YEAR BOOK for that reason. There is currently escalating inter-

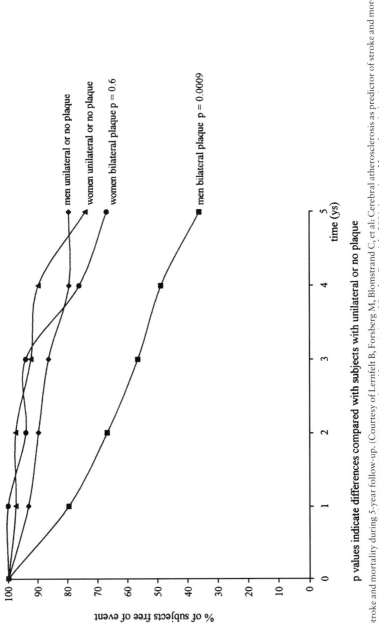

men unilateral or no plaque

women unilateral or no plaque

women bilateral plaque p = 0.6

men bilateral plaque p = 0.0009

time (ys)

% of subjects free of event

p values indicate differences compared with subjects with unilateral or no plaque

FIGURE 2.—Stroke and mortality during 5-year follow-up. (Courtesy of Lernfelt B, Forsberg M, Blomstrand C, et al: Cerebral atherosclerosis as predictor of stroke and mortality in representative elderly population. *Stroke* 33:224-229, 2002. Reproduced by permission of *Stroke*. Copyright 2001 American Heart Association.)

est among the Vascular Societies (SVS/AAVS) in establishing screening programs for vascular disease. I will always defend a patient's right to purchase health care that doesn't hurt them. I will, however, balk at using taxpayers' money for unselected carotid screening. The yield of high-grade lesions of unselected patients, in my opinion, remains too low to justify screening.

G. L. Moneta, MD

Collateral Ability of the Circle of Willis in Patients With Unilateral Internal Carotid Artery Occlusion: Border Zone Infarcts and Clinical Symptoms
Hendrikse J, Hartkamp MJ, Hillen B, et al (Univ Med Ctr Utrecht, The Netherlands)
Stroke 32:2768-2779, 2001   12–4

Background.—Postocclusive diminished arterial pressure is present in patients with occlusion of the internal carotid artery (ICA). Collateral blood flow is maintained by the circle of Willis to assure cerebral perfusion at a level that will accommodate metabolic demands. When collateral compensation mechanisms are inadequate, low-flow infarcts in border zone regions of the brain may occur. Previous studies have shown that patients with asymptomatic ICA occlusion have a more well-preserved hemodynamic status of the brain compared than patients with symptoms associated with ICA occlusion. However, the role of the circle of Willis in this respect is not fully understood. Whether the presence of border zone infarcts is associated with the collateral ability of the circle of Willis was investigated by evaluating patients with and without symptoms with unilateral occlusion of the internal carotid artery.

Methods.—The study enrolled 51 patients (35 with symptoms and 16 without) and 53 control subjects. All of the patients had unilateral occlusion of the ICA and contralateral stenosis between 0% and 69%. Magnetic resonance (MR) angiography was used to investigate the direction of flow on the side of the ICA occlusion and the size of the component vessels in the circle of Willis.

Results.—Twenty-six patients without border zone infarcts (92%) had collateral flow via the circle of Willis, compared with 25 patients (60%) with border zone infarcts. This increased collateral flow in patients without border zone infarcts was caused by the high prevalence of collateral flow via the posterior communicating artery in these patients. However, no statistically significant relationship was observed between the pattern of collateral flow via the circle of Willis and the presence of clinical symptoms. Symptom-free patients with ICA occlusion did demonstrate an increased diameter of the anterior communicating artery.

Conclusions.—The presence of collateral blood flow through the posterior communicating artery in the circle of Willis in patients with unilateral ICA occlusion is associated with a low prevalence of border zone infarcts.

There is no increased collateral function of the circle of Willis in symptom-free patients with an ICA occlusion.

▶ The posterior communicating artery "is where it is at" in the circle of Willis. Of the arteries constructing the "circle," large posterior communicating arteries promote relative protection against cerebral infarction in patients with an occluded cervical ICA.

G. L. Moneta, MD

Hemodynamic and Metabolic Changes in Transient Ischemic Attack Patients: A Magnetic Resonance Angiography and ¹H-Magnetic Resonance Spectroscopy Study Performed Within 3 Days of Onset of a Transient Ischemic Attack

Bisschops RHC, Kappelle LJ, Mali WPTM, et al (Univ Med Ctr Utrecht, The Netherlands)

Stroke 33:110-115, 2002   12–5

Background.—The annual risk of death from all vascular causes, nonfatal stroke, or nonfatal myocardial infarction is 7% to 12% for patients who have a transient ischemic attack (TIA). About 50% of these patients have ischemia from arteriosclerosis of the cerebrovascular arteries, 25% from intracranial small-vessel disease, and 20% from embolism originating in the heart. Cerebral perfusion is decreased in the affected hemisphere of TIA patients who do not have severe carotid artery lesions. This decrease persists up to 90 days after the onset of symptoms. TIA patients were assessed for systemic low blood flow to the brain or altered intracranial flow distribution secondary to abnormal anatomic changes of the circle of Willis. Metabolic changes in the brain were also evaluated.

Methods.—Clinical and neurologic data were collected for 44 patients with TIA who were prospectively enrolled and assessed within 3 days of the onset of symptoms. These patients and a control group of 57 subjects underwent the following tests: MRI; quantitative flow measurements of the internal carotid artery (ICA), middle cerebral artery(MCA), and basilar (BA) artery; magnetic resonance angiography (MRA) of the circle of Willis; and ¹H-MR spectroscopy (¹H-MRS).

Results.—Compared with control subjects, patients with TIA had no significant alterations in the flow of any of the arteries assessed, nor did the volume of flow differ between symptomatic and asymptomatic ICA and MCA for these individuals. In addition, those patients with hemispheric TIAs (hTIAs) and those with non-hTIAs showed no differences in volume flow. No significant differences were noted in the completeness of the circle of Willis on MRA between control subjects and patients. Patients with TIA had significant decreases in the N-acetylaspartate (NAA)/choline ratio in the symptomatic hemisphere as compared with the asymptomatic one. A significantly increased choline/creatine ratio in the symptomatic hemisphere in comparison with that in the asymptomatic was also noted in the patient group in comparison with those of the control subjects. Slight increases in the lactate/ NAA ratio were also noted between the asymptomatic hemisphere and that of the control individuals. Comparing hTIA and non-hTIA patients, the NAA/choline ratio in the symptomatic hemisphere was significantly decreased, but the lactate/NAA ratio was increased. No correlation was noted between metabolic ratios in the symptomatic or asymptomatic hemisphere and independent clinical risk factors (hypertension, diabetes mellitus, hypercholesterolemia, and smoking). Patients who had a history of a previous TIA had significant decreases in the NAA/choline ratio in both hemispheres in comparison with patients who only had 1 TIA. On diffusion-weighted imaging, 47% of the patients had an acute ischemic lesion, but these patients showed no differences in their NAA/choline, NAA/creatine, choline/ creatine, or lactate/NAA ratios.

Conclusions.—Patients with TIA had decreased NAA/choline ratios in the noninfarcted white matter of the symptomatic hemisphere, but none of them exhibited changes in cerebral blood flow, alterations in the circle of Willis, or changes in the intracranial distribution of flow to the brain when compared with normal individuals. The metabolic damage that results from TIA lasts as long as 3 days after the symptoms begin and are not limited to areas close to the ischemic lesions or even the symptomatic hemisphere. Patients with non-hTIAs had no metabolic changes.

▶ Brain metabolism, at least as measured by MR techniques, is altered after a TIA for at least 3 days, even though clinical symptoms resolve much earlier. These alterations in metabolism are not associated with continued reduced blood flow to the brain. It is unclear if these MR techniques of measuring brain metabolism actually measure anything important. At least in the short term, these changes in metabolism are probably not important, as the patient's clinical symptoms had resolved. However, it will be interesting to learn from future studies if the extent of metabolic derangements in the brain correlates with long-term cognitive function.

G. L. Moneta, MD

Matrix Metalloproteinase Expression After Human Cardioembolic Stroke: Temporal Profile and Relation to Neurological Impairment
Montaner J, Alvarez-Sabín J, Molina C, et al (Vall d'Hebron Hosp, Barcelona)
Stroke 32:1759-1766, 2001   12–6

Background.—Matrix metalloproteinases (MMPs) participate in many physiologic remodeling processes, but the uncontrolled expression of these enzymes can result in tissue destruction and inflammation. Studies in animal models suggest that MMPs are involved in the pathophysiologic state of cerebral ischemia. To test this hypothesis for humans in vivo, the temporal profile of MMP expression was investigated for patients with acute ischemic stroke.

Methods.—The study included 39 patients who had peripheral blood samples drawn for serial MMP-2 and MMP-9 determinations, using an enzyme-linked immunosorbent assay (ELISA). All patients had cardioembolic strokes involving the middle cerebral artery (MCA) area and were evaluated within the first 12 hours of stroke onset. Transcranial Doppler recordings were obtained and National Institutes of Health Stroke Scale (NIHSS) scores recorded at baseline, 12, 24, and 48 hours. All patients had CT scans to measure infarct volume at admission and at 48 hours. Subcutaneous low-molecular-weight heparin was given as prophylaxis for deep vein thrombosis.

Results.—Patients with a good neurologic status at the end of the study were those with decreased MMP-9 levels at any time period. No correlation was noted between MMP-2 and NIHSS scores at any time, but a close relation apparently existed between MMP-9 and the final NIHSS score. In the multiple logistic regression analysis, only MMP-9 was associated with the final NIHSS score. Overall, 14 patients improved during the study period, 10 remained stable, and 15 deteriorated. The improving group had lower MMP-2 and MMP-9 levels than the unimproved group. The mean MMP-9 levels were positively correlated with infarct volume, and when recanalization occurred, final MMP-2 and MMP-9 levels were significantly lower.

Conclusion.—For patients studied during the acute phase of stroke, an association was noted between MMP upregulation and neurologic impairment. Higher MMP-9 levels were associated with deterioration, and lower levels were strongly associated with neurologic improvement during the first 48 hours. Overexpression of MMP-9 was also associated with infarct size and the time and location of MCA occlusion.

▶ MMPs running amok are turning out to be ubiquitous bad actors in patients with vascular disease. These enzymes participate in normal remodeling of extracellular matrix, but their uncontrolled expression results in inflammation and destruction of tissue. They have been implicated in the pathogenesis of aneurysmal degeneration. In this study, stroke severity and infarct volume correlated with MMP-9 upregulation. The rapid growth of interest over the last few years in the role of MMPs in vascular disease appears justified. We all may have to become "MMP-ologists" before it is all over.

G. L. Moneta, MD

Hyperhomocysteinemia and Other Inherited Prothrombotic Conditions in Young Adults With a History of Ischemic Stroke
Madonna P, de Stefano V, Coppola A, et al (Università degli studi di Napoli "Federico II", Naples, Italy)
Stroke 33:51-56, 2002   12–7

Background.—Genetic factors that have theoretically predisposed young adults to stroke and those who have suffered stroke are thrombophilia and moderate hyperhomocysteinemia. Specifically, the gene for homozygous

C677T 5,10-methylenetetrahydrofolate reductase (MTHFR) has been linked to coronary artery disease, peripheral artery disease, and venous thrombosis. The roles of homozygous C677T MTHFR gene mutation and risk of cerebrovascular disease were assessed in young adults who had a history of ischemic arterial stroke.

Methods.—The study included 66 male and 66 female patients (age, 6 months to 50 years; mean age, 34.8 years) when the initial stroke occurred. All had been referred between January 1997 and December 1999 for their history of young adult ischemic stroke; prevalence of factor V Leiden, prothrombin (FII) G20210A, and C677T MTHFR gene mutations; and fasting serum total homocysteine levels. Results were compared with those of 262 healthy control individuals (117 males and 145 females).

Results.—The patient group was more likely to smoke currently and have hypertension, diabetes, and hyperlipidemia than was the control group. No statistical difference in frequency of heterozygosity was found between patients and control subjects for VF Leiden and FII G20210A gene mutations, for homozygosity of the C677T mutation of the MTHFR gene, or for prevalence of the associations of FV Leiden and FII variant with the *TT* genotype of MTHFR. Patients had significantly higher fasting serum total homocysteine levels than control subjects, and the latter showed a significant difference between sexes that was not present in the patient population. Patients homozygous for the MTHFR mutation had significantly higher total homocysteine levels than either heterozygotes or wild-type homozygotes of the patient population or the control group. When patients with major thrombophilic factors were excluded, significant differences remained in total serum homocysteine levels. The MTHFR genotype was the first variable entered into the multiple regression analysis to detect the main determinants of homocysteine levels; sex was the second variable.

Conclusions.—No significantly higher prevalence was shown for either FV Leiden or the 20210A FII variant for the patient population in comparison with the control group. Total homocysteine serum levels, however, were significantly higher for patients who suffered ischemic stroke than for the control population, even when patients with major thrombophilic factors were excluded from the assessment. Homozygosity for the *TT* variant of MTHFR mutation did not prove to be a risk factor for arterial ischemic stroke for the patients studied. Higher serum homocysteine levels were found in those with the *TT* genotype than in either the *CC* or the *CT* genotypes. The strongest variable entered into the multiple regression analysis of the principal factors determining moderate hyperhomocysteinemia was the MTHFR genotype.

▶ In a young person with ischemic stroke, the hypercoagulable problem that mattered was hyperhomocysteinemia, and not factor V Leiden or the prothrombin gene mutation. It therefore appears reasonable to check homocysteine levels in young adults with ischemic stroke and treat the homocysteine level if elevated. I would still, however, do a complete hypercoagulable panel.

Other studies have found other markers of hypercoagulability to also be associated with ischemic stroke.

G. L. Moneta, MD

Outcome of Stroke Patients Without Angiographically Revealed Arterial Occlusion Within Four Hours of Symptom Onset

Tomsick TA, for the EMS Bridging Trial (Univ of Cincinnati, Ohio; et al)
AJNR Am J Neuroradiol 22:685-690, 2001   12–8

Background.—Stroke patients without an angiographically detected arterial occlusion may not be given a thrombolytic agent to avoid the danger of inducing an intracerebral hemorrhage and in the belief that no added benefit accrues to its use. But angiograms are not able to discern occlusion in small cerebral arteries, and, therefore, cerebral infarction and long-term neurologic disability can result. The patients assessed were participants in the Emergency Management of Stroke (EMS) bridging trial who showed no angiographically apparent evidence of arterial occlusion. The EMS trial was designed to investigate the safety and potential efficacy of combined IV and intra-arterial thrombolytic therapy with recombinant tissue plasminogen activator (rtPA) for patients who suffered acute ischemic stroke. The imaging and long-term clinical outcomes were evaluated.

Methods.—The 35 patients included in the study randomly received either IV rtPA (n = 17)or placebo (n = 18); then cerebral angiography was performed in 34 patients.

Results.—Ten patients of the 34 who had angiography had no evidence of intracerebral arterial occlusion, and 3 had received IV rt-PA while 7 received IV placebo. Normal carotid arteriographic results were obtained in 2 patients who were believed to have carotid distribution ischemia, and spin-echo MR imaging done later found posterior circulation infarctions that did not show up on MR angiography. In 8 of the 10 patients who had no angiographic evidence of arterial occlusion within 4 hours of the onset of symptoms, new cerebral infarctions were found on follow-up brain imaging. Inconclusive MR findings were noted on the other 2 patients. Two patients had asymptomatic hemorrhagic conversion detected on the seventh day after symptom onset (1 in each treatment group). Small-vessel occlusion was suspected in 3 patients, cardiac embolism in 2 patients, and coronary catheter-induced embolism in 1 patient; the other 4 causes remained unknown. Groin oozing was found in 1 patient receiving IV rtPA therapy, but neither large groin or retroperitoneal hematoma occurred in the 10 patients for whom no clots were visible angiographically. One patient died within 3 months of metastatic breast cancer; no other deaths occurred among the 10 patients with no clot detected.

Conclusions.—Clinically significant brain infarctions occurred in 8 of the 10 EMS trial patients who had no angiographically detected clot within 4 hours of symptom onset. New infarctions were found in 7 with the use of CT and in 1 with the use of MR imaging. MR studies also detected ischemic abnormalities whose age could not be pinpointed in 2 patients; a result consistent with the symptoms being reported. Long-term functional disability can be expected in at least half of the patients. Negative angiograms were obtained early, possibly because of very early irreversible ischemic damage, despite recanalization or because of ongoing ischemia that is secondary to occlusion in penetrating arterioles or in the microvasculature that is not visible.

▶ Nearly one third of patients with ischemic stroke and who undergo cerebral angiography within 4 hours of onset of symptoms will have no visible intracranial intraarterial thrombosis. There is controversy as to whether such patients should still be treated with thrombolytic agents, as it suggested tiny clots in end arteries may not be visible with cerebral angiography. I don't know what the right answer is, but the concept of infusing a lytic agent directly into the brain in a patient with a fresh stroke and no specific target makes me nervous.

G. L. Moneta, MD

Validation of a Weight-based Nomogram for the Use of Intravenous Heparin in Transient Ischemic Attack or Stroke

Toth C, Voll C (Univ of Saskatchewan, Saskatoon, Canada)
Stroke 33:670-674, 2002   12–9

Background.—Patients presenting with transient ischemic attack (TIA) or stroke are often treated with heparin therapy either as a bridge to anticoagulation with warfarin or as primary therapy in patients with suspected intracranial arterial dissection, crescendo TIAs, or suspected hypercoagulable states. Fixed dosing of IV heparin provides a variable degree of anticoagulation between different patients, which may be due to a heparin-resistance phenomenon, heparin-neutralizing proteins, and nonlinear pharmacodynamics. These factors make it difficult to achieve a therapeutic range for heparin dosing and can lead to subtherapeutic and supratherapeutic anticoagulation levels. An attempt was made to validate the use of a weight-based nomogram for heparin-adjusted therapy during hospitalization of patients with TIA or stroke.

Methods.—A specially designed weight-based heparin nomogram was compared with the traditional method of physician-ordered heparin therapy for patients admitted with TIA or stroke in a prospective, single-blinded, randomized, clinical trial (Fig 1). The goal was not to evaluate the efficacy of heparin therapy but to examine the use of the nomogram for labor requirements, costs of monitoring, safety, length of heparin therapy, and user friendliness.

Results.—The pretreatment clinical factors were similar for patients randomly assigned to the nomogram (101 patients) and to usual care (105 patients). The patients treated by nomogram achieved a therapeutic range of anticoagulation sooner than patients who received usual care (13.4 hours vs 17.9 hours). In addition, the fraction of time during which anticoagulation was therapeutic was significantly greater in patients receiving nomogram

<u>HEPARIN-ADJUSTED NOMOGRAM FOR STROKE/TRANSIENT ISCHEMIC</u>
ATTACK
PHYSICIAN'S ORDERS

DATE	TIME	PROCESSED AT/BY:

1. Medication is provided intravenously. No intramuscular injections.
2. APTT, INR, and CBC must be drawn prior to start of therapy.
3. CBC must be drawn at least every three days during therapy.
4. If patient has a transient ischemic attack, a bolus of intravenous heparin may be given at the discretion of the admitting physician. Suggested IV heparin bolus is 50U/kg to a maximum of 5000U. If a bolus is desired, this must be indicated:
   ☐ Give _____ U IV heparin as a bolus.
5. Initial dosing for continuous infusion of intravenous heparin:

WEIGHT (kg)	INITIAL INFUSION
☐ <50	500U/hr = 10mL/hr
☐ 50-59	600U/hr = 12mL/hr
☐ 60-69	700U/hr = 14mL/hr
☐ 70-79	800U/hr = 16mL/hr
☐ 80-89	900U/hr = 18mL/hr
☐ 90-99	1000U/hr = 20mL/hr
☐ 100-109	1100U/hr = 22mL/hr
☐ 110-119	1200U/hr = 24mL/hr
☐ >119	1400U/hr = 28mL/hr

6. APTT is to be drawn six hours after heparin therapy initiation.
7. Adjusted heparin therapy as according to APTT based on sliding scale:

APTT (seconds)	STOP INFUSION	RATE CHANGE	REPEAT APTT
< 40	---	Increase by 250 U/hr	6 hours
40 – 49	---	Increase by 150 U/hr	6 hours
50 – 59	---	Increase by 100 U/hr	6 hours
60 – 90	---	---	Next a.m.
91 – 100	---	Decrease by 100 U/hr	6 hours
101 – 120	---	Decrease by 150 U/hr	6 hours
> 120	60 minutes	Decrease by 250 U/hr	6 hours

8. If significant bleeding occurs, stop heparin and call physician to reassess.
   Physician's signature: _____   Date: _____

FIGURE 1.—Weight-based nomogram used for heparin therapy in nomogram patients. (Courtesy of Toth C, Voll C: Validation of a weight-based nomogram for the use of intravenous heparin in transient ischemic attack or stroke. *Stroke* 33:670-674, 2002. Reproduced with permission of *Stroke*. Copyright 2002 American Heart Association.)

therapy (74%) than those receiving usual care (67%). The nomogram patients also had significantly fewer supratherapeutic coagulation results, dose-adjustment mistakes, calls to house staff regarding anticoagulation, and total complications than non-nomogram patients. There were no significant differences between the 2 groups in the times required for discontinuation of heparin and discharge from the hospital. Both house and nursing staffs expressed a preference for nomogram use.

Conclusions.—The heparin nomogram is a user-friendly method for maintenance of heparin infusion. The nomogram provides fewer total complications related to heparin therapy, fewer mistakes in dosage adjustment, and decreased labor on the part of house staff and nursing staff.

▶ I am not sure why this article was published. The authors acknowledge there is no proven efficacy of heparin in the treatment of TIA or stroke, and yet they went to significant efforts to evaluate how to best use an unproven therapy. Why encourage continuation of likely ineffective therapy?

G. L. Moneta, MD

A Comparison of Warfarin and Aspirin for the Prevention of Recurrent Ischemic Stroke
Mohr JP, for the Warfarin-Aspirin Recurrent Stroke Study Group (Columbia Presbyterian Med Ctr, New York; et al)
N Engl J Med 345:1444-1451, 2001   12–10

Introduction.—The recurrence rate for patients with ischemic stroke treated prophylactically after a noncardiogenic ischemic stroke with 1 or more of a wide variety of platelet-antiaggregant drugs, especially aspirin, is about 8%. Warfarin, which is effective and superior to aspirin in the prevention of cardiogenic embolism, was compared with aspirin in a multicenter, double-blind, randomized trial to determine whether it is also superior in the prevention of recurrent ischemic stroke in patients with a prior noncardio-embolic ischemic stroke.

Methods.—The effects of warfarin (at a dose adjusted to create an international normalized ratio [INR] of 1.4-2.8) and aspirin (325 mg/d) on the combined major end point of recurrent ischemic stroke or death from any cause within 2 years were compared.

Results.—Both study groups had similar baseline risk factors. In the intention-to-treat analysis, no significant differences were observed between the treatment groups in any measured outcomes. The major end point of death or recurrent ischemic stroke was reached in 196 of 1103 patients (17.8%) in the warfarin group and in 176 of 1103 in the aspirin group (16%; $P = .25$; hazard ratio comparing warfarin with aspirin, 1.13; 95% confidence interval, 0.92-1.38). The rates of major hemorrhage were low (2.22 per 100 patient-years and 1.49 patient-years in the warfarin and aspirin groups, respectively). There were no significant treatment-related differences in the rate of or time to the major end point or major hemorrhage according to the cause of the initial stroke.

Conclusion.—During a 2-year evaluation period, no differences were observed between aspirin and warfarin in the prevention of recurrent ischemic stroke or death or in the incidence of major hemorrhage. Both warfarin and aspirin may be considered reasonable therapeutic alternatives.

▶ Since there is no difference between aspirin (325 mg per day) and warfarin (INR, 1.4-2.8) for prevention of recurrent ischemic stroke, it doesn't take a rocket scientist to stumble to the fact that aspirin should be the preferred drug;

it is, after all, easier to use. Perhaps the corollary is not so immediately obvious: in patients unable to tolerate aspirin, warfarin works just as well with no difference in major hemorrhagic complications.

G. L. Moneta, MD

Parity and Carotid Artery Atherosclerosis in Elderly Women: The Rotterdam Study
Humphries KH, Westendorp ICD, Bots ML, et al (Univ of British Columbia, Vancouver, Canada; Erasmus Med Centre Rotterdam, The Netherlands; Univ Med Ctr, Utrecht, The Netherlands)
Stroke 32:2259-2264, 2001   12–11

Background.—The relationship between parity and risk of cardiovascular disease is inconclusive, but findings favor the hypothesis that the risk increases with increasing parity. Potential mechanisms for the association between parity and cardiovascular disease are pregnancy-related changes in lipoprotein levels and glucose metabolism. The association between parity and the presence of carotid atherosclerosis was studied in postmenopausal women who participated in the Rotterdam Study.

Methods.—Included in the population-based study were 4878 women, aged 55 years and older. Carotid atherosclerosis was assessed by carotid duplex US and defined as the presence of plaques at 1 or more sites. Intima-media thickness (IMT) was also measured. Participants had blood drawn for glucose and cholesterol measurements.

Results.—Parity in the study group ranged from 0 to 16 children; 21.5% of the women were nulliparous. Positive associations were found between parity and body mass index, total/HDL cholesterol ratio, insulin resistance, age at menopause, and socioeconomic status. Compared with nulliparous women, the women with children had a 36% higher risk for carotid artery atherosclerosis; the risk was 64% higher for women with 4 or more children. With increased parity, a trend was observed to an increased mean and maximum IMT, and this finding remained significant even after adjustment for covariate factors.

Conclusion.—A positive association between parity and the risk of carotid artery plaques was found in this cohort of postmenopausal women. Parity has adverse effects on lipid and glucose metabolism, and these effects persist long after childbearing has ceased. The magnitude of the observed association was not reduced by adjustment for known cardiovascular risk factors, including insulin resistance and current lipid levels.

▶ The authors found a modest association between parity and the risk of carotid atherosclerosis in old females. The association held up despite correction for lipid levels, weight, smoking, alcohol intake (all of which were higher in multiparous vs nulliparous females), and socioeconomic status (lower in multiparous females). I am not really convinced by these data. I understand the math, but the babies were born many years before the data were collected. I would think all the variables that were controlled for in this study would actually be impossible to truly control for over such a long period of time. If my wife gets carotid disease, I won't blame it on my children . . . she might, but I won't.

G. L. Moneta, MD

Carotid Stenosis: Factors Affecting Symptomatology
Liapis CD, Kakisis JD, Kostakis AG (Athens Univ, Greece)
Stroke 32:2782-2786, 2001   12–12

Background.—An open prospective study was done to identify factors that affect symptomatology in patients with carotid stenosis.

Methods.—The status of 332 patients with internal carotid artery stenosis in 442 arteries was followed up between 1988 and 1997. Color Duplex US was performed every 6 months. The mean follow-up time was 44 months.

Findings.—Significant progression of stenosis was observed in 18.5% of arteries. Such progression was more common in younger patients, in patients with coronary artery disease, and in those with echolucent plaques. A trend toward higher frequency of stroke in their history was seen in men, hypertensive patients, and patients with echolucent plaques. Neurologic events occurred in 12.4% of patients during follow-up. These events were associated with severity of carotid disease, history of neurologic events, progression of stenosis, echolucent plaques, and hypertension.

Conclusions.—These data show that variables other than extent of stenosis and history of neurologic events are also important for determining high-risk carotid plaque. Hypertension, echolucent plaques, and progressive lesions appear to be associated with an increased risk of neurologic events. Clinicians should consider such factors when making decisions about carotid stenosis treatment.

▶ Previous studies have shown an association between severity of carotid stenosis, progression of carotid stenosis, and a history of neurologic symptoms with the development of new neurologic symptoms. I don't for one minute trust a retrospective analysis of the echogenicity of carotid plaques, and neither should have the editors of *Stroke*. Sorry, that part of this article is a "no sale."

G. L. Moneta, MD

In Vivo Accuracy of Multispectral Magnetic Resonance Imaging for Identifying Lipid-Rich Necrotic Cores and Intraplaque Hemorrhage in Advanced Human Carotid Plaques

Yuan C, Mitsumori LM, Ferguson MS, et al (Univ of Washington, Seattle; Marina Ferguson Inc, Seattle; Mountain-Whisper-Light Statistical Consulting, Seattle; et al)
Circulation 104:2051-2056, 2001   12–13

Background.—High-resolution MRI can identify plaque constituents in human carotid atherosclerosis. Differential contrast-weighted images, specifically a multispectral MR technique, were used to improve the accuracy of lipid-rich necrotic core and acute intraplaque hemorrhage identification in vivo.

Methods.—Eighteen patients undergoing carotid endarterectomy were examined preoperatively by MRI by means of a protocol that produced 4 contrast weightings including T1, T2, proton density, and 3-dimensional time of flight. The MR images of the vessel wall were assessed for a lipid-rich necrotic core or intraplaque bleeding. In a double-blind fashion, 90 cross sections were compared with matched histologic sections of the excised specimen.

Findings.—The overall accuracy of multispectral MRI was 87%, with a sensitivity and specificity of 85% and 92%, respectively. Agreement between MRI and histologic findings was good, at 0.69.

Conclusion.—Multispectral MRI can accurately detect the lipid-rich necrotic core in carotid atherosclerosis in vivo. The sensitivity and specificity of this modality are high. The technique offers a noninvasive way to assess the pathogenesis and natural history of carotid atherosclerosis and allows direct evaluation of the effect of pharmacologic therapy on plaque lipid composition.

▶ This must be complicated research—18 patients and 10 authors, 1.8 patients per author. The study demonstrates lipid-rich areas of carotid plaque can be identified by MRI. The authors contend MRI will allow assessment of the effects of lipid lowering agents on plaque composition. This seems a bit of a stretch as no data are presented indicating MRI can result in calculations of volume of lipid-rich areas. The data indicate MRI can indicate lipid-rich areas are present, but not their volume.

G. L. Moneta, MD

Identification of Fibrous Cap Rupture With Magnetic Resonance Imaging Is Highly Associated With Recent Transient Ischemic Attack or Stroke

Yuan C, Zhang S-x, Polissar NL, et al (Univ of Washington, Seattle; Mountain-Whisper-Light Statistical Consulting, Seattle; VA Puget Sound Health Care System, Seattle)

Circulation 105:181-185, 2002   12–14

Background.—An important role in acute ischemic events, such as stroke and transient ischemic attack (TIA), is postulated for rupture of a fibrous cap that overlies the thrombogenic necrotic core of an atherosclerotic plaque. The ability to assess the state of the fibrous cap may improve patient assignment to medical or surgical management and allow monitoring of the progression of disease or therapeutic intervention. High-resolution MRI can distinguish between intact, thick fibrous caps and thin, ruptured caps. A protocol of multiple contrast-weighted high-resolution MR images of the carotid artery was used to assess the relationship between characteristics of the carotid plaque fibrous cap and the patient's neurologic symptoms.

Methods.—The study included 53 consecutive patients (49 male; mean age, 71 years), who were all scheduled to undergo carotid endarterectomy. Twenty-eight subjects had a recent history of TIA or stroke on the side appropriate to the index carotid lesion; 25 patients were asymptomatic. On high-resolution MRI, fibrous caps were categorized as intact-thick, intact-thin, or ruptured.

Results.—No statistically significant differences were noted between the symptomatic and asymptomatic patients with respect to mean age, number with a history of smoking, diabetes, hypertension, hypercholesterolemia, or family history of atherosclerosis. Preoperative carotid duplex scanning of the index carotid artery detected no significant differences in mean peak systolic velocity (PSV). Eleven patients had intact thick fibrous caps, 12 had intact thin caps, and 30 had ruptured fibrous caps. Among those with a thin fibrous or ruptured cap, a statistically significant higher percentage were symptomatic patients; In addition, a recent TIA or stroke was present 10 times more often than among those with thick fibrous caps. Only 9% of patients who had thick fibrous caps had symptoms in contrast to 50% of those who had symptoms with thin caps and 70% of those who were symptomatic with ruptured caps. Those with ruptured fibrous caps were 23 times more likely to have suffered recent ischemic neurologic symptoms. The odds ratios were 6 for thin caps and 18 for ruptured caps in comparison to thick caps when logistic regression analysis controlling for PSV was performed.

Conclusions.—The evidence strongly suggests that the status of the fibrous cap shown on high-resolution MRI correlates with the occurrence of recent ischemic neurologic events. This noninvasive method of detecting atherosclerotic plaques at risk of rupture before ischemic complications develop offers significant clinical applications.

▶ Carotid plaques may have a "fibrous cap" overlying a presumably necrotic portion of the plaque. Theoretically, cap rupture allows access of plaque contents to the flow stream resulting in a TIA or stroke. In this study, MRI identified ruptured carotid plaque fibrous caps in patients with carotid plaques thought to be symptomatic. The obvious next step is to determine which fibrous caps will break down and lead to symptoms. Given the marginal therapeutic benefit of treatment of asymptomatic carotid stenosis, work such as this is important in hopefully eventually allowing us to be more selective in our application of carotid endarterectomy in asymptomatic patients.

G. L. Moneta, MD

Expression of Tissue Factor in High-Grade Carotid Artery Stenosis: Association With Plaque Destabilization

Jander S, Sitzer M, Wendt A, et al (Heinrich-Heine-Univ, Düsseldorf, Germany; Johann Wolfgang Goethe-Univ, Frankfurt am Main, Germany)
Stroke 32:850-854, 2001   12–15

Background.—The procoagulant protein tissue factor (TF) appears to play a role in thromboembolic complications associated with advanced atherosclerosis. Whether TF expression in high-grade stenoses of the internal carotid arterry (ICA) correlates with clinical features of plaque destabilization was investigated.

Methods.—Thirty-six consecutive patients undergoing surgery for high-grade ICA stenosis were studied. Clinical evidence of plaque instability was provided by the recent occurrence of ischemic symptoms attributable to stenosis and detection of cerebral microembolism by using transcranial Doppler US monitoring of the ipsilateral middle cerebral artery. Immunocytochemically, endarterectomy specimens were stained for TF expression and macrophage and T-cell infiltration.

Findings.—Morphologic analysis showed that TF immunoreactivity was codistributed with plaque inflammation and localized mainly to CD68+ macrophages. Expression of TF was significantly associated with plaque infiltration by macrophages and T cells (Table 2). Plaques that stained extensively for TF were more common in symptomatic than in asymptomatic pa-

TABLE 2.—Relationship Between TF Expression and Ischemic Symptoms

| TF+ Section Area, Median | Ipsilateral Ischemic Symptoms Within Past 120 Days | | | |
| | Absent | | Present | |
	n	%	n	%
<20%	3	33	1	4
20-40%	5	56	14	52
>40%	1	11	12	44

Note: TF expression was determined semiquantitatively in each plaque section, and the median of TF+ section area was calculated for each entire plaque. Mann-Whitney U test revealed a significant association between TF expression and the occurrence of ischemic symptoms ($P = .016$).

(Courtesy of Jander S, Sitzer M, Wendt A, et al: Expression of tissue factor in high-grade artery stenosis association with plaque destabilization. *Stroke* 32:850-854, 2001.)

tients, and plaques that showed little TF expression were more common in asymptomatic than in symptomatic patients. The correlation between TF expression and cerebral microembolism occurrence was significant.

Conclusions.—Increased TF expression in high-grade ICA stenoses is associated with plaque destabilization. This occurrence was shown clinically both by a history of previous ischemic symptoms and the detection of microemboli in long-term transcranial Dopper US monitoring of the ipsilateral middle cerebral artery.

▶ The previous 2 articles (Abstracts 12–13 and 12–14) looked at rupture of the carotid bifurcation fibrous caps in the production of symptoms associated with carotid atheroma. This article sought to explain why the plaques rupture, and concludes tissue factor may play a role. The hypothesis goes along with the increasingly postulated role of inflammation in atherosclerosis, as tissue factor is induced by activated macrophages and T cells. In addition, tissue factor could serve to link atherosclerosis and thrombosis.

G. L. Moneta, MD

Increased Prevalence of Carotid and Femoral Atherosclerosis in Renal Transplant Recipients
Cofan F, Nuñez I, Gilabert R, et al (Univ of Barcelona)
Transplant Proc 33:1254-1256, 2001   12–16

Background.—Renal transplant recipients (RTRs) are at increased risk for cardiovascular disease. The most important cardiovascular risk factors in this population are hyperlipemia, hypertension, diabetes, and vascular disease during dialysis. US findings of carotid atherosclerosis may be useful in predicting the development of cardiovascular disease in RTRs with no clinical evidence of such disease.

Methods.—High-resolution B-mode US of the carotid and common femoral arteries was performed in 70 RTRs and 70 age- and sex-matched control subjects. All RTRs were without clinical evidence of cardiovascular disease. The US parameters analyzed included mean and maximum intima-media thickness (IMT) and data on atherosclerotic plaques. Both RTRs and control subjects also underwent a complete evaluation of nonlipid cardiovascular risk factors.

Results.—Compared with control subjects, RTRs had a greater prevalence of hypertension and dyslipidemia and significantly higher serum concentrations of total cholesterol, LDL-cholesterol, triglycerides, ApoB, and Lp(a). Current smoking was more frequent in the control group. In transplanted patients, the IMT of the carotid and femoral arteries was significantly greater than that of control subjects, and the prevalence of arteriosclerotic plaque was much higher in both carotid and femoral arteries of RTRs (74% and 79% vs 13% and 29%, respectively, in controls).

Conclusion.—High-resolution B-mode US demonstrated that a high proportion of RTRs with no clinical evidence of cardiovascular disease had carotid and femoral arteriosclerosis. Compared with a matched control population, the RTRs had greater carotid and femoral IMT and a higher prevalence of atherosclerotic plaques. Carotid B-mode US is recommended as a routine examination during renal transplantation follow-up.

▶ I have always regarded renal transplant patients, especially those transplanted for complications of diabetes or hypertension, as not being much different from dialysis patients. It is not surprising they have more detectable atherosclerosis.

G. L. Moneta, MD

Cost of Identifying Patients for Carotid Endarterectomy
Benade MM, Warlow CP (Univ of Edinburgh, Scotland)
Stroke 33:435-439, 2002   12–17

Background.—Reports of the costs of carotid endarterectomy (CEA) usually consider only the cost of the preoperative investigations and the procedure for the individual patient; the cost incurred in selecting a patient from a referred "pool" of potential candidates, or the "total direct program cost," is often ignored. The pool of potential candidates consists of those patients who are experiencing symptoms suggesting a transient ischemic attack (TIA) or mild stroke within the distribution of the carotid artery. The total direct program cost includes the cost of workup of these potential CEA patients as well as the cost of the procedure. A retrospective study was used to estimate the total direct program cost of CEA at a large major teaching hospital in Edinburgh, Scotland.

Methods.—The study group included patients with TIAs and mild strokes who were referred to the neurovascular clinics for assessment, investigation, and possible CEA. The workup in these patients was defined as the clinical consultation, carotid duplex, a follow-up visit, and a catheter angiogram as indicated. Data collected routinely from the neurovascular clinics during 1 year were used to estimate the workup cost for patients who might be suitable candidates for CEA. The cost of the CEA procedure was prospectively estimated in a concurrent study. To determine the total direct program cost of CEA, estimated costs were applied to the proportions assessed at the different levels of investigation.

Results.—A total of 790 patients were enrolled in the study. Carotid duplex US was ordered in 401 patients (51%), and among them, duplex imaging identified 78 (10%) with carotid stenosis 70% or greater. Overall, 26 of 790 patients (3.3%) had catheter angiogram, and 18 of 790 (2.3%) had CEA. The total direct program cost for investigation of this cohort was approximately £207,000, with 68% of the cost incurred before surgery.

Conclusions.—Significant expense is associated with the identification of suitable patients for carotid surgery, and more than 30% of this cost is attributable to the initial consultation at neurovascular clinics. In Scotland, the cost of preventing 1 stroke by CEA is about £100,000 (1997-1998 prices) when all the costs involved in the workup of a cohort of potential CEA patients are included.

▶ "Cost" studies are always difficult to evaluate. True costs vary so much from country to country, and among institutions, that I have never found them of much interest. What is interesting here, however, is that of 790 patients with possible symptomatic carotid disease, only 18 came to endarterectomy. That fact alone indicates a lot of money will be spent to identify patients for carotid endarterectomy.

G. L. Moneta, MD

Association of Surgical Specialty and Processes of Care With Patient Outcomes for Carotid Endarterectomy
Hannan EL, Popp AJ, Feustel P, et al (State Univ of New York, Rensselaer, NY; Albany Med College, New York; Mount Sinai School of Medicine, New York)
Stroke 32:2890-2897, 2001   12–18

Background.—Carotid endarterectomy has been shown to be effective for the treatment of both symptomatic and asymptomatic carotid occlusive disease. However, the appropriate use of carotid endarterectomy is controversial, and studies have found large temporal and geographic variations in practice patterns. As with many other invasive surgical procedures, patient outcomes for carotid endarterectomy have been found to be associated with the volume of procedures performed in a hospital as well as the volume performed by the surgeon.

The variations in practice patterns and outcomes underscore the need for a study of the processes of care that are associated with adverse outcomes. The effects of the processes of care and surgical specialty on adverse outcomes for carotid endarterectomy were investigated.

Methods.—This retrospective study gathered data from a voluntary carotid endarterectomy registry containing 3644 patients who underwent carotid endarterectomy from April 1997 to March 1999 in a number of New York hospitals. By means of a multivariable statistical model, significant independent patient risk factors were identified and the association of processes of care and surgical specialty with outcomes were evaluated after adjustment for differences in patient risk factors.

Results.—The rate of overall adverse outcome, which was defined as in-hospital death or stroke, was 1.84%. The use of 1 or more specific processes of care (eversion endarterectomy, protamine, or shunts) was found to be associated with lower odds of an adverse outcome relative to patients undergoing carotid endarterectomy without these processes. In addition, patients whose surgical procedures were performed by vascular surgeons had reduced odds of experiencing an adverse outcome. The processes of care and surgical specialty were found to be highly correlated.

Conclusion.—The processes of care and surgical specialty are closely correlated and are significant determining factors for adverse outcomes in patients undergoing carotid endarterectomy.

▶ Articles such as this will certainly get one's attention. The finding vascular surgeons have better outcomes with carotid endarterectomy than neurosurgeons is potentially misleading. One cannot brand a vascular surgeon better than a neurosurgeon simply by title. Each surgeon should be judged by his or her outcomes regardless of training or background. Training and technique may increase one's odds of being competent, but in the end it is results that matter.

G. L. Moneta, MD

Geographic Variation in the Rate of Carotid Endarterectomy in Canada
Feasby TE, Quan H, Ghali WA (Univ of Calgary, Alta, Canada; Calgary Health Region, Alta, Canada)
Stroke 32:2417-2422, 2001   12–19

Background.—The rate of carotid endarterectomy (CEA) began to rise in the 1990s. There has, however, after publication of serveral large randomized trials of CEA been little published regarding the use of this procedure in Canada. Since the early 1990s, there has been nothing regarding the utilization of CEA nationally in Canada. The rate and regional variations in the rate of CEA in Canada for 1994 through 1997 were investigated. In this report, the rate of CEA utilization was evaluated by province and census divisions.

Methods.—For 1994 through 1997, discharge data were obtained from all hospitals in Canada, with the exception of Quebec, from the Canadian Institute for Health Information. The rates and the variations in these rates were then calculated for each province and territory and for each census division.

Results.—The national age- and sex-adjusted rate for CEA in persons 40 years or older rose from 31.7 per 100,000 persons in 1994 to 40.5 per 100,000 persons in 1997. The provincial rates for 1997 varied from 25.7 in Saskatchewan to 82.8 in Prince Edward Island. The variation in rates among census divisions was even more pronounced, from a low of 0 in several divisions to a high of 179.

Conclusions.—The recent slight increase in the utilization of CEA in Canada may be a reflection of the release of new efficacy results for CEA, particularly for asymptomatic carotid stenosis. However, the utilization rates for CEA in Canada are still far below those for CEA in the United States. The significant variation in utilization rates by regions may be a reflection of differing views on the appropriateness of indications for CEA, such as for asymptomatic carotid stenosis, as well as the inconsistency of current clinical practice guidelines.

▶ The authors found marked geographic variation in CEA rates in Canada. This type of information must drive health planners crazy. Despite the fact CEA is among the best-studied procedures, this variation in usage exists. While one can speculate as to reasons for geographic variation, it all boils down to inappropriate use in some regions, and under use in others. A focused exam of clinical practice where the rate of CEA seems either high or low is indicated.

G. L. Moneta, MD

Silent Cerebral Infarction: Risk Factor for Stroke Complicating Carotid Endarterectomy
Fürst H, Hartl WH, Haberl R, et al (Ludwig-Maximilian Univ, Munich; Univ of Edinburgh, Scotland)
World J Surg 25:969-974, 2001   12–20

Background.—Some patients with significant carotid artery disease are asymptomatic, yet their imaging studies reveal areas of hypodensity consistent with cerebral infarction. Whether these "silent" cerebral infarcts increase the risk of perioperative stroke and death during carotid endarterectomy (CEA) was prospectively examined.

Methods.—The subjects were 663 patients less than 80 years of age with stenosis of the internal carotid artery (ICA) who underwent CEA during a 5-year period. About 45% of patients had asymptomatic stenosis, defined as more than 95% stenosis of the ICA without symptoms. The other 55% had symptomatic stenosis, defined as more than 70% stenosis of the ICA in association with transient ischemic attack. Preoperatively, all patients underwent CT to identify and characterize any "silent" cerebral infarctions. Perioperative stroke and death were correlated with the presence or absence of "silent" cerebral infarction in the operated ICA territory.

Results.—CT identified silent cerebral infarcts in the territory of the operated ICA in 182 patients (27.4%). The incidence of silent infarction was significantly higher in the patients with symptomatic stenosis (124 of 297, or 41.8%) than in those with asymptomatic stenosis (58 of 366, or 15.8%). Compared with the patients without silent infarction, patients with silent infarction were significantly older (69.2 vs 67.6 years), significantly more likely to be male (79.7% vs 67.8%), and significantly more likely to have contralateral ICA disease (32.4% vs 25.2%) or an ipsilateral high-grade (but not threadlike) ICA stenosis (14.3% vs 8.9%).

Multivariate analysis indicated that the risk of silent infarction was predicted by clinical symptoms (relative risk [RR], 2.1), male sex (RR, 2.1), and age above the median (RR, 1.7). Perioperatively, 20 patients (3.0%) had a major stroke, and 4 patients (0.6%) died; all deaths were related to stroke. Strokes were equally common in the symptomatic and asymptomatic patients (3.8% vs 2.0%). However, strokes were significantly more common in the patients with silent cerebral infarction than in the remaining patients (16 patients, or 8.8% vs 4 patients, or 0.8%). Multivariate analysis indicated that the presence of a silent cerebral infarction was the only significant independent predictor of perioperative major stroke for both symptomatic (RR, 12.9) and asymptomatic (RR, 7.9) patients.

Conclusion.—The risk of major perioperative stroke was markedly higher in the patients with silent cerebral infarction in the territory of the operated ICA than in patients without CT evidence of ischemia in that area. Because the risk of major perioperative stroke or death did not differ significantly between the asymptomatic and symptomatic groups, preoperative CT should be used for risk classification in all patients undergoing CEA.

▶ This is a very interesting article that is unfortunately buried in a moderately obscure journal. The authors found that all the usual factors that may increase the risk for perioperative stroke with CEA (contralateral occlusion, diabetes, gender, and whether stenosis was asymptomatic or associated with transient ischemic attack) did not predict perioperative stroke complicating CEA. Perioperative stroke was strongly predicted by silent cerebral infarction detected on routine preoperative CT scanning. The implication is that such patients in response to CEA behave like patients with clinically evident preoperative stroke. There may be a higher risk for such patients with CEA, but there is also the possibility they will derive greater benefit from CEA.

G. L. Moneta, MD

Early Versus Delayed Carotid Endarterectomy After a Nondisabling Ischemic Stroke: A Prospective Randomized Study
Ballotta E, Da Giau G, Baracchini C, et al (Univ of Padua, Italy)
Surgery 131:287-293, 2002   12–21

Introduction.—Many retrospective and some prospective trials have analyzed the outcome of early and delayed carotid endarterectomy (CEA) after a recent minor or nondisabling stroke. However, the optimal timing for this procedure remains unknown. The perioperative death and stroke rates of CEA performed within 30 days (early group) or more than 30 days (delayed group) after a nondisabling ischemic stroke were prospectively compared for patients with carotid bifurcation disease.

Methods.—Of 86 patients who experienced a minor stroke during a 4-year evaluation period, 45 were randomly assigned to an early CEA group and 41 to a delayed CEA group. Preoperative cerebral CT, duplex US screening, and angiography of the supra-aortic trunks were performed in all patients. All CEAs were carotid eversion endarterectomies performed by the same surgeon. Deep anesthesia was used with continuous ECG monitoring for selective shunting. The incidences of perioperative death and stroke were compared.

Results.—No perioperative deaths occurred in either group. No patients in the delayed group experienced recurrent strokes. The incidence of perioperative stroke was similar in the 2 groups (1/45, 2%; 1/41, 2%). Follow-up ranged from 6 to 50 months (mean, 23 months). Both groups were similar in survival rates at 1, 2, and 3 years.

Conclusion.—The timing of CEA does not appear to impact its benefit. Early CEA after a nondisabling ischemic stroke had safety, mortality, and stroke rates comparable to patients with delayed CEA.

▶ The "early" patients in this study were not all that "early." *Early* was defined as less than 30 days after stroke and the median time to operation was 18 days (15-30) in the early group. That the patients did well after waiting a minimum of 2 weeks is not surprising. Some might say that the most useful information in this article is that no additional preop strokes occurred in either group, even waiting up to 120 days to perform endarterectomy. But, of course, the total number of patients is small, and I wouldn't use the information here to justify waiting. Perhaps the best usage of this paper is to line the bird cage.

G. L. Moneta, MD

Early Carotid Endarterectomy for Critical Carotid Artery Stenosis After Thrombolysis Therapy in Acute Ischemic Stroke in the Middle Cerebral Artery
McPherson CM, Woo D, Cohen PL, et al (Univ of Cincinnati, Ohio)
Stroke 32:2075-2080, 2001   12–22

Background.—When to perform carotid endarterectomy (CEA) after a patient has had a stroke is as yet unclear, with reports indicating adverse events after both early and delayed CEA. Acute ischemic stroke can be effectively treated with tissue plasminogen activator (tPA), but patients risk recurrent stroke when a high-grade cervical carotid stenosis is still present after tPA therapy. Performing CEA can reduce the risk of stroke in cases of high-grade cervical carotid stenosis, but the safety of performing CEA after tPA therapy is undetermined. Five patients had early CEA (within less than 48 hours) because of the presence of persistent high-grade cervical carotid stenosis after they had received tPA therapy for acute ischemic stroke affecting the region of the middle cerebral artery (MCA). The safety of this procedure was evaluated.

Methods.—The patients were 4 men and 1 woman (age, 45-64 years) who had an MCA stenosis of more than 99% on the symptomatic side after having undergone tPA therapy. All exhibited neurologic deficits traced to the MCA stenosis. Angiograms had been done, and 3 patients were given intra-aortic tPA, after which CEA was performed. Follow-up extended for 5 to 22 months.

Results.—All patients showed obvious improvement after tPA therapy and after CEA, which was performed under general anesthesia and electro-encephalographic monitoring. In 1 patient, CEA was done within 45 hours; in another, within 26 hours; in 2 others, within 23 hours; and in 1 other, within 6 hours. No intraoperative or postoperative complications developed, and patients were discharged after 3 or 4 days, except the 1 woman whose stay was prolonged because myocardial infraction and respiratory failure had occurred when she suffered her stroke before surgery. No ischemic cerebrovascular events occurred during follow-up, even for the patient whose hospitalization was prolonged.

Conclusions.—When a carotid artery stenosis persists despite tPA therapy, it is apparently safe to perform CEA within 48 hours. The patients for whom this would be most appropriate have mild stable neurologic deficits and show no significant area of stenosis on CT or MRI. Any risk of complications attending early surgery is outweighed by the benefits of CEA for these cases.

▶ CEA for very high-grade cervical internal carotid artery stenosis (greater than 99%) was performed in 5 patients without complication, and within 2 days of the patients undergoing thrombolytic therapy for acute middle cerebral artery stroke. There are a number of limitations of this study: the numbers are small, the post thrombolysis deficits were mild, and no brain imaging information was provided, so we don't know the size of the infarct. The NASCET Study only 1 of 58 patients with nondisabling stroke and preocclusive internal carotid arteries, and who were managed medically had another stroke within 30 days. Therefore, while CEA can be done very early after stroke, it may not actually need to be done early. Certainly, a middle of the night operation is not required.

G. L. Moneta, MD

Carotid Endarterectomy in Women: Challenging the Results From ACAS and NASCET
Mattos MA, Sumner DS, Bohannon WT, et al (Southern Illinois Univ, Springfield)
Ann Surg 234:438-446, 2001   12–23

Background.—The number of carotid endarterectomies (CEAs) performed in the United States substantially increased after reports of randomized trials clearly showed the procedure to reduce the risk of stroke. But because the majority of trial participants have been men, the short- and long-term benefits of CEA in women are less certain. Using data from a 21-year period, investigators evaluated and compared short- and long-term outcomes in women and men after CEA.

Methods.—During the study period (March 1976 to October 1997), 1113 patients who underwent 1249 CEAs had data included in the computerized cerebrovascular surgery registry at Southern Illinois University School of Medicine. Nearly all patients underwent endarterectomy with normocapnic, normotensive general anesthesia. Patch angioplasty was performed selectively by some surgeons and routinely by others. Demographic data and risk factors were available for 413 women (465 CEAs) and 655 men (739 CEAs). The mean follow-up was 48.6 months for women and 50.9 months for men.

Results.—The mean age at CEA was similar for men (68.0 years) and women (68.5 years). Compared with men, women were less likely to have evidence of coronary artery disease and were more likely to be hypertensive and to have a significantly higher incidence of diabetes. The use of shunts, patching, tacking sutures, and severity of carotid stenoses did not differ significantly between men and women. When symptomatic and asymptomatic groups were compared, perioperative stroke rates were similar, and surgical death rates were nearly identical for men and women. Overall, 7 early deaths occurred within 30 days after CEA; 4 patients (3 men and 1 woman) died of cardiac-related complications. Long-term survival rates (at 1, 5, and 8 years) were higher for asymptomatic women compared with men and for symptomatic women compared with men.

Conclusion.—The findings of this review challenge conclusions from the Asymptomatic Carotid Endarterectomy Study and the North American Symptomatic Carotid Endarterectomy Trial. Men and women should have comparable benefits and outcomes (including early and late survival, stroke-free, or stroke-free death rates) after CEA.

▶ I have never regarded females as being at a higher risk with CEA than males. It is always nice to have some data to confirm your prejudices.

G. L. Moneta, MD

Carotid Endarterectomy in Patients 55 Years of Age and Younger
Rockman CB, Svahn JK, Willis DJ, et al (New York Univ)
Ann Vasc Surg 15:557-562, 2001   12–24

Background.—Carotid endarterectomy (CEA) is not often performed in younger patients (aged <55 years), and late complications have been reported to occur more often in this age group than among elderly patients. A series of CEAs performed on younger adults was reviewed to assess whether these patients are at increased risk of recurrent stenosis and to determine reasons for failure of the primary operation.

Methods.—From 1985 through 1994, 94 patients underwent a total of 109 CEAs. A control group selected for comparison of outcomes consisted of 222 patients aged 55 years or more who underwent 256 CEAs from 1991 through 1993. Potential risk factors analyzed included sex, hypertension, diabetes, smoking, and cardiac disease. Follow-up duplex scans were obtained at varying intervals.

Results.—Young and older patients did not differ significantly in sex distribution or the presence of hypertension, diabetes, or cardiac disease. Younger patients, however, were significantly more likely to have a positive history of cigarette smoking (67.8% versus 45.0% for the older group). Indications for surgery also differed significantly between the 2 age groups, with preoperative stroke more common in younger (29.4%) versus older (17.2%) patients. The mean duration of clinical follow-up was 48.1 months in younger patients and 41.2 months in older patients. During follow-up, younger patients were significantly more likely to experience a late failure of CEA, including total occlusion of the operated artery or recurrent stenosis, requiring redo surgery.

Conclusion.—Because patients younger than 55 years are at increased risk for a late failure of CEA, careful patient selection and regular noninvasive follow-up examination are mandatory for this age group. Recommended are an early scan, within 3 months after surgery, and repeat scans every 6 months thereafter.

▶ CEA was as safe, but not as durable, when performed in patients younger than 55 versus those older than 55. This study is not the first to come to this conclusion, but it does remind us that arterial surgery in young patients often just doesn't work out as well as in older patients.

G. L. Moneta, MD

Reoperations for Carotid Artery Stenosis: Role of Primary and Secondary Reconstructions
Archie JP Jr (Wake Med Ctr; Raleigh, NC)
J Vasc Surg 33:495-503, 2001   12–25

Background.—Do a patient's clinical characteristics or the type of primary carotid endarterectomy (CEA) performed affect the outcomes after secondary CEA? Do outcomes differ depending on the type of secondary CEA performed (patch reconstruction or interposition bypass grafting)? These questions were examined by reviewing 1 surgeon's experience.

Methods.—Between August 1981 and June 1999, 66 patients (29 men and 37 women; mean age, 68 years) underwent 69 reoperative CEAs (3 were bilateral). The author had performed the primary CEA in 29 patients (29 procedures, representing 1.9% of 1514 primary CEAs), while other surgeons had performed the primary CEA in 37 patients (including all 3 patients requiring bilateral secondary CEA). Indications for secondary CEA included asymptomatic recurrent stenosis of 70% or greater in 36 patients (52%), transient ischemic attack in 19 (27%), stroke in 8 (12%), and global ischemia in 6 (9%). Secondary procedures included saphenous vein patching in 39 patients (57%), Dacron patching in 20 (29%), polytetrafluoroethylene patching in 1 (1%), and interposition bypass grafting in 9 (13%). After secondary CEA, all patients were followed up at least annually to determine the incidence of re-restenosis, stroke, and death.

Results.—Secondary procedures were significantly less common after primary patching than after primarily closed CEA (1.6% vs 6.2%). The mean time from primary CEA to reoperation was significantly shorter after Dacron patching than after vein-patched CEA (16 vs 84 months). The incidence of secondary CEA and the timing of reoperation were slightly (but not significantly) worse in men and in smokers. The rate of restenosis in the distal common carotid artery was near linear, while restenosis of the internal carotid artery segment had a bimodal distribution, with peaks during the first 3 years and after 7 years. None of the patients died within 30 days of reoperation, but 2 patients (2.9%) experienced a stroke (1 major, 1 minor).

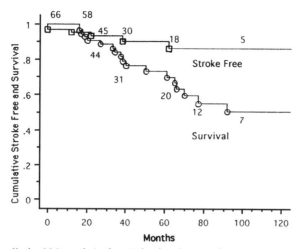

FIGURE 4.—Kaplan-Meier analysis of survival and stroke rates after secondary carotid artery operations. SE is 6.7% at 5 years and 9.3% at 10 years for survival. SE is 4.3% at 5 years and 5.9% at 10 years for
stroke. (Courtesy of Archie JP Jr: Reoperations for carotid artery stenosis: Role of primary and secondary
reconstructions. *J Vasc Surg* 33:495-503, 2001.)

During a mean follow-up of 50 months, Kaplan-Meier estimates of cumulative survival were 74% and 54% at 5 and 10 years, respectively (Fig 4).
Stroke-free estimates at 5 and 10 years were 90% and 86%, respectively. After the secondary CEA, re-restenosis developed in 29 patients (44%), including 17 (25%) with 25% restenosis or greater, 9 (13%) with 50% restenosis
or greater, and 3 (4%) with 70% restenosis or greater. The type of secondary
procedure did not significantly affect the rates of stroke or re-restenosis after
secondary CEA.

Conclusion.—Secondary CEA is required more commonly after primarily
closure of the CEA site than after patching. Perioperative mortality and
stroke rates after secondary procedures are similar to those after primary
procedures. However, in this study, survival after secondary CEA was significantly worse than survival after primary CEA, even after controlling for
age. Stroke and re-recurrence rates after secondary CEA were similar to
those in the literature, and both the current study and results from the literature suggest that outcomes are similar after secondary CEA with the use of
vein or Dacron patching, but that polytetrafluoroethylene appears to be better than vein or Dacron patching for interposition bypass grafting.

▶ In Dr Archie's hands, reoperative carotid surgery is quite safe and associated with little in the way of technical complications. The operations are also durable (see Fig 4). There is genuine concern whether these types of results are
generalizable; thus, the increasing use of carotid stents in patients with recurrent stenosis. While it seems in some centers any excuse is sufficient to de-
ploy a carotid stent, restenosis may be a reasonable indication in institutions
where the results of redo carotid surgery may not be optimal. Of course, rather

than have an experimental, nonreimbursable procedure, the patients could be referred to a surgeon skilled in reoperative surgery. That would work too.

G. L. Moneta, MD

Redo Carotid Endarterectomy Versus Primary Carotid Endarterectomy
AbuRahma AF, Jennings TG, Wulu JT, et al (West Virginia Univ, Charleston; Camcare Health Education and Research Inst, Charleston, WVA; Boehringer Ingelheim Pharmaceuticals, Inc, Ridgefield, Conn)
Stroke 32:2787-2792, 2001   12–26

Background.—Carotid endarterectomy (CEA) has long been one of the most commonly performed procedures in the United States, and recent studies have confirmed the benefits of this procedure for patients with specific levels of carotid artery stenosis. The incidence of recurrent carotid stenosis after primary CEA has been reported to range from 10% to 25%. It is generally agreed that reoperation for significant recurrent carotid artery stenosis is indicated in patients with symptomatic disease. Surgery has also been recommended by several authors for more than 80% asymptomatic restenosis. Recently carotid stenting has been recommended for the treatment of carotid stenosis because of the perception that reoperation is accompanied by a higher complication rate than primary CEA. The early and late results of reoperation versus primary CEA were compared.

Methods.—Reoperations for recurrent carotid stenosis performed by a single surgeon over 7 years were compared with primary CEA. All of the reoperations employed polytetrafluoroethylene (PTFE) or vein patch closure, so only primary CEA procedures that used these same patch closures were included. Estimation of stroke-free survival rates and freedom from $\geq 50\%$ recurrent stenosis was done with a Kaplan-Meier life-table analysis.

Results.—There was a total of 547 primary CEAs, of which 256 had PTFE or saphenous vein patch closure, and 124 reoperations had PTFE or vein patch closure during the study period. Demographic characteristics for both groups were similar. Indications for reoperation and primary CEA were symptomatic stenosis in 78% and 58% of the patients and $\geq 80\%$ stenosis in 22% and 42% of the patients, respectively. The 30-day perioperative stroke rates for reoperation and primary CEA were 4.8% versus 0.8%, and the transient ischemic attack rates for reoperation and primary CEA were 4% versus 1.1%. There were no perioperative deaths in either group. Cranial nerve injury was noted in 17% of the reoperation patients, compared with 5.3% in primary CEA patients. However, for the most part, these injuries were transient. The mean hospital stay was 1.8 days for reoperation compared with 1.6 days for primary CEA. Cumulative rates of stroke-free survival and freedom from 50% or greater recurrent stenosis at 1, 3, and 5 years were 96%, 91%, and 82% and 98%, 96%, and 95%, respectively, for reoperation and 94%, 92%, and 91% and 98%, 96%, and 96%, respectively, for primary CEAs. These cumulative rates were not significantly different for the 2 groups.

Conclusions.—Perioperative stroke and cranial nerve injury rates are higher for reoperation than for primary CEA. However, reoperations are durable, and the stroke-free survival rates for the 2 procedures are similar. These findings should be considered when one is recommending carotid stenting versus reoperation; it would appear that reoperation remains the standard of care for recurrent carotid artery stenosis in most patients with an acceptable level of risk.

▶ I guess if you are in the South and need reoperative carotid surgery it may be better to go to Raleigh than Charleston (see Abstract 12–25).

G. L. Moneta, MD

Determinants of Carotid Microembolization
Golledge J, Gibbs R, Irving C, et al (Imperial College School of Medicine, London; Bristol Royal Infirmary, London)
J Vasc Surg 34:1060-1064, 2001   12–27

Introduction.—Previous studies report that female sex, preoperative symptoms, and cerebral infarction are risk factors for perioperative stroke for patients undergoing carotid endarterectomy. Mechanisms responsible for perioperative stroke are intraoperative and postoperative thromboembolism (60%), ischemia during carotid artery clamping (20%), and intracranial hemorrhage (20%). Transcranial Doppler US scanning (TCD) was performed preoperatively and intraoperatively during carotid endarterectomy to investigate the relationship between the risk factors for stroke and perioperative microembolization.

Methods.—Transcranial Doppler US scanning was possible in 190 (81%) of 235 patients entered into the study. Scanning was performed to detect microemboli, as signaled by high-intensity transient signals, and to monitor middle cerebral artery velocity. Patient characteristics recorded included age, sex, the presence of symptoms, and history of stroke, hypertension, and diabetes. The operations were performed at 2 hospitals; all employed a general anesthetic under normotensive and normocapnic conditions. Risk for complications was assessed in hospital and at a 6-week follow-up examination. A neurologic deficit immediately after the procedure was defined as an intraoperative stroke.

Results.—Microemboli (ME) were detected in 28 patients (15%) preoperatively, in 79 (42%) during carotid artery dissection, and in 98 (52%) after closure of the artery. ME during carotid dissection were highly predicted by the presence of preoperative ME, whereas ME after closure of the carotid artery were only predicted by the occurrence of emboli during dissection of the carotid artery. The presence of 10 or more closure emboli were more common in women and in patients with symptoms and were highly predicted by the occurrence of ME during carotid dissection. In addition, 10 or more closure emboli were found in 3 of 6 patients who had a perioperative stroke; these 3 patients had preoperative evidence of cerebral infarction and an intraoperative middle cerebral artery velocity of less than 40 cm/s.

Conclusion.—Data obtained with TCD suggest that patients undergoing carotid endarterectomy are at increased risk of perioperative stroke because of higher rates of thromboembolism or increased susceptibility. Perioperative microembolization is more common in women and in patients with carotid artery disease.

▶ Intraoperative and perioperative TCD monitoring continues to be technology in search of an application. It makes for interesting research, but it is basically too cumbersome and expensive to be used routinely in most centers. Also, the predictive values to identify clinical events are so low it is impossible to know what to do with the information in an individual patient.

G. L. Moneta, MD

Assessment of Silent Embolism From Carotid Endarterectomy by Use of Diffusion-Weighted Imaging: Work in Progress
Forbes KPN, Shill HA, Britt PM, et al (Barrow Neurological Inst, Phoenix, Ariz)
AJNR Am J Neuroradiol 22:650-653, 2001   12–28

Background.—Carotid endarterectomy (CEA), performed to decrease the risk of subsequent stroke, may itself result in postoperative neurologic deficit. Transcranial Doppler studies suggest that cerebral embolism occurs during the majority of CEA procedures, and some emboli may cause clinically silent infarction. The risk of asymptomatic infarction from CEA was investigated by the use of diffusion-weighted imaging.

Methods.—Included in the prospective study were 12 men and 6 women with a median age of 68 years. All were scheduled for CEA for carotid stenosis, which was symptomatic in 9 patients. Participants were evaluated with diffusion-weighted imaging at a median of 2.5 hours before surgery and 15 hours after surgery. In all cases, single-shot echo-planar imaging was performed with a maximum diffusion sensitivity of b = 1000 s/mm^2 applied to 3 orthogonal planes. Images were independently interpreted by 2 radiologists blinded to operative status and detailed clinical findings.

Results.—Seventeen patients had normal neurologic examination results preoperatively. The remaining patient had a National Institutes of Health (NIH) Stroke Scale score of 6 before CEA, reflecting a hemiparesis on the contralateral side. After surgery, 1 patient had an increase in the NIH Stroke Scale score from 0 to 1, but this change was attributed to mild postoperative confusion. No patient had diffusion-weighted imaging evidence of silent embolism.

Conclusion.—The findings in this small series of patients with carotid stenosis indicate that CEA is a safe procedure, carrying a low risk of complications, including that of clinically silent cerebral infarction. Compared with clinical assessment, diffusion-weighted imaging is more sensitive to perioperative cerebral infarction.

▶ No silent perioperative cerebral infarcts occurred in this small series. Other investigators, however, have found silent perioperative cerebral infarction to be relatively common.[1] As in all cases of small series with widely different results, the truth probably lies somewhere in between. The clinical significance of silent perioperative cerebral infarction, however, remains unknown.

G. L. Moneta, MD

Reference

1. Muller M, Reiche W, Langenscheidt P, et al: Ischemia after carotid endarterectomy: Comparison between transcranial Doppler sonography and diffusion-weighted MR imaging. *AJNR Am J Neuroradiol* 21:47-54, 2000.

Dextran Reduces Embolic Signals After Carotid Endarterectomy
Levi CR, Stork JL, Chambers BR, et al (John Hunter Hosp, Newcastle, Australia; Monash Univ, Melbourne, Australia; Natl Stroke Research Inst, Melbourne, Australia)
Ann Neurol 50:544-547, 2001   12–29

Background.—Thromboembolism accounts for 38% to 68% of perioperative neurologic events associated with carotid endarterectomy (CEA). Transcranial Doppler (TCD) is ideally suited for detection of cerebral emboli. Dextran is a polysaccharide that reduces platelet adhesion to vascular grafts and improves the patency of lower limb arterial bypass grafts. Whether dextran reduces embolic signals in the early postoperative period after CEA was investigated.

Methods.—A group of 150 patients undergoing CEA were randomly assigned to receive either IV 10% dextran 40 or placebo. TCD monitoring of the ipsilateral middle cerebral artery was used to detect embolic signals.

Results.—TCD detected embolic signals at 1 hour or earlier postoperatively in 57% of patients in the placebo group and 42% of those in the dextran group. At 2 to 3 hours postoperatively, embolic signals were present in 45% of patients in the placebo group and 27% in the dextran group. Embolic signal counts were 64% less in patients in the dextran group.

Conclusions.—In patients undergoing CEA, the IV infusion of 10% dextran 40 reduces embolic signals within 3 hours of the procedure.

▶ One is left to wonder what the perioperative stroke rate was in these patients. In patients on preoperative aspirin, I am not convinced dextran is useful for anything other than a volume expander. We don't use it on our vascular surgical service. Again, the information in this study is hard to extrapolate to routine clinical practice.

G. L. Moneta, MD

Serum S100B Protein Levels Are Correlated With Subclinical Neurocognitive Declines After Carotid Endarterectomy

Connolly ES Jr, Winfree CJ, Rampersad A, et al (Columbia Univ, New York)
Neurosurgery 49:1076-1083, 2001   12–30

Background.—Many patients experience subtle cognitive injuries after carotid endarterectomy (CEA) that can be assessed by neuropsychometric tests (NPMTs). Other indicators of severe neurologic injury include neuron-specific enolase (NSE; a glycolytic enzyme present in neurons and neuroendocrine cells) and S100B (a calcium-binding protein involved in neuronal and glial cell-cell communication and intracellular signal transduction). The possible correlations between NSE and S100B levels and NPMT results in patients with cognitive injury after CEA were examined.

Methods.—The subjects were 55 patients undergoing elective CEA; 2 patients experienced postoperative stroke and were excluded. The remaining 53 patients underwent a battery of NPMTs at 24 hours before and at 24 hours after surgery. Tests were administered more than 3 hours after any analgesic or sedative medications had been given. Venous blood samples were drawn preoperatively; just before clamping of the internal carotid artery; and at 24, 48, and 72 hours after surgery for measuring levels of NSE and S100B. NSE and S100B levels were compared between the patients whose preoperative and postoperative NPMT scores did not change (41 patients; uninjured group) and those whose postoperative scores declined significantly (12 patients; injured group).

Results.—Demographic data did not differ significantly between the injured patients (68% men; mean age, 70.7 years) and the injured group (50% men; mean age, 72.7 years). Baseline NSE and S100B levels were also similar between the 2 groups. NSE levels did not differ significantly from baseline at any time point in either group. S100B levels, however, were significantly higher than baseline in the injured group during clamping and at 24, 48, and 72 hours after surgery, but did not differ significantly from baseline in the uninjured group. The greatest increase in S100B levels in the injured patients was measured at 24 hours after surgery.

Conclusion.—About 25% of these patients undergoing CEA experienced subtle, yet significant, neurocognitive declines in the absence of overt stroke. Serum S100B levels increased significantly in the patients whose NPMT scores declined significantly after surgery. Given the short half-life of S100B, it would be interesting to see whether earlier measurements of S100B would correlate more strongly with postoperative NPMT results and thus become a useful biochemical marker of cerebral injury after CEA.

▶ It is disturbing that with detailed testing subtle cognitive dysfunction is evident in otherwise neurologically normal patients 24 hours after CEA. A marker of brain injury indicating glial cell death (serum S100B protein levels) was elevated postoperatively in the patients with cognitive dysfunction. These serum S100B protein levels declined rapidly but were still elevated over baseline at 72 hours postoperatively. The levels of this protein also were increased in the "injured" patients intraoperatively. The data remind one of the neuropsychiatric deficits detected after cardiopulmonary bypass. The clinical significance of all this is unknown. I am not prepared to say CEA results in a loss of IQ points. I am reasonably sure, however, the operation doesn't make the patient any smarter either. In this situation, a tie is a victory.

G. L. Moneta, MD

Mechanisms of Intracerebral Hemorrhage After Carotid Endarterectomy
Henderson RD, Phan TG, Piepgras DG, et al (Mayo Clinic, Rochester, Minn)
J Neurosurg 95:964-969, 2001   12–31

Background.—Fewer than 1% of patients undergoing carotid endarterectomy (CEA) suffer an intracerebral hemorrhage (ICH), yet this development accounts for up to one fourth of all neurologic complications occurring postoperatively and carries high rates of morbidity and mortality. The clinical and radiologic findings in patients who developed ICH after CEA were reviewed to evaluate the risk factors leading to ICH, with the objective of determining the factors that differed between patients who had an ICH after CEA and those who had not.

Methods.—A computerized record search was used to identify patients undergoing a CEA at the Mayo Clinic between January 1990 and December 1999 who had an ICH; 12 such patients were found, and 44 control subjects were chosen from among patients who underwent CEA and had US and MRI of the carotid artery during the same decade as those in the group who had an ICH. Assessments included evaluations of known cerebrovascular risk factors, perioperative electroencephalographic studies, and cerebral blood flow (CBF) studies. Possible underlying mechanisms were sought among the clinical histories and imaging of ischemic events along with the ICH.

Results.—An increase in CBF of more than 100% occurred in 5 of 8 patients with ICH who had CBF studies performed. ICH after CEA generally occurred within the first week; it was noted in symptomatic patients after reopening of severe arterial obstruction, and was ipsilateral to the CEA. Differences were noted between the ICH and control groups with respect to the number of patients who had the CBF double after CEA and to the mean change in CBF before and after CEA. In 7 patients, cerebral hyperperfusion syndrome (HPS) contributed to the development of ICH. When HPS was a major contributing factor, hemorrhage occurred 3 to 8 days after CEA, and the ICH occurred in the anterior circulation but did not usually bleed directly into the infarcted area. Three patients showed clinical symptoms of HPS. Four patients suffered a perioperative cerebral ischemic event, and 6 had anticoagulation therapy—these factors also contributing to the subsequent ICH. Of the 12 patients suffering ICH, a moderate outcome was achieved in 5 patients, and 7 patients died.

Conclusions.—ICH occurred ipsilateral to the CEA and occurred in the first week after CEA in most cases. It was usually caused by hyperperfusion, a perioperative cerebral ischemic event, anticoagulation therapy, or multiple mechanisms. A doubling of the CBF is a risk factor for subsequent ICH.

▶ This is a sufficiently large series of CEAs (2747) with a sufficiently large number of postoperative ICHs (n = 12) that is actually worth reading. There was no clear clinical risk factor identified for ICH. Because of the peculiar use of intraoperative ^{133}Xe measured cerebral blood flow by the neurosurgeons at the Mayo Clinic, the authors were able to document increased cerebral blood flow compared with controls in the patients with ICH. Intraoperative stroke, euphemistically termed "operative cerebral ischemic event" by the authors, also appeared associated with postoperative ICH, as did postoperative use of heparin.

G. L. Moneta, MD

Remifentanil Conscious Sedation During Regional Anaesthesia for Carotid Endarterectomy: Rationale and Safety

Marrocco-Trischitta MM, Bandiera G, Camilli S, et al ("Istituto Dermopatico dell Immacolata," Rome)
Eur J Vasc Endovasc Surg 22:405-409, 2001   12–32

Background.—The optimal anesthetic modality in patients undergoing carotid endarterectomy (CEA) is controversial. Overall, regional anesthesia may be associated with a lower morbidity and mortality rate than general anesthesia, but general anesthesia has been widely and successfully used for CEA with very low perioperative complication rates. Apparent differences between the 2 techniques may be a product of differences in patient populations. Regional anesthesia can be used to assess mental status during carotid artery cross-clamping. Mental status evaluation significantly reduces the requirement for shunting and provides early detection of perioperative neurologic events. Objections to regional anesthesia include anxiety and discomfort to the patient that result from being awake during surgery and patient movement during the procedure. Remifentanil is a potent μ-opioid agonist with an ultrashort half-life and duration of effect. The safety and efficacy of remifentanil during regional anesthesia for CEA were prospectively evaluated.

Methods.—A consecutive series of 28 patients underwent CEA with combined superficial and deep cervical plexus block supplemented with continuous intravenous 0.04 $\mu g \cdot kg^{-1} \cdot min^{-1}$ remifentanil infusion. The Observer's Assessment of Alertness Scale (OAA/S) was used to monitor the depth of sedation, with 5 signifying awake and alert and 1 signifying asleep. Patients self-assessed the degree of pain, discomfort, and anxiety they experienced according to a horizontal visual analog scale.

Results.—Comfort and analgesia were rated as satisfactory by all patients, and there was no need in any patient for local anesthetic supplementation. None of the patients had an OAA/S score lower than 4. There were no incidents of respiratory depression. Four patients required selective shunting. None of the patients were converted to general anesthesia. There were no permanent neurologic deficits, cardiopulmonary complications, or deaths.

Conclusions.—Remifentanil can be used to supplement regional anesthesia in patients undergoing CEA to provide comfort and analgesia without interfering with the evaluation of mental status in these patients.

▶ Remifentanil is an opiate agonist with a very short half-life that, at low doses, does not supposedly alter mental status. It appears it can be safely used to perhaps increase patient comfort without affecting mental status during regional anesthesia for CEA. It can also be used during general anesthesia for CEA. In such cases after the general anesthetic, the patients appear to wake up faster, thereby facilitating postoperative neurologic assessment in the operating room.

G. L. Moneta, MD

Carotid Dissection With and Without Ischemic Events: Local Symptoms and Cerebral Artery Findings

Baumgartner RW, Arnold M, Baumgartner I, et al (Univ Hosp, Zurich, Switzerland; Univ Hosp, Bern, Switzerland)
Neurology 57:827-832, 2001   12–33

Background.—Extracranial internal carotid artery dissection (ICAD) has been recognized as 1 of the most frequent causes of ischemic stroke for patients aged less than 50 years. In most patients, ICAD causes permanent or transient ischemia of the brain or retina and is often preceded by local signs and symptoms on the side of dissection. These signs and symptoms of ICAD include headache, neck pain, Horner syndrome, pulsatile tinnitus, and palsy of the cranial nerves. However, in some patients, ICAD causes no cerebral or retinal ischemia, but manifests only local signs and symptoms or remains clinically asymptomatic. Whether spontaneous dissections of the cervical ICAD with and without ischemia of the brain differ in the prevalence of vascular risk factors, local neurologic signs and symptoms, and stenoses and occlusions of the cerebral arteries was investigated.

Methods.—A consecutive series of 181 patients with 200 ICADs were prospectively studied. The diagnosis of ICAD was based on US, MRI, or catheter angiography. Vascular risk factors, presenting and ischemic signs and symptoms, and US findings in the carotid and basal cerebral arteries were evaluated.

Results.—Ischemic events occurred in 145 ICADs, and these events had a higher prevalence of hypercholesterolemia, more than 80% stenoses and occlusions of the internal carotid artery, and had intracranial obstructions. The 55 ICADs without ischemic events had a higher prevalence of Horner syndrome, cranial nerve palsy, and normal ICA findings (Table 4).

Conclusions.—These findings suggest that ICADs that cause high-grade stenosis and occlusion are more likely to lead to intracranial obstructions

TABLE 4.—Cerebrovascular Findings in 55 Latency-Matched Carotid Dissections With and 55 Carotid Dissections Without Ischemic Events

Artery	Finding	Ischemic Events, n (%)		P Value for Ischemia vs No Ischemia
		Yes (n = 55)	No (n = 55)	
Extracranial internal carotid artery	Normal	3 (5)	16 (29)	<.01
	Stenosis ≤50%	3 (5)	9 (16)	NS
	Stenosis >50%	5 (11)	8 (15)	NS
	Stenosis >80% and occlusion	43 (81)	22 (40)	<.0001
Intracranial arteries*	Stenosis or occlusion	9 (16)	2 (4)	<.05
Median latency (range)	Symptom onset, ultrasonography	10 d (4-114 d)	10 d (0-125 d)	NS

*Middle and anterior cerebral arteries.
(Courtesy of Baumgartner RW, Arnold M, Baumgartner I, et al: Carotid dissection with and without ischemic events: Local symptoms and cerebral artery findings. *Neurology* 57:827-832, 2001. Copyright American Academy of Neurology. Used with permission of Lippincott-Raven Publishers.)

and cerebral and retinal ischemic events. In contrast, ICADs not associated with luminal narrowing manifest more local signs and symptoms.

▶ This is an enormous series of patients with carotid dissection. In addition to the findings detailed in the abstract regarding association with cerebral ischemia, it is interesting that the classic findings of carotid dissection are not all that classic. Overall, about 65% of patients had headache, 20% neck pain, and less than 50% Horner's syndrome. Overall, an excellent review of carotid dissection.

G. L. Moneta, MD

Skull Base Resection With Cervical-to-Petrous Carotid Artery Bypass to Facilitate Repair of Distal Internal Carotid Artery Lesions
Eliason JL, Netterville JL, Guzman RJ, et al (Vanderbilt Univ, Nashville, Tenn)
Cardiovasc Surg 10:31-37, 2002   12–34

Background.—Numerous methods enable exposure of the distal extracranial internal carotid artery (ICA), but the only way to reach the last centimeter of the ICA before it enters the carotid canal is by resecting the mastoid process at the skull base. An approach to treating isolated distal extracranial ICA lesions via resection of the mastoid process and bypass grafting was described.

 Technique.—The technique of lateral skull base resection with cervical-to-petrous carotid artery saphenous vein bypass, in brief, is as follows. A curvilinear incision extending to the posterior aspect of the earlobe is made to expose and isolate the jugular vein, ICA, and cranial nerves (CNs) X–XII. Exposure is widened by resecting the posterior belly of the digastric muscle and the level II jugular nodes. The ICA can be exposed up to the skull base by excising the stylohyoid and stylopharyngeus muscles and resecting the styloid process.
 If these steps allow sufficient access to the ICA lesion, vascular repair can be completed. If not, more distal exposure of the ICA is obtained by bringing up the cervical incision around the earlobe anterior to the ear, up into the temporal region, and forward to the hairline (Fig 4). A temporary flap is raised and the zygomatic arch is identified. To preserve the temporal branch of CN VII, the deep temporal fascia is incised, but the remainder of the nerve is left intact. The temporomandibular joint is then bluntly moved forward out of its fossa and held in place by retractors to expose the glenoid fossa. The glenoid is resected with the aid of an operative microscope to expose the first vertical portion of the petrous ICA and the second horizontal portion of the intrapetrous ICA (Fig 5).
 The skull base resection is extended to the dura if the entire petrous carotid artery needs to be exposed. The chorda tympani nerve and eustachian tube are divided, and the ICA is drilled free. A reversed

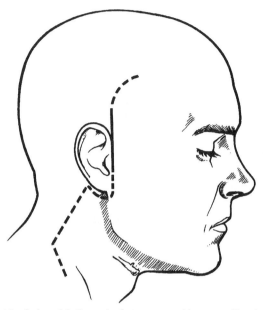

FIGURE 4.—Incision for lateral skull resection for petrous carotid exposure. (Reprinted by permission of the publisher from Eliason JL, Netterville JL, Guzman RJ, et al: Skull base resection with cervical-to-petrous carotid artery bypass to facilitate repair of distal internal carotid artery lesions. *Cardiovasc Surg* 10:31-37, 2002. Copyright 2002 by Elsevier Science Inc.)

saphenous vein graft harvested from the groin is anastomosed to the origin of the ICA, with spatulation onto the common carotid artery. Distal anastomosis to the vertical portion of the petrous ICA can be accomplished through the cervical incision. Distal anastomosis to the horizontal portion can be performed through a small opening in the lateral skull base. This approach has been used in 5 patients with skull base ICA lesions who were operated on between 1993 and 1999.

Results.—The patients ranged in age from 51 to 80 years. All 5 patients had aneurysmal changes; changes were nonspecific atherosclerotic in 3 cases and dysplastic in 2 cases. The mean operative time was 7.2 hours. Preoperative neurologic symptoms occurred in 2 patients with transient ischemic attack (TIA), 2 with dysphagia, and 1 with Horner's syndrome with vascular headache. TIAs, Horner's syndrome, and 1 case of dysphagia resolved completely after surgery; the other case of dysphagia improved after surgery.

Postoperatively, all 5 patients experienced paresis in the distribution of CN VII (transient in 4 cases), permanent loss of the eustachian tube (resulting in mild hearing loss), and permanent loss of the chorda tympani nerve (which caused taste alteration in 1 patient). In addition, there were 2 cases of transient CN IX deficit and 2 cases of transient CN XI deficit. The 1 patient with residual paresis experienced a minor intraoperative stroke that resulted in arm weakness and seizure; however, at 1 year, arm weakness had resolved.

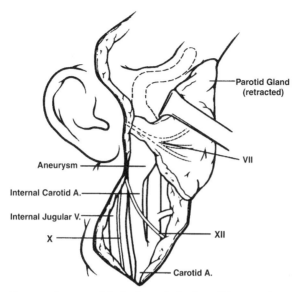

Parotid Gland
(retracted)

VII

Aneurysm

Internal Carotid A.

Internal Jugular V.

X

XII

Carotid A.

FIGURE 5.—Exposure after temporal flap has been raised and mandible retracted anteriorly. (Reprinted by permission of the publisher from Eliason JL, Netterville JL, Guzman RJ, et al: Skull base resection with cervical-to-petrous carotid artery bypass to facilitate repair of distal internal carotid artery lesions. *Cardiovasc Surg* 10:31-37, 2002. Copyright 2002 by Elsevier Science Inc.)

Duplex US at a mean of 45.8 months of follow-up identified no graft occlusions, nor were there any ipsilateral strokes or deaths during follow-up.

Conclusion.—Skull base resection with a cervical-to-petrous carotid artery saphenous vein bypass graft provides a valuable option for patients with skull base ICA lesions.

▶ This appears a useful technique for the very occasional patient with an ICA lesion at the skull base. I wouldn't, however, do this without a surgeon who routinely works in this area. In our hospital, that would be an ear, nose, and throat surgeon with special interest in head and neck cancer.

G. L. Moneta, MD

Procedural Safety and Short-term Outcome of Ambulatory Carotid Stenting
Al-Mubarak N, Roubin GS, Vitek JJ, et al (Lenox Hill Heart and Vascular Inst of New York)
Stroke 32:2305-2309, 2001   12–35

Background.—Elective carotid stenting is a less invasive endovascular alternative to carotid endarterectomy, and the stenting procedure has been reported to be successful in preventing stroke for patients with occlusive carotid artery disease. The procedural safety and short-term outcomes of patients with ambulatory carotid stenting were investigated.

Methods.—Between April 1999 and January 2001, 98 of 341 carotid stenting procedures were able to be completed on 92 patients (66 men, 26 women; mean age, 70 years) in an ambulatory setting. All patients had previous duplex US or MR angiographic evidence of severe carotid artery stenosis. Procedures were performed for patients in the conscious state without general anesthesia or sedation. The patients were observed for approximately 6 hours after carotid stenting and had neurologic evaluations before intervention and before discharge, which required that specific criteria be met. Short-term follow-up (mean, 6 months) was completed in 96% of the 92 ambulatory patients.

Results.—Most patients (72%) were asymptomatic, but the remaining patients had neurologic symptoms related to the treated artery within 3 months before the procedure. Suture-mediated vascular closure devices achieved successful access site hemostasis for 96 patients; manual compression was used for 2. Transient bradycardia occurred in 38% of procedures and transient hypotension in 14%, but no patient experienced sustained hemodynamic instability. During follow-up, no deaths, neurologic events, or major access site complications occurred, and no repeated procedures were required.

Conclusion.—After carotid stenting, patients at low risk for postprocedural complications can be identified and safely discharged home on the same day. Early discharge requirements are the absence of neurologic events within 6 hours after a successful intervention and successful vascular access site hemostasis.

▶ The envelope continues to be pushed by the zealots.

G. L. Moneta, MD

Technical Aspects and Current Results of Carotid Stenting
d'Audiffret A, Desgranges P, Kobeiter H, et al (Centre Hospitalier Universitaire Henri-Mondor, Paris)
J Vasc Surg 33:1001-1007, 2001   12–36

Introduction.—Recent reviews have attempted to give objective summaries of currently available data. These reviews cannot provide data concerning the impact of new technology. An experience with carotid stenting (CS) is reviewed with a focus on the procedure's technical evolution. Immediate and intermediate results are reported since the first (1995) carotid angioplasty with a stent.

Methods.—Between September 1995 to February 2000, 77 patients with 83 arterial lesions (68 internal carotid artery [ICA]; 15 common carotid artery [CCA]) were selected for CS. These patients were categorized into 3 consecutive periods, based on patient selection, material, and technical skills. For ICA lesions, period 1 was made up of 11 patients treated via direct carotid puncture with balloon expandable stents; in period 2, 42 patients were treated via a femoral approach with the use of self-expandable stents; in pe-

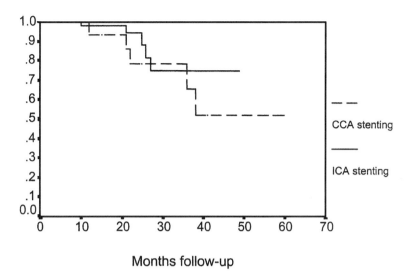

Months follow-up

FIGURE 4.—Cumulative survival rate free of restenosis and neurologic events in patients with common carotid artery (CCA) or internal carotid artery (ICA) stenting. (Courtesy of d'Audiffret A, Desgranges P, Kobeiter H, et al: Technical aspects and current results of carotid stenting. *J Vasc Surg* 33:1001-1007, 2001.)

riod 3, 15 patients were treated with a monorail system and cerebral protection devices. CCA lesions were treated via carotid puncture in 5 patients and via the femoral approach in 10 patients. Cerebral protection devices were used in 2 patients who underwent the femoral approach.

Results.—The overall immediate success rate, defined as successfully treated stenosis with no neurologic events, was 89.7% and 100% for ICA and CCA lesions, respectively. All neurologic events occurred in periods 1 and 2 and included reversible events, minor strokes, and major strokes in 4.4%, 1.5%, and 2.9% of patients. During periods 1, 2, and 3, the rates of surgical conversion were 18%, 9.5%, and 0%, respectively; the rates of a transient ischemic attack with a reversible ischemic neurologic deficit were 0%, 7%, and 0%, respectively; the minor and major stroke rates were 0%, 7%, and 0%, respectively. The use of intra-arterial thrombolysis cleared all major strokes. At discharge, the success rate, which was considered the absence of conversion and neurologic events, was 82%, 76%, and 100% during periods 1, 2, and 3, respectively. The rates for freedom from neurologic deficits were 100%, 97.6%, and 100% for periods 1, 2, and 3, respectively. Differences were not significant for the life-table analysis of survival free of symptoms and recurrent stenosis for CCA and ICA stenting (Fig 4). During follow-up, 6 significant asymptomatic restenoses were identified with duplex scanning. One patient needed reintervention.

Conclusion.—Technical skills and technological improvements, including low-profile balloons and catheters, cerebral protection devices, and intra-arterial rescue techniques, may decrease the rate of neurologic events associated with CS. Technical improvements need to undergo careful consideration before initiation of randomized trials comparing CS and carotid endarterectomy.

▶ The authors provide a chronology of CS at their institution over about a 5-year period. The authors feel current results are better than earlier results, although no statistical analysis is provided. I wonder how this slipped by the editors of *JVS*?

G. L. Moneta, MD

Endovascular Treatment of Severe Symptomatic Stenosis of the Internal Carotid Artery: Early and Late Outcome
Baudier J-F, Licht PB, Røder O, et al (Odense Univ, Denmark)
Eur J Vasc Endovasc Surg 22:205-210, 2001   12–37

Background.—Carotid thromboendarterectomy (CEA) is currently the preferred treatment for symptomatic stenosis exceeding 70% in the internal carotid artery. This approach has been associated with a 17% decrease in the risk of ipsilateral stroke after 2 years. Carotid percutaneous transluminal angioplasty (CPTA) has several advantages over CEA, including a shorter treatment duration, no need for general anesthesia, avoidance of surgical stress, and avoidance of possible surgical complications such as peripheral nerve lesions and hemorrhage. A 6-year experience with CPTA was reported.

Methods.—Fifty-four patients undergoing CPTA between 1993 and 1999 were included in the retrospective analysis. Eighteen had stent deployment and 36 did not. All but 1 patient had had focal hemispheric neurologic symptoms. In the same time period, 284 patients underwent CEA. The 54 patients treated with CPTA were selected based on the carotid angiogram. The only inclusion criterion for endovascular treatment was short, concentric, smooth stenosis exceeding 70% with no ulceration or severe calcification.

Findings.—In the first 30 days after treatment, CPTA was considered technically successful in 93% of the patients. Eighteen percent of the patients had a neurologic event related to the procedure and 2% had a major stroke. One stent became occluded within 30 days of the procedure. At a median follow-up of 34 months, 13% of patients had recurrent symptoms. Color-duplex examination in 45 patients indicated internal carotid artery occlusion in 5% of patients and restenosis of more than 70% in 22%. The recurrence of neurologic symptoms and restenosis rate did not differ significantly between patients treated with and without stents.

Conclusions.—In this group of selected patients, CPTA was associated with mortality and stroke rates comparable to that of CEA. However, CPTA was also associated with a high risk of transient neurologic events and incidence of restenosis after 3 years.

▶ This is one of the few carotid angioplasty series I am aware of in which virtually all (53 of 54) patients had symptomatic carotid lesions. In addition, the lesions are what one would consider ideal for CPTA: short, concentric, smooth lesions without ulceration or severe calcification. Despite this, the total procedural neurologic event rate was 18%, and there was a high restenosis rate. Stents made no difference in the periprocedure complication rate or restenosis rate. The results are probably honest; no one fudges poor results. At the very least, they suggest protection devices should be strongly considered in patients with symptoms referable to their carotid lesion.

G. L. Moneta, MD

Multicenter Evaluation of Carotid Artery Stenting With a Filter Protection System

Al-Mubarak N, Colombo A, Gaines PA, et al (Lenox Hill Heart and Vascular Inst, New York; Centro Cuore Colombus-Interventional Cardiology, Milan, Italy; Sheffield Vascular Inst, England)

J Am Coll Cardiol 39:841-846, 2002   12–38

Background.—Neurologic events can complicate the performance of carotid artery stenting (CAS) and may result from embolized friable thrombotic and atherosclerotic components from the obstructive carotid artery lesions. Some "distal protection" strategies have been used to capture this debris and reduce the risk. A temporary intravascular filter was placed to capture embolized debris in the distal internal carotid artery (ICA) during CAS, and patient outcomes were assessed to determine the feasibility and safety of this strategy.

Methods.—CAS with filter protection (Fig 1) was performed in 162 patients (164 hemispheres; age, 51-85 years; mean age, 68 years) between September 1999 and July 2001. Prospective protocols were followed at 3 institutions to evaluate the process and patient outcomes.

Results.—During the 3 months before CAS was performed, 48% of patients had symptoms that could be attributed to the treated artery. For 99% of the patients, angiographic success was achieved, with successful placement and retrieval of the filter in 94% of patients. Eight percent of cases required a predilation and/or "buddy wire" to ease placement of the filter, and placement failed in 5% of cases. When the filter was placed successfully, flow through the ICA was preserved. None of the filters failed, and 35% of them retrieved macroscopically visible fragments (fibrin, cholesterol clefts, organized thrombi, and red and white blood cell aggregates). Three percent of patients had a non–flow-limiting spasm that resolved after the filter was removed; 2% had spasm that limited flow. No clinical sequelae developed in these cases, nor were there vascular dissections. Minor strokes developed in 1% of patients, 1 in a patient for whom filter placement failed. Complete recovery was achieved within 48 hours. Of the 154 patients who had successful deployment of the filter, only 1 embolic neurologic event occurred. After 30 days, the combined rate of strokes and deaths was 2% (4 events), including 2 minor strokes and 2 deaths. All of the other patients were asymptomatic and suffered neither neurologic events nor myocardial infarction.

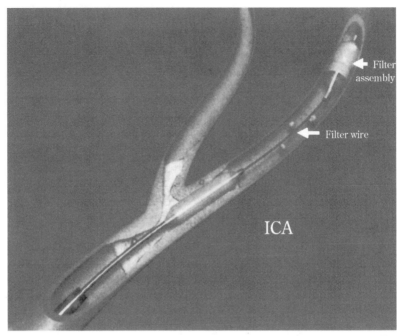

FIGURE 1.—Application of the NeuroShield filter system during carotid artery stenting. The filter is mounted on a filter wire that is used to cross the lesion and deliver interventional balloon and stent catheters. *Abbreviation: ICA*, Internal carotid artery. (Courtesy of Al-Mubarak N, Colombo A, Gaines PA, et al: Multicenter evaluation of carotid artery stenting with a filter protection system, *J Am Coll Cardiol* 39:841-846, 2002. Reprinted with permission from the American College of Cardiology.)

Conclusions.—The use of the filter protection system during CAS was found to be both safe and feasible for the majority of patients. No major embolic events occurred, and the risk of atheroembolic complications when the filter was placed successfully was low.

▶ A bigger series with a different filter; apparently good results.

G. L. Moneta, MD

Balloon-Protected Carotid Artery Stenting: Relationship of Periprocedural Neurological Complications With the Size of Particulate Debris
Tübler T, Schlüter M, Dirsch O, et al (Ctr for Cardiology and Vascular Intervention, Hamburg, Germany; Univ Hosp, Essen, Germany; Cardiovascular Ctr Bethanien, Frankfurt, Germany; et al)
Circulation 104:2791-2796, 2001   12–39

Background.—A catheter-based protection system initially developed for saphenous vein graft interventions to reduce the risk of distal embolization has been modified and made available for carotid angioplasty and stenting. In this system, occlusion of the vessel distal to the target lesion with an inflat-

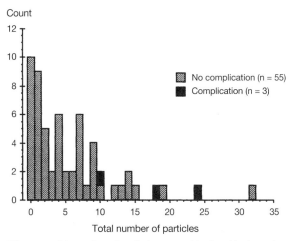

FIGURE 1.—Histogram of the total number of relevant particles found in the aspirates collected in 55 procedures without PNCs (*hatched bars*) and 3 procedures associated with PNCs (*black bars*). Note that although particle numbers of the latter are located at the upper end of the distribution, they are completely contained within the range of the former. *Abbreviation: PNC,* Periprocedural neurologic complication. (Courtesy of Tübler T, Schlüter M, Dirsch O, et al: Balloon-protected carotid artery stenting: Relationship of periprocedural neurological complications with the size of particulate debris. *Circulation* 104:2791-2796, 2001.)

able balloon allows the capture of particulate debris with an aspiration catheter. Some patients, however, experience periprocedural neurologic complications despite balloon protection. Scant data are currently available regarding the type, number, and size of the particles retrieved during protected carotid artery stenting. Whether a correlation exists between captured particle characteristics and the patients' neurologic outcome was investigated.

Methods.—This 4-center, phase I study included 54 patients (mean age, 69 years) who underwent 58 carotid artery stenting procedures, with the PercuSurge GuardWire system used for distal protection. Aspirated debris were subjected to histologic and cytologic evaluation. Stent placement was successful in all of the patients.

Results.—The mean balloon occlusion time was 10.4 minutes. Three patients experienced periprocedural neurologic complications, including 2 strokes, 1 of which resolved in less than 48 hours, and 1 transient ischemic attack. Relevant particles were found in 48 aspirates (83%) (Fig 1). The median number of particles, their maximum diameter, and the maximum area of these particles were all significantly higher in the aspirates obtained during procedures associated with periprocedural neurologic complications compared with aspirates obtained during procedures with no periprocedural complications. However, a significant degree of overlap was noted in the distributions of the number and maximum diameter of particles associated with the patients with periprocedural complications versus those with no complications, which made it impossible to make any predictive inferences. A maximum particle area of more than 800,000 μm^2 was found to be associated with a 60% chance of having a periprocedural neurologic complication.

Conclusions.—Periprocedural neurologic complications occurred in 5.2% of patients who underwent carotid artery stenting despite balloon protection. The results demonstrate that the maximum area of aspirated particles is an indicator of increased risk for these complications.

▶ Still another filter. A few neurologic events were associated with stent placement in this study. It appears the more particles captured, the more likely some will get through. It will take a while to figure out what cerebral protection device works best. I get the feeling that with all these filters someone thinks there is money to be made here.

G. L. Moneta, MD

Initial Experience of Platelet Glycoprotein IIb/IIIa Inhibition With Abciximab During Carotid Stenting: A Safe and Effective Adjunctive Therapy
Kapadia SR, Bajzer CT, Ziada KM, et al (Cleveland Clinic Found, Ohio)
Stroke 32:2328-2332, 2001   12–40

Background.—Platelet activation at the site of intervention during carotid stenting contributes to the risk of a number of adverse events, including thrombosis, ischemic complications, and restenosis. Glycoprotein (GP) IIb/IIIa inhibitors have reduced ischemic complications during coronary interventions, but may increase the risk of intracranial hemorrhage when used in carotid stenting. Adjuvant therapy with abciximab, used for platelet GP IIb/IIIa inhibition, was evaluated for its safety and efficacy for patients at high surgical risk undergoing carotid stenting.

Methods.—Abciximab was administered to 128 consecutive patients. A 0.25 mg/kg bolus was given before the lesion was crossed with guidewire, and a 0.125 µg/kg per minute infusion was given for 12 hours. Patients received a heparin bolus of 50 U/kg, and activated clotting time was maintained between 250 to 300 seconds. Aspirin and thienopyridine were also administered. End points of the study were any major or minor stroke, intracranial hemorrhage, and neurologic death within 30 days. A control group consisted of 23 consecutive patients who underwent carotid stenting without adjunctive use of abciximab.

Results.—Patients in the abciximab and control groups were similar in clinical characteristics, comorbidities, and age and sex distribution. Adverse procedural events were more frequent in the control group (8%) than in the abciximab group (1.6%). In the control group, 1 major stroke and 1 death occurred, in contrast to the abciximab group where only 1 minor stroke and 1 retinal infarction occurred. During the 30-day period after hospital discharge, 1 female patient who had been treated with abciximab was found to have a small intracranial hemorrhage at the site of a previous stroke; she recovered with conservative management.

Conclusion.—The adjunctive use of abciximab for carotid stenting was safe and effective for this high-risk study population. Abciximab did not increase the risk of intracranial bleeding; the overall event rate, however, was low in both study and control groups.

▶ I don't understand why at some centers all of the sudden there are so many patients at "high surgical risk" for carotid endarterectomy. Does anyone really think the patients have changed that much in the last few years? Aside from that, I am not sure how to reconcile the results of this article with the previous one, other than the debris may consist of bits of plaque and newly formed platelet aggregates as well.

G. L. Moneta, MD

Diffusion-Weighted MR Imaging After Angioplasty or Angioplasty Plus Stenting of Arteries Supplying the Brain
Jaeger HJ, Mathias KD, Drescher R, et al (Staedtische Kliniken Dortmund, Germany; Univ Witten/Herdecke, Dortmund, Germany)
AJNR Am J Neuroradiol 22:1251-1259, 2001   12–41

Background.—In recent years, procedures for interventional revascularization of vessels supplying the brain have been developed as an alternative to medical and/or surgical treatment. However, concerns have been expressed regarding the safety of such interventions because of the risk of cerebral embolization during the procedure. The most sensitive tool for detecting early cerebral ischemia is diffusion-weighted MRI. This has been used to detect structural damage to the brain resulting from silent embolism during cerebral angiography and stenting at the carotid bifurcation. A high incidence of hyperintense lesions on diffusion-weighted images of the brain has been observed after stenting at the carotid bifurcation. The hypothesis that diffusion-weighted MR imaging of the brain can demonstrate new diffusion abnormalities after angioplasty or angioplasty plus stenting of arteries supplying the brain in areas other than at the carotid bifurcation was investigated.

Methods.—Diffusion-weighted MR images of the brain were obtained 24 hours before and 24 hours after 37 revascularization procedures in 32 patients. The procedures included interventions at the distal internal carotid artery, the external carotid artery, the common carotid artery, the innominate artery, the vertebral artery, and the proximal subclavian artery.

Results.—After 8 of the 37 procedures (22%), new hyperintensities were visible on the diffusion-weighted MR images. In 6 of the 8 procedures, the hyperintensities occurred in the vascular territory supplied by the treated vessel. Thirty-five new cerebral lesions were visible, 33 of them (94%) in vascular territory supplied by the treated vessel. No patients in whom new diffusion abnormalities were found had new neurologic symptoms or deficits. No new lesions were seen after procedures performed at the subclavian artery.

Conclusions.—Diffusion-weighted MR imaging of the brain is useful for assessing the effects of modification of procedural technique and/or the use of cerebral protection devices such as stents when these lesions occur.

▶ This article looks at MRI-determined abnormalities in the brain after angioplasty of extracranial cerebral arteries other than the internal carotid at the cervical-carotid bifurcation. There were a lot of MRI abnormalities after stenting (22%), but none were associated with clinical neurologic events. Nevertheless, it would be interest to know if these MR abnormalities could be decreased by cerebral protection devices.

G. L. Moneta, MD

Recanalization Results After Carotid Stent Placement
Berkefeld J, Turowski B, Dietz A, et al (Johann Wolfgang Goethe-Univ of Frankfurt am Main, Germany)
AJNR Am J Neuroradiol 23:113-120, 2002   12–42

Background.—The implantation of self-expanding stents is used increasingly as an alternative to carotid endarterectomy, and high technical success rates with carotid stent placement have been documented. Angiographic recanalization results are commonly reported in terms of the resolution of stenosis or luminal gain. However, the anatomic details of stent placement in the vascular lumen and the adaptation of carotid stents to the vessel wall are only occasionally cited. The immediate and longer-term anatomic results of the implantation of self-expanding carotid stents were investigated.

Methods.—In a retrospective study, preoperative and postoperative angiograms and duplex sonograms were evaluated in 40 consecutive carotid stent procedures in 39 patients with a mean age of 67 years. All the patients had high-grade ($\geq 70\%$) internal carotid artery (ICA) stenoses. Angiograms and duplex sonograms were evaluated to assess the expansion of the vascular lumen, apposition of the stent, and geometric changes in the ICA after stent placement. Rolling-membrane and carotid Wallstents were implanted in 22 patients, and Easy Wallstents in 18.

Results.—Eleven of 40 arteries (28%) showed optimal widening of the lumen and apposition of the stent. Minor shortcomings of stent reconstruction included residual stenoses in 16 patients, free stent filaments not attached to the vessel wall in 21 patients, and stent-induced kinking of the ICA in 6 patients. There was 1 death, for peri-interventional morbidity and mortality rates of 3%. One high-grade restenosis, 1 ipsilateral stroke, and 2 ipsilateral transient ischemic attacks were observed during a median follow-up of 24 months.

Conclusions.—Suboptimal anatomic results are common with the use of self-expanding Wallstents for endovascular treatment of atherosclerotic carotid artery stenosis. Despite this, there were no major complications or long-term sequelae obviously related to these anatomic defects, with the exception of 1 symptomatic restenosis.

▶ Self-expanding wall stents were associated with frequent suboptimal anatomic results at the time of carotid angioplasty and stent placement. On the
other hand, with a median follow-up of 24 months, there was not much restenosis in these vessels. Perhaps cervical stenting is so good you don't need
optimal anatomic results to achieve a low restenosis rate?

G. L. Moneta, MD

13 Grafts and Graft Complications

Long-term Outcome of Revised Lower-Extremity Bypass Grafts
Landry GJ, Moneta GL, Taylor LM Jr, et al (Oregon Health Sciences Univ, Portland)
J Vasc Surg 35:56-63, 2002   13–1

Background.—Reversed lower-extremity vein grafts (LEVGs) often need to be revised to maintain patency. The outcomes of such revisions after more than 5 years have not been well documented. Patients undergoing surgical LEVG revisions were followed up for up to 10 years.

Methods and Findings.—Between 1990 and 2000, 1498 LEVG procedures were performed at the authors' center. Three hundred thirty surgical graft revisions were required in 259 extremities in 245 patients. Patients were followed up for a median of 38 months. The assisted primary patency rate of all grafts was 87.4% at 5 years (Table 7). The 5-year limb salvage rate for patients undergoing surgery for limb salvage indications was 88.7%. The patient survival rate at 5 years was 72.4%. The assisted primary patency rate of all grafts, the limb salvage rate for patients undergoing surgery for limb salvage indications, and the survival rate of all patients at 7 years after the original bypass grafting procedure were 85.7%. 83.4%, and 67.8%, respectively. At 10 years, these rates were 80.4%, 75.4%, and 53.4%, respectively.

TABLE 7.—Assisted Primary Patency of Revised Lower-Extremity Bypass Grafts

Interval (Months)	Cumulative Patency	Interval Patency	SE	Occluded	Withdrawn	At Risk
0-6	.9880	.9880	.0069	3	20	259
7-12	.9573	.9693	.0132	7	29	236
13-24	.9309	.9736	.0174	5	33	200
25-36	.9058	.9749	.0942	4	30	162
36-48	.8735	.9677	.0257	4	28	128
48-60	.8735	1.0000	.0257	0	24	96
61-84	.8570	.9835	.0301	1	21	72
85-108	.8345	.9775	.0368	1	20	50
109-120	.8035	.9690	.0466	1	12	29

(Courtesy of Landry GJ, Moneta GL, Taylor LM Jr, et al: Long-term outcome of revised lower-extremity bypass grafts. *J Vasc Surg* 35:56-63, 2002.)

In the first year after the original procedure, 180 revisions were performed. One hundred ten were performed between the first and fifth year, and 40 were done after 5 years. Seventy-eight percent of the grafts revised in the first year had lesions in the graft. Lesions were found in the native arterial inflow of 10% and in the native arterial outflow in 12%. In revisions performed between 1 and 5 years, 63% of the lesions were located in the graft, 20% in the inflow, and 17% in the outflow. After 5 years, these proportions were 62%, 19%, and 19%, respectively.

Conclusion.—Excellent assisted primary patency and limb-salvage rates can be obtained for as long as 10 years for patients undergoing LEVG revision. At between 5 and 10 years after the original procedure, overall patency and limb salvage rates in this series declined by only 7%. Thirty-four percent of revisions needed were done between the first and fifth year after the original procedure, and 11% were done after 5 years. An aggressive regimen of duplex scanning surveillance of LEVGs is warranted for the life of the graft.

▶ Vein grafts just plain stay open if you keep after them. Of course, it is a pain for the doctor and the patient to stay after them, as apparently they never lose the propensity to develop a stenosis.

G. L. Moneta, MD

Bipedicle Fasciocutaneous Flaps for Inframalleolar Vascular Graft Coverage at the Ankle/Foot
Sood R, Flannagan RP, Lalka S, et al (Indiana Univ, Indianapolis)
Ann Plast Surg 47:511-516, 2001   13–2

Background.—Improvements in vascular surgical techniques have made inframalleolar arterial bypass an accepted surgical modality for limb salvage. However, distal wound complications from these procedures are common and are associated with diabetes, advanced limb ischemia, and bypass grafting to the dorsalis pedis artery. In patients for whom primary closure of the foot incision is not possible, immediate and reliable tissue coverage must be provided to preserve postoperative vessel patency and foot viability. The use of bilateral pedicle fasciocutaneous flaps for immediate coverage in these challenging wounds is described.

Methods.—Intraoperative consult in 9 patients (11 ankles) revealed saphenous vein grafts at either the medial ankle or the dorsum of the foot in which primary closure of the wound resulted in the reduction or occlusion of blood flow. These patients were treated with longitudinally oriented bipedicle fasciocutaneous flaps raised with widths of 2 to 4 cm and lengths ranging from 12 to 18 cm, with Doppler confirmation of discrete fascial perforators. Split-thickness skin grafts were placed in the wake of the flaps.

Results.—Patient follow-up ranged from 2 to 78 months. All of the wounds healed, with salvage of 10 of 11 limbs (Fig 1).

Conclusions.—The use of bipedicle flaps allows the reconstruction of soft tissue defects with the transposition of local tissues of similar qualities,

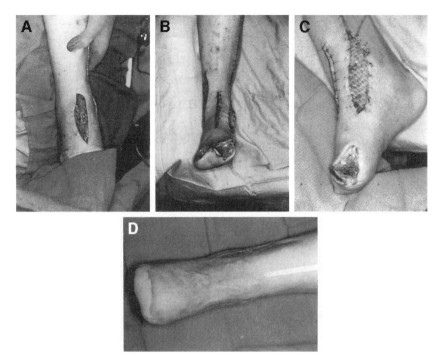

FIGURE 1.—Patient 1 (D. M.) **A,** Intraoperative consult with exposed dorsal vein graft. **B,** Tension-free coverage of vein graft with medial rotation of bipedicle fasciocutaneous flaps. **C,** The wake of the fasciocutaneous flaps covered with skin grafts. **D,** Healed dorsal incision and skin graft sites 16 months postoperatively. (Courtesy of Sood R, Flannagan RP, Lalka S, et al: Bipedicle fasciocutaneous flaps for inframalleolar vascular graft coverage at the ankle/foot. *Ann Plast Surg* 47:511-516, 2001.)

which avoids the need for more complex distant tissue reconstruction. Vascular perfusion, even in the ischemic lower extremity, is enhanced by the inclusion of the deep fascia with the flap. This type of flap derives its reliability from standard principles of angiosome anatomy rather than traditional concepts of length-to-width ratios.

▶ All surgeons doing very distal bypasses should be aware of this technique to achieve coverage of exposed pedal grafts. No one likes to have the patient's graft blow out in the cafeteria.

G. L. Moneta, MD

Comparative Decades of Experience With Glutaraldehyde-Tanned Human Umbilical Cord Vein Graft for Lower Limb Revascularization: An Analysis of 1275 Cases

Dardik H, Wengerter K, Qin F, et al (Englewood Hosp, NJ)
J Vasc Surg 35:64-71, 2002   13–3

Background.—Experimental work with human umbilical vein as an alternative to the autologous saphenous vein began in the early 1970s. Clinical trials began in 1974 for the use of glutaraldehyde-tanned umbilical vein graft (UVg). The experience of a single group with the UVg graft for revascularization of the lower extremity over 28 years is reported. Results comparing the decades from 1975 to 1985 and from 1990 to 2000 are emphasized.

Methods.—A total of 283 lower extremity bypass grafting procedures were performed in 230 patients (264 limbs) from 1990 to 2000, with UVg used as the predominant or sole graft material. Findings documenting this group's experience with 907 reconstructions from 1975 to 1985 served as a baseline comparison for the second decade of experience with UVg. Reconstructions were classified on the basis of the distal anastomotic site with or without distal arteriovenous fistulas. The primary and secondary graft patency rates were determined for each category. Cumulative palliation, which combines outcomes graft failure, amputation, and death, also was determined.

Results.—The results from 1990 to 2000 demonstrated a continuing improvement in patency rates for UVg grafts in revascularization of the lower extremity (Fig 5). A comparison of complications showed no changes between the first and second decades in the low incidence rates of infection,

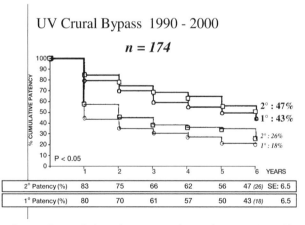

FIGURE 5.—Comparative cumulative graft patency rates for crural reconstructions with use of umbilical vein graft during decades from 1975 to 1985 (*bold lines*) and from 1990 to 2000 (*light lines and italics*). Differences between curves were statistically significant (*P* < .05). *Abbreviations: UV,* Umbilical vein graft; *SE,* standard error. (Courtesy of Dardik H, Wengerter K, Qin F, et al: Comparative decades of experience with glutaraldehyde-tanned human umbilical cord vein graft for lower limb revascularization: An analysis of 1275 cases. *J Vasc Surg* 35:64-71, 2002.)

stenosis, dissection, and pseudoaneurysm. Findings in the first decade showed a 2.9% rate for aneurysm surgery, with an incidence rate of biodegradation of 57%. Findings for the second decade have shown no aneurysms. There was no significant change between the 2 decades in the limb salvage rate of 6 years or in the types of bypass grafts.

Conclusions.—This study confirms the fact that favorable results can be obtained from the use of glutaraldehyde-tanned human UVg for revascularization of the lower limb. Concerns regarding biodegradation and aneurysm formation, even after 5 years, are unfounded. The use of UVg can improve patency and limb salvage rates in conjunction with lower nonthrombotic failure rates, increasing performance of associated endovascular procedures, use of tourniquets, and the addition of distal arteriovenous fistulas for crural bypass grafting. However, prospective randomized studies comparing the role of all graft materials still are needed.

▶ This is a difficult article to comment upon. My only experience with umbilical vein grafts for lower extremity bypass has been to take them out, either for infection or degeneration or to perform a secondary procedure where one has thrombosed. Of course, this is also my primary experience with polytetrafluoroethylene infrainguinal grafts as well. Overall, Dr Dardik and colleagues make a valid point that his current results with umbilical vein grafts are not all that bad. I do note, however, routine arteriovenous fistulas are used for tibial bypasses, all patients are placed on warfarin, and special care must be used for vessel control, and everyone agrees the grafts are difficult to use and virtually impossible to thrombectomize. It is these factors rather than graft degeneration that gets me to reach for polytetrafluoroethylene, when autologous vein is truly not available.

G. L. Moneta, MD

Technical Details With the Use of Cryopreserved Arterial Allografts for Aortic Infection: Influence on Early and Midterm Mortality

Vogt PR, Brunner-LaRocca H-P, Lachat M, et al (Univ Hosp Zurich, Switzerland)
J Vasc Surg 35:80-86, 2002   13–4

Introduction.—The use of cryopreserved arterial allografts has become a distinct technique for treating mycotic aneurysms and prosthetic graft infections of the thoracic aorta and abdominal aorta. This is a safe, single-step in situ technique that limits extensive perivascular debridement and preserves healthy autologous tissue. The use of cryopreserved arterial allografts for aortic infections was evaluated.

Methods.—Between 1990 and 1999, 49 patients underwent in situ repair with cryopreserved arterial allografts. Of these, 21 patients (43%) had mycotic aneurysms, and 28 (57%) had prosthetic graft infections of the thoracic aorta and abdominal aorta that included pelvic and groin vessels. Seventeen patients (35%) experienced aortobronchial, aortoesophageal, or aortoenteric fistulas.

Results.—Allograft-associated technical problems were observed in 8 patients (16%) and included an intraoperative rupture caused by allograft friability; allograft-enteric fistula from ligated allograft side branches rupturing 8, 18, and 48 months after implantation; anastomotic failure caused by inappropriate mechanical stress; anastomotic stricture after partial replacement of infected prosthetic grafts; allograft failure caused by inappropriate wound drainage; and a recurrence of infection after inappropriate duration of antifungal treatment. Seven of the 8 technical problems (87%) occurred in the initial 10 patients (80%) in this cohort. One technical failure occurred in the remaining 39 patients in the series (2.6%; $P = .0002$) and was caused by various technical adaptations, including critical selection of allografts, the use of allograft strips supporting large anastomoses, sealing with antibiotic-impregnated fibrin glue, and a change in the technique of allograft side-branch ligature. The overall 30-day mortality rate was 6%; it was 2.6% for the last 39 patients, and no recurrent infection or allograft-associated late death occurred.

Conclusion.—The in situ repair of cryopreserved allografts provides excellent early and late results in the treatment of aortic infections. Distinct allograft-related problems need to be overcome to improve outcomes in patients who have major vascular infections.

▶ It took a while to get this paper in print. Originally presented at the Joint Vascular Meetings in June 2000, it didn't show up in print until 18 months later. The bottom line of this article is that cryopreserved allografts are difficult to use well. It is not like in situ graft replacement with a prosthetic graft, a procedure, by the way, I also try to avoid. Nor are the problems with these cryopreserved allografts and infected fields the same as the more familiar problems with extra anatomic bypass and graft excision. Implantation of cryopreserved grafts for infection is probably not a procedure for the occasional graft or aortic infectionologist. Graft infections, in general, probably should be treated at major centers. They occur too infrequently for most surgeons to achieve adequate experience in their management.

G. L. Moneta, MD

Endovascular Repair of Bleeding Aortoenteric Fistulas: A 5-Year Experience
Burks JA Jr, Faries PL, Gravereaux EC, et al (Mount Sinai School of Medicine, New York)
J Vasc Surg 34:1055-1059, 2001   13–5

Background.—Aortoenteric fistula (AEF) is an uncommon but catastrophic complication of aortic reconstruction that is uniformly fatal when untreated. The conventional surgical management of AEF is associated with a perioperative mortality rate of 25% to 90%, and major complications are common. Several recent case studies have reported the endovascular management of AEFs in high-risk patients with lower perioperative morbidity

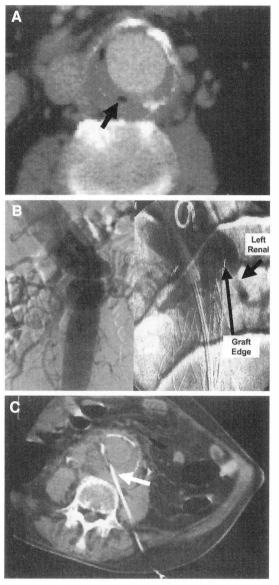

FIGURE 3.—**A,** Air surrounding a previously placed aortic graft (*arrow*). **B,** Predeployment (**left**) and postdeployment (**right**) intraoperative angiography. A Talent tube graft was placed just below the renal arteries, excluding the earlier proximal anastomosis that was the site of the aortoenteric fistula. **C,** Percutaneous drainage catheter (*arrow*) placed with CT guidance immediately after graft deployment. (Courtesy of Burks JA Jr, Faries PL, Gravereaux EC, et al: Endovascular repair of bleeding aortoenteric fistulas: A 5-year experience. *J Vasc Surg* 94:1055-1059, 2001.)

and mortality rates than traditional surgery. The experience with endovascular management of primary and secondary AEFs was reviewed with the objective of determining whether endovascular repair in selected patients can result in lower morbidity rates than traditional surgical management.

Methods.—During a 5-year period, 7 high-risk patients with bleeding and an AEF documented by radiologic or endoscopic findings were treated with coil embolization or an endovascular aortic stent graft. One patient underwent CT-guided percutaneous catheter drainage of an infected perigraft collection (Fig 3). Patients were followed up for an average of 27 months, which included a physical examination, complete blood count, and contrast-enhanced helical CT scanning at 3, 6, and 12 months, and then, annually. All patients were treated with IV antibiotics perioperatively and then were given lifelong oral antibiotics at discharge.

Results.—One patient died during surgery, caused by fungal sepsis, and 1 patient required laparotomy and bowel resection, resulting from persistent sepsis after stent-graft placement. One patient had 3 bouts of recurrent sepsis, all of which were successfully treated by changing antibiotics. Three patients later died of causes unrelated to AEF or the surgical procedure. Three patients were alive and well at an average of 36 months after the procedure and had no clinical or radiologic evidence of recurrent bleeding or infection.

Conclusions.—Endovascular management of AEFs for selected patients is feasible and successful. Endovascular treatment may be the preferred modality for the management of select patients with bleeding and no indications of sepsis. For high-risk patients with gross infection, endovascular repair of aortoenteric fistula may be useful as a bridge to more definitive treatment after the patient's condition has stabilized.

▶ The only thing you can conclude from this article is that if you are willing to totally disregard basic surgical principles, you can place an endovascular graft for aortoenteric fistula.

G. L. Moneta, MD

Superficial Femoral-Popliteal Vein as a Conduit for Brachiocephalic Arterial Reconstructions

Modrall JG, Joiner DR, Seidel SA, et al (Univ of Texas, Dallas)
Ann Vasc Surg 16:17-23, 2002   13–6

Introduction.—The revascularization of brachiocephalic arteries with the use of prosthetic graft provides excellent patency for most reconstructions. For complex brachiocephalic reconstructions, including redo operations or reconstructions for infection, autogenous conduit may be preferred. The saphenous veins may be absent or inadequate for use as a bypass conduit. The indications and intermediate-term outcomes of superficial femoral-popliteal vein (SFPV) as an alternative conduit for brachiocephalic reconstructions were investigated.

Methods.—The study included 71 patients who underwent carotid, subclavian, or axillary artery reconstruction (excluding endarterectomy) between November 1994 and July 2000. Of these, 13 (19%) of the bypasses were subclavian-to-carotid artery transpositions, and 32 (44%) were performed with the use of prosthetic graft. The saphenous vein was used as the bypass conduit in 8 (12%) bypasses. The SFPV was used as the conduit in 18 (25%) patients (9 men, 9 women; ages, 30-79 years; mean age, 62.1 years). The primary indications for the use of the SFPV as a conduit for brachiocephalic reconstruction were (1) inadequate or absent saphenous vein in 13 patients (72%); (2) infected or grossly contaminated operative fields in 3 (17%) patients; and (3) failed prosthetic grafts in 3 patients (17%).

Results.—The mortality rate at 30 days was 5.5% and the neurologic event rate was 5.5%. At a mean follow-up of 26 months, no incidences of graft thromboses or graft infections were noted. The revision-free primary patency rate was 92% for the SFPV at 48 months, and the assisted primary patency rate was 100%.

Conclusion.—The SFPV is a safe, durable conduit for brachiocephalic reconstructions.

▶ The superficial femoral vein, or femoral vein as it is more properly called, has proved to be an excellent arterial substitute when large caliber autogenous arterial substitutes are needed. We have used it for treatment of an occasional infected aortic graft, infected femorofemoral grafts, as a femoral interposition graft in trauma, and as a conduit for brachiocephalic reconstructions in contaminated fields. So far, no significant problems.

G. L. Moneta, MD

14 Vascular Trauma

Traumatic Renal Artery Dissection Identified With Dynamic Helical Computed Tomography
Dobrilovic N, Bennett S, Smith C, et al (Univ of Cincinnati, Ohio)
J Vasc Surg 34:562-564, 2001   14–1

Background.—Renal vascular injury is reported to occur in 3% to 14% of patients with renal trauma. Among these injuries are stretch injuries to the vascular pedicle, which may result in renal artery avulsion or intimal tear with dissection and stenosis. The latter injury is usually asymptomatic and is diagnosed only after the vessel has thrombosed. Early diagnosis, however, is associated with a high rate of renal salvage. Two cases of renal artery intimal dissection with stenosis recognized by a delayed nephrogram during dynamic helical CT scan for evaluation of blunt trauma were presented.

Case 1.—Man, 25, was unrestrained while driving and was ejected from his sport utility vehicle during a head-on, rollover collision. He was hypotensive at the scene, with a Glasgow Coma Scale score of 3, and was immediately intubated. At the emergency department, the patient was tachycardic but normotensive. Dynamic helical CT of the abdomen revealed a grade II splenic laceration, left transverse process fractures of L1 through L5 vertebrae, and a small left perinephric hematoma. There was diminished enhancement of the left kidney compared with the right kidney (Fig 1). Subsequent arteriography identified an intimal dissection with stenosis, which was corrected with deployment of a 154 Palmaz stent. Duplex scanning confirmed excellent flow through the stented portion of the artery 10 months after stent placement.

Case 2.—Woman, 40, was the restrained front-seat passenger in a vehicle that sustained a high-speed lateral impact on the passenger side. She experienced several hypotensive episodes during transport to an outside hospital and responded to IV fluid administration before transfer to the authors' facility. Abdominal CT scan identified multiple bilateral rib fractures, displaced transverse process fractures of the right L1 through L4 vertebrae, and a grade III liver laceration. Review of the nephrogram on CT scan revealed reduced enhancement on the left, which was suggestive of decreased perfusion. Selective angiography identified an intimal dissection in the midpor-

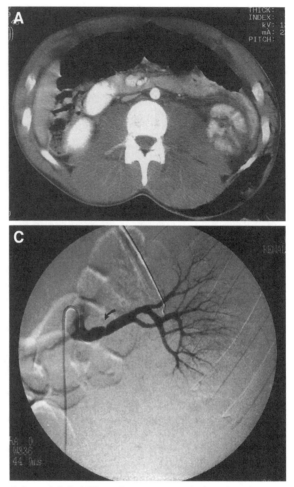

FIGURE 1.—**A,** Dynamic helical CT reveals numerous irregular linear hypodensities scattered throughout left renal parenchyma. This appearance can be mistaken for multiple lacerations or contusions. **C,** Arteriography identified arterial dissection (*arrow*) with stenosis in midportion of left renal artery. (Courtesy of Dobrilovic N, Bennett S, Smith C, et al: Traumatic renal artery dissection identified with dynamic helical computed tomography. *J Vasc Surg* 34:562-564, 2001.)

tion of the left renal artery, producing a 95% stenosis. The luminal diameter was restored with a 154 Palmaz stent with normal perfusion.

Conclusions.—Blunt trauma is the most common mechanism producing trauma to the renal artery and is known to produce acute thrombosis. In both of these patients, the observation of asymmetric renal enhancement raised suspicion of decreased flow resulting from an arterial injury. An intimal dissection with stenosis in each vessel was demonstrated on angiography; in both patients, endovascular stent placement restored renal perfusion. This unique pattern of renal enhancement during dynamic CT imaging is considered a sign of severe renal arterial injury requiring evaluation with arteriography.

▶ The routine use of CT scanning in the evaluation of blunt abdominal trauma is leading to earlier diagnosis of some renal artery injuries that otherwise would not have been discovered. We also have treated 2 patients with renal injuries diagnosed by CT scanning. Endovascular stent placement allows minimally invasive treatment for patients who don't otherwise require laparotomy.

G. L. Moneta, MD

Focal Arterial Injuries of the Proximal Extremities: Helical CT Arteriography as the Initial Method of Diagnosis
Soto JA, Múnera F, Morales C, et al (Universidad de Antioquia, Medellín, Colombia)
Radiology 218:188-194, 2001   14–2

Background.—Direct contrast material-enhanced arteriography is typically used to evaluate arterial integrity in patients with extremity trauma. The use of helical CT arteriography as the initial diagnostic examination in patients thought to have focal arterial injuries in the proximal extremities was reported.

Methods.—A total of 142 arterial segments in the proximal extremity portions of 139 patients were studied by helical CT arteriography during 19 months. The CT arteriograms were interpreted on site by radiologists in charge of emergent procedures. Subsequently, 2 radiologists provided a consensus interpretation on retrospective review.

Findings.—Studies were nondiagnostic in 3.6% of patients, who then had conventional arteriography. In the remaining 137 arterial segments, CT arteriography showed arterial injuries in 61 segments and normal arteries in 76. Fifty-five of these segments were treated initially with surgery, and 4 with endovascular intervention. Seventy-eight segments were observed, 77 of which remained stable at 3 to 18 months. No differences were seen between on-site and consensus interpretations. The sensitivity and specificity of CT arteriography were 95.1% and 98.7%, respectively.

Conclusions.—In most patients thought to have focal arterial injuries of the proximal portions of the extremities, helical CT arteriography can be used as the initial diagnostic procedure. Further research is needed to determine how this examination can be combined with other noninvasive assessments.

▶ In this study, helical CT scanning was highly accurate in identifying focal arterial injuries in the proximal portion of the extremities. The examination still requires a radiologist to process the images, but apparently image processing can be done in about 10 minutes. If you are fortunate enough to work in an institution where radiologists are present after 4:30 in the afternoon, this technique should be useful in the evaluation of potential arterial injuries.

G. L. Moneta, MD

Surgical Intervention for Complications Caused by Femoral Artery Catheterization in Pediatric Patients

Lin PH, Dodson TF, Bush RL, et al (Emory Univ, Atlanta, Ga; Baylor College of Medicine, Houston)

J Vasc Surg 33:1071-1078, 2001   14–3

Background.—The femoral artery is the preferred access site for diagnostic or therapeutic catheterization. However, there is a risk of complications, including occlusion, hemorrhage, dissection, and pseudoaneurysm formation, with the use of the femoral artery. Therapeutic principles in adult iatrogenic injury to the groin have been well characterized in the literature, but these injuries and their management in children have not been well defined. The risk factors and surgical management of complications resulting from catheterization of the femoral artery in pediatric patients were evaluated.

Methods.—The hospital records of all children who underwent operative repairs for complications caused by femoral artery catheterization from January 1986 to March 2001 were reviewed. Determination of risk factors associated with iatrogenic femoral artery injury was accomplished with a prospective cardiac data bank containing 1674 catheterization procedures during the study period.

Results.—There were 36 operations in 34 patients (age range, 1 week to 17.4 years) in whom iatrogenic complications developed after either diagnostic or therapeutic femoral artery catheterization. Nonischemic complications included femoral artery pseudoaneurysm (4 patients), arteriovenous fistulas (5 patients), uncontrollable bleeding, and expanding hematoma (4 patients). Operative repairs were successful in all patients with nonischemic iatrogenic femoral artery injuries. In contrast, ischemic complications occurred in 21 patients, including 14 patients with acute femoral ischemia. These 14 patients underwent surgical interventions that included femoral artery thrombectomy with primary closure (6 patients), saphenous vein patch angioplasty (6 patients), and resection with primary anastomosis (2 patients). Chronic femoral artery occlusion for more than 30 days occurred in 7 patients, with symptoms including either severe claudications or gait disturbance or limb growth impairment. Operative treatments for these patients included ileofemoral bypass grafting, femorofemoral bypass grafting, and femoral artery patch angioplasty. Over a mean follow-up period of 38 months, there were no incidents of limb loss, and 84% of the children with ischemic complications eventually gained normal circulation. The factors that were correlated with an increased risk of iatrogenic groin complications requiring surgical management were age under 3 years, therapeutic intervention, 3 or more catheterizations, and the use of a 6F or larger guiding catheter.

Conclusions.—Excellent outcomes may be obtained from surgery for nonischemic complications of femoral artery catheterization, but acute femoral occlusion in children under 2 years of age often results in less satisfactory outcomes. Claudication in children caused by chronic limb ischemia can be successfully treated with operative intervention. Significant iatrogenic groin complications were associated with the variables of young age, therapeutic intervention, earlier catheterization, and the use of a large guiding catheter.

▶ This article focuses on pediatric patients who required either acute or late operation for a complication of femoral artery catheterization. It is important to note that these are patients who eventually required operation. As such, the article should not be construed as indicative that all femoral artery occlusions after femoral catheterization in pediatric patients require operation. At our institution, we examined 58 children from 5 to 14 years after undergoing diagnostic femoral artery catheterization before the age of 5 years. Arterial occlusion was present in 37% of limbs (24 of 65) in which catheterization had been performed. Leg growth retardation was present, however, in only 4 limbs. Only 1 patient had symptoms of arterial occlusion (claudication), and only 1 patient had symptoms with reference to the leg growth retardation (gait disturbance). Based on these data, we concluded children having diagnostic femoral artery catheterization should be monitored for arterial occlusion, and those detected should be monitored for leg growth retardation. However, arterial repair in the absence of clinical symptoms does not appear to be indicated.[1]

G. L. Moneta, MD

Reference

1. Taylor LM Jr, Troutman R, Feliciano P, et al: Late complications after femoral artery catheterization in children less than five years. *J Vasc Surg* 11:297-306, 1990.

Percutaneous Ultrasound-Guided Thrombin Injection for the Treatment of Pseudoaneurysms
Powell A, Benenati JF, Becker GJ, et al (Miami Cardiac and Vascular Inst, Fla)
J Am Coll Surg 194:S53-S57, 2002   14–4

Background.—Increased percutaneous intervention for coronary and peripheral arterial disease and increased numbers of catheter-based diagnostic procedures has resulted in an increased prevalence of postcatheterization pseudoaneurysms (PSAs). The treatment of PSAs has been revolutionized by the introduction of US-guided compression. However, the success rate for this procedure is as low as 42% and can be lower for patients receiving anticoagulation therapy. Procedural pain leads to early termination and procedure failure in up to 10% of patients, and long procedure times of 10 to 300 minutes result in both patient and physician dissatisfaction with the procedure. Thrombin has been widely used for local hemostasis for years. It serves to propagate the final pathway of the coagulation cascade by initiating fibrinogen to form thrombin and has been successfully used to treat PSAs. The basis for and the technique of US-guided thrombin injection for the treatment of pseudoaneurysms are described.

Methods.—Gray-scale and color-flow imaging are used to investigate the PSA to clarify the relationship of the PSA to the native vessels. The site and the US probe are then prepared and draped according to standard sterile techniques. Local anesthesia may be used. Thrombin is reconstituted to concentrations of 1000 U/mL to 100 U/mL. Under direct visualization, the thrombin is slowly injected with a 19- to 25-g needle of appropriate lengths and 1 mL syringes. The injection process is imaged with either gray-scale or color-flow US. The needle tip must be visualized with certainty within the PSA. Once total thrombosis is suspected, a detailed interrogation of the PSA is necessary to assess for any residual flow. Typical total injection volumes range from 0.3 to 3 mL independent of the thrombin concentration utilized. The patient is placed on bed rest for 4 to 6 hours, and a repeat ultrasonogram is performed the next day. A postprocedure US evaluation is then obtained at 1 to 2 weeks.

Literature Review.—A literature review of 12 studies with 319 patients was performed; 309 of the 319 patients were successfully treated with thrombin injection, for an overall procedural success rate of 97%. There were complications in 3 patients (0.94%). None resulted in limb loss, but complications requiring urgent surgery, lytic therapy, or systemic anticoagulation have been reported. A significant percentage of the patients either were fully heparinized or were being treated with antiplatelet agents. The success rate of the thrombin injection was considered to be independent of anticoagulation status. No independent predictors of failure were reported, but there was a trend toward an increased failure rate with larger-size PSA.

Conclusions.—US-guided thrombin injection is a highly successful procedure in the appropriate setting and has a low overall complication rate in the treatment of patients with postcatheterization pseudoaneurysms.

▶ For those of you having lived in a cave for the last 5 years, this is a nice "how-to" article to get you up to speed in the percutaneous treatment of pseudoaneurysms secondary to arterial cannulation.

G. L. Moneta, MD

Multiinstitutional Experience With the Management of Superior Mesenteric Artery Injuries
Asensio JA, Britt LD, Borzotta A, et al (Univ of Southern California, Los Angeles; Eastern Virginia Med School, Norfolk; Emanuel Hosp, Portland, Ore; et al)
J Am Coll Surg 193:354-366, 2001   14–5

Background.—Injuries to the superior mesenteric artery (SMA) are rare but frequently lethal injuries with very high morbidity and mortality. This study reviewed a multi-institutional experience with SMA injuries. Fullen's classification based on anatomic zone and ischemia grade was evaluated for its predictive value, and the American Association for the Surgery of Trauma—Organ Injury Scale (AAST-OIS) for abdominal vascular injury was correlated with mortality. Finally, independent risk factors predictive of death were identified, with a description of current trends for the management of this injury in the United States.

Methods.—A retrospective multi-institutional study of patients who sustained SMA injuries was conducted in 34 trauma centers in the United States over 10 years. Outcome variables were analyzed with univariate methods at first, then with multivariate analysis using stepwise logistic regression to identify a set of risk factors significantly associated with mortality.

Results.—A total of 250 patients were enrolled, with a mean Revised Trauma Score (RTS) of 6.44 and a mean Injury Severity Score (ISS) of 25. Surgical management of these patients included ligation in 175 of 244 patients (72%), first-degree repair in 53 of 244 patients (22%), autogenous grafts in 10 of 244 patients (4%), and prosthetic grafts of PTFE in 6 of 244 patients (2%). The overall mortality rate was 97 of 250 patients (39%). Mortality rate versus Fullen's zones was 76.5% for zone I, 44.1% for zone II, 27.5% for zone III, and 23.1% for zone IV. Mortality rate versus Fullen's ischemia grade was 64.7% for grade I. Mortality rate versus AAST-OIS for abdominal vascular injury was 16.4% for grade I, 25.5% for grade II, 40% for grade III, 53.6% for grade IV, and 89.5% for grade V. Independent risk factors for mortality identified on logistic regression analysis included transfusion of greater than 10 units of packed red blood cells, intraoperative acidosis, dysrhythmias, injury to Fullen's zone I or II, and multisystem organ failure.

Conclusions.—Injuries to the SMA are extremely lethal. Fullen's anatomic zones, ischemia grade, and AAST-OIS abdominal vascular injuries are well correlated with mortality. Significant predictors of mortality include AAST-OIS injury grades IV and V, high intraoperative transfusion requirements, and presence of acidosis and dysrhythmias. These predictive factors for mortality must be considered in the surgical management of these injuries.

▶ The main conclusion of this article is that proximal SMA injuries are bad, while distal SMA injuries are not so bad. Most of us already knew that.

G. L. Moneta, MD

Vascular Complications in Anterior Thoracolumbar Spinal Reconstruction

Oskouian RJ Jr, Johnson JP (Univ of Virginia, Charlottesville; Univ of California, Los Angeles)
J Neurosurg: Spine 96:1-5, 2002   14–6

Background.—Operative procedures done through an anterior approach to the spine carry a risk of vascular injury, but the magnitude of the risk associated with anterior thoracic or lumbar spine approaches is undetermined. In addition, while intraoperative vascular complications are obvious, delayed ones are less apparent. The incidence of vascular complications and effective management strategies in these cases were evaluated in patients undergoing anterior thoracic and lumbar reconstructive spinal surgery.

Methods.—The incidence, causes, and management of vascular injuries and complications were documented retrospectively for 207 patients (112 women; mean age, 56.7 years).

Results.—Twelve patients had vascular complications develop, and 2 died. Seven had direct vascular injuries, and 1 died. Five patients had deep vein thrombosis, and 1 died of a massive pulmonary embolus. Seven patients suffered direct vascular injury caused by surgical techniques and error: 5 acute venous injuries and 2 arterial injuries that were delayed in development. Five patients suffered acute intraoperative vessel injuries: 3 cases of common iliac vein injury and 2 of inferior vena cava injury. Three injuries were linked to mobilization of a densely scarred retroperitoneum (the result of previous surgery) and 2 to tuberculous and bacterial osteomyelitis (1 each). No acute arterial injuries to the aorta or aortoiliac arterial system occurred, but delayed vascular complications that were arterial in origin developed in 2 patients who had transthoracic surgery for symptomatic vertebral fractures. The overall incidence of vascular complications was 5.8%, and mortality was 1%.

Conclusions.—Vascular complications occur rarely in patients who have anterior spinal reconstruction procedures. Venous injury, while uncommon, is associated with mobilization of the common iliac vein at L4-5, particularly when previous anterior spinal surgery has been performed or the patient has osteomyelitis. Patients who are elderly and have underlying vascular disease are more likely to develop arterial injuries, though these also are rare. The surgeon must recognize and treat all complications promptly to minimize potential morbidity and mortality.

▶ Anterior approaches to the thoracolumbar spine occasionally result in vascular injury, usually venous injury. This potential complication is probably underemphasized by surgeons doing this type of work. When the injuries are venous, and the result is deep venous thrombosis, many patients appear to sue their doctor. I know of at least 6 such suits in my area of the country. I advise surgeons to speak frankly with their patients regarding this potential complication.

G. L. Moneta, MD

Unpredictability of Cerebrovascular Ischemia Associated With Cervical Spine Manipulation Therapy: A Review of Sixty-Four Cases After Cervical Spine Manipulation
Haldeman S, Kohlbeck FJ, McGregor M (Univ of California, Irvine; Southern California Univ, Los Angeles; Univ of California, Los Angeles; et al)
Spine 27:49-55, 2002   14–7

Introduction.—The growing acceptance of mobilization and manipulation of the cervical spine has prompted the need to examine its effectiveness and its potential side effects and complications, of which the most serious is the risk of cerebrovascular accidents (CVAs). Nearly 117 cases of postmanipulation CVAs have been reported in the English literature. Possible risk factors include age, sex, migraine headaches, hypertension, diabetes, taking birth control pills, cervical spondylosis, and smoking. It is frequently assumed that complications may be avoided by clinically screening patients and by positioning the head and neck to assess the patency of the vertebral arteries. Patient characteristics, potential risk factors, the nature of complications, and neurologic sequelae were defined retrospectively from a review of medicolegal records.

Methods.—Sixty-four previously unpublished medicolegal records describing cerebrovascular ischemia after cerebral spine manipulation were independently reviewed by 3 researchers. Descriptive statistics were determined for patient characteristics and complications.

Results.—It was not possible to determine factors from the clinical history and physical examination of affected patients that would have helped a physician attempting to identify the patient at risk of cerebral ischemia after cervical manipulation.

Conclusion.—CVAs after manipulation seem to be unpredictable and need to be considered an inherent, idiosyncratic, and rare complication of this treatment approach.

▶ This is an interesting review of 64 medical legal cases of cerebrovascular ischemia after cervical spine manipulation therapy. The key points are that the patients generally present with symptoms of head and neck pain, and that the onset of symptoms is within 2 days of manipulation in 94% of cases, and within 30 minutes in 75% of cases. There are no particular risk factors that can be identified for the complication, and therefore the complication is unpredictable. Given the number of chiropractors out there and the number of manipulations performed, this complication is obviously, and fortunately, uncommon.

G. L. Moneta, MD

Vertebral Artery Injury in Cervical Spine Trauma

Parbhoo AH, Govender S, Corr P (Univ of Natal, Congella, South Africa)
Injury 32:565-568, 2001   14–8

Background.—Vertebral artery injuries that occur with cervical spine trauma rarely cause symptoms and can been missed until vertebrobasilar ischemia develops. Among the lesions that can occur are dissection, thrombosis, tears of the intima, ruptures, and arteriovenous fistulas. The incidence and natural history of vertebral artery injuries were assessed with use of MRI and MR angiography (MRA) in patients who had sustained trauma to the cervical spine.

Methods.—Of the 47 patients studied (mean age, 35 years; age range, 21-73 years), 30 had been in motor vehicle collisions and 17 had fallen from a height. Three patients had burst fractures, 14 had bifacet dislocations, and 30 had unifacet dislocations. None showed signs or symptoms of vertebrobasilar insufficiency. Both MRI and MRA were performed, and the results were reviewed by 2 independent radiologists. MRA was repeated in 4 patients after 3 years to evaluate any recanalization.

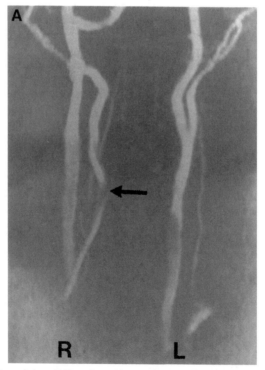

FIGURE 1.—Coronal view of MR angiographic scan; the *arrow* demonstrates dissection of right vertebral artery and an occluded left vertebral artery. (Reprinted from Parbhoo AH, Govender S, Corr P: Vertebral artery injury in cervical spine trauma. *Injury* 32:565-568, 2001. Copyright 2001, with permission from Elsevier Science.)

Results.—Vertebral artery injuries were found in 12 patients, and 1 of these was bilateral. All were diagnosed as loss of normal flow void on axial MRI and were confirmed on MRA. Ten of the patients had unifacet dislocations, 1 had a burst fracture, and 1 had a bifacet dislocation (Fig 1). No evidence indicating recanalization was found on MRA after 3 years in 4 patients.

Conclusions.—Patients with unifacet dislocations were more likely to have vertebral artery injuries in association with blunt cervical trauma. No signs or symptoms indicating vertebrobasilar insufficiency were present, perhaps because adequate collateral circulation to the basilar system had developed and prevented ischemia from occurring. No specific treatment was undertaken, and, in the 4 patients evaluated at a 3-year follow-up, no evidence of recanalization was found.

▶ This article is a factoid of vertebral artery injury. Vertebral artery injury occurs in one fourth of patients with fractures or dislocation of the cervical spine. The artery, once occluded, does not recanalize, and neurological symptoms referable to injury are rare, but when they do occur, presentation is often delayed. In the latter respect, vertebral artery and carotid injuries after trauma appear to act in similar fashion with delayed presentation being a frequent finding.

G. L. Moneta, MD

15 Venous Thrombosis and Pulmonary Embolism

The PORtromb Project: Prothrombin G20210A Mutation and Venous Thromboembolism in Young People
Mansilha A, Araújo F, Sampaio S, et al (S João Univ, Oporto, Portugal)
Cardiovasc Surg 10:45-48, 2002   15–1

Background.—Many studies have linked a single mutation in the 3' untranslated region of the prothrombin gene (G20210A) to venous thromboembolism (VTE). Whether this mutation is a significant risk factor for VTE in the general Portuguese population was studied by comparing its frequency in healthy patients to that in patients with VTE.

Methods.—The subjects were 40 unrelated patients seen with a first episode of VTE when they were under the age of 40 years (14 males and 26 females; age range, 17-40 years). The control subjects were 100 blood donors with no history of VTE. Both groups provided blood samples for polymerase chain reaction analysis to identify any mutation in the 20210A alleles of the prothrombin gene.

Results.—Five of the 40 patients (12.5%) had the G20210A mutation in the prothrombin gene. This was not significantly different from the incidence of the mutation found in the control subjects (5 of 100, or 5%). Nonetheless, patients were almost 3 times as likely as control subjects to carry the G20210A mutation (odds ratio, 2.71).

Conclusion.—Compared with studies from other Northern European countries, the prevalence of the prothrombin gene mutation 20210A in this study was higher in these Portuguese subjects, as had been reported in an earlier study. However, carriage of the G20210A mutation was not significantly higher in these young patients with VTE than in the controls. Thus, the G20210A mutation of the prothrombin gene appears to confer, at most, a marginally increased risk for VTE in the Portuguese population.

▶ Again, blood doesn't clot without a reason.

G. L. Moneta, MD

Acute Renal Vein Thrombosis, Oral Contraceptive Use, and Hyperhomocysteinemia

Chan HHW, Douketis JD, Nowaczyk MJM (McMaster Univ, Hamilton, Ont, Canada)
Mayo Clin Proc 76:212-214, 2001   15–2

Background.—Hyperhomocysteinemia and the use of oral contraceptives (OCs) appear to be relatively weak risk factors for venous thromboembolism (VTE). A patient with acute renal vein thrombosis who had recently started taking an OC and who was subsequently found to have marked hyperhomocysteinemia is reported.

> *Case Report.*—Woman, 21, sought medical attention for acute onset of right-sided flank pain accompanied by gross hematuria. The pain had been present for 24 hours. Previously, she had been healthy, and her only medication was an OC begun 6 months earlier. Venacavogram revealed thrombosis of the right renal vein. Extensive coagulation evaluation revealed marked hyperhomocysteinemia and no evidence of any other known hypercoagulable state. Further testing identified no inborn error of vitamin B_{12} or folate metabolism. The OC was stopped, and the patient was given 7 days of IV heparin with warfarin. In addition, she received folic acid, vitamin B_6, and subcutaneous vitamin B_{12} treatment. During a 2-year follow-up, the patient remained on warfarin and vitamin therapy. She had no further episodes of VTE.

Conclusions.—Oral contraceptives and hyperhomocysteinemia may interact synergistically in the pathogenesis of thrombosis. When venous thrombosis develops in OC users in the absence of other risk factors, clinicians should investigate for an underlying prothrombotic biochemical disorder.

▶ It is well-known that risk factors for venous thromboembolism are additive. How the enhanced effects of multiple weak risk factors work at the biochemical level is, however, not known but likely varies with the combination of risk factors. Not all components of Virchow's triad are equal. I bet hypercoagulability is the most important.

G. L. Moneta, MD

Venous Thromboembolism in Childhood: A Prospective Two-Year Registry in The Netherlands

van Ommen CH, Heijboer H, Büller HR, et al (Univ of Amsterdam; Free Univ, Amsterdam)

J Pediatr 139:676-681, 2001   15–3

Background.—Venous thromboembolism (VTE) is rarely seen in children, and its incidence, morbidity, and mortality rates are undetermined. A prospective registry of VTE was made for The Netherlands, outlining the current incidence, signs and symptoms, diagnostic tests, risk factors, therapy, and complications seen in children from birth through age 18 years.

Methods.—Using monthly notification cards, the Dutch Pediatric Surveillance Unit instituted a surveillance system to detect various pediatric illnesses in The Netherlands. Questionnaires were completed for patients who were identified. The incidence of VTE was determined with the use of population age-distribution data.

Results.—A total of 99 patients were entered into the registry, and the annual incidence was calculated to be 0.14 cases per 10,000 children. In 47% of cases, the patient was a neonate, and 26 were preterm (Fig 1). In the neonates, 94% of the cases of VTE were related to a central venous catheter and were located in the upper venous system. In more than a third of cases, the children were free of symptoms. Among older children, VTE was related to the catheter in one third of cases and was generally found in the lower venous system. Usually (in 85% of cases), thrombosis developed while the child was in the hospital. It was diagnosed by echocardiography in 53% and by US in 43% of neonates. Older children generally received diagnoses with use of US alone or combined with other modalities (69% of cases). At least 1 clinical risk factor was found in 98% of all patients, and 2 risk factors were found in 74% of neonates and in 81% of older children. Older children were more likely to have congenital prothrombotic disorders than were neonates. Vari-

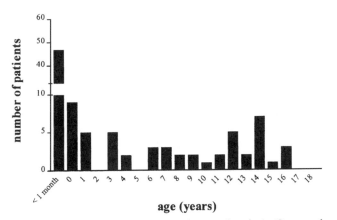

FIGURE 1.—Age distribution of pediatric patients with venous thrombosis. (Courtesy of van Ommen CH, Heijboer H, Büller HR, et al: Venous thromboembolism in childhood: A prospective two-year registry in The Netherlands. *J Pediatr* 139:676-681, 2001.)

ous forms of treatment were used, including supportive care, removal of catheters, and antithrombotic therapy (eg, urokinase and vitamin K antagonists or heparin and vitamin K antagonists in most cases). Two children died of VTE. Morbidity that developed included bleeding and recurrent thrombosis (each found in 7% of cases).

Conclusions.—Among the general Dutch population of children from birth through age 18 years, the incidence of VTE is 0.14 per 10,000, and more than a third of the cases are asymptomatic. Neonates are affected more than older children, and hospitalized children, particularly those with central venous catheters or combined risk factors, are especially at risk.

▶ Ninety-eight percent of children with VTE have a reason for the venous thrombosis, whether it be an indwelling catheter, the primary risk factor in neonates, or a relative hypercoagulable state, the primary risk factor in older children. The study again emphasizes that in children, as well as adults, blood does not clot without a reason.

G. L. Moneta, MD

Anomalies of the Inferior Vena Cava in Patients With Iliac Venous Thrombosis

Obernosterer A, Aschauer M, Schnedl W, et al (Karl-Franzens Univ, Graz, Austria)

Ann Intern Med 136:37-41, 2002

15–4

Background.—During embryogenesis, the normal inferior vena cava is converted from 3 sets of paired veins to a unilateral right-sided system that consists of the postrenal, renal, prerenal, and hepatic segments. However, if the originally paired structures do not unite, anomalies of the inferior vena cava may result. The prevalence of these anomalies has been estimated at 0.07% to 8.7% of the general population. These anomalies become apparent in infants when combined with heart failure or visceral malformation. Anomalies in adults are commonly discovered as incidental findings in abdominal surgery or in radiologic workup. However, there have been case reports of patients with anomalies of the inferior vena cava that became symptomatic because of deep venous thrombosis of the iliac veins. Anomalies of the inferior vena cava were identified in consecutive patients with deep venous thrombosis in the lower extremities.

Methods.—This prospective consecutive case series enrolled 97 patients with deep venous thrombosis. All the patients underwent sonography, venography, or both for the diagnosis of deep venous thrombosis, as well as MR angiography to image the inferior vena cava. The primary outcome measure was the identification of anomalies of the inferior vena cava on MR angiography.

Results.—Thrombotic occlusion of iliac veins was evident in 31 of 97 patients. Five of these patients had an anomaly of the inferior vena cava. The anomalies included a missing inferior vena cava, a hypoplastic hepatic segment, and missing renal or postrenal segments. Patients with anomalies of the inferior vena cava were significantly younger (mean age, 25 ± 6 years) than the 92 patients who did not have these anomalies (mean age, 53 ± 19 years). The thrombotic occlusion was evident in 2 patients with anomalies.

Conclusions.—Thrombosis involving the iliac veins in a patient aged 30 years or younger should prompt suspicion of an anomaly of the inferior vena cava. Patients may be at higher risk if they have both an anomaly and thrombosis.

▶ I had not previously thought of looking for a caval anomaly in patients with iliac vein thrombosis. I suppose if you find one, it should be considered a risk for recurrent deep venous thrombosis. Perhaps such patients should be on lifelong warfarin therapy after their first episode of iliac vein thrombosis.

G. L. Moneta, MD

Fondaparinux Compared With Enoxaparin for the Prevention of Venous Thromboembolism After Elective Major Knee Surgery

Bauer KA, for the Steering Committee of the Pentasaccharide in Major Knee Surgery Study (Veterans Affairs Boston Healthcare System; et al)
N Engl J Med 345:1305-1310, 2001   15–5

Background.—Venous thromboembolism is a frequent, life-threatening postoperative complication of total knee replacement surgery. The prevalence rate for venographically verified postoperative deep vein thrombosis is 40% to 84%, and the prevalence rate for pulmonary embolism is 2% to 7%. Thromboprophylaxis that is effective in patients undergoing hip replacement surgery, such as low-dose or low molecular weight heparin or warfarin, is not as effective in patients undergoing knee replacement. Fondaparinux is the first of a new class of synthetic antithrombotic agents that may prove to be more effective in the prevention of venous thromboembolism after elective major knee surgery.

Methods.—The effectiveness and safety of 2.5 mg of fondaparinux once daily for thromboprophylaxis were compared with that of 30 mg of enoxaparin twice daily in a double-blind study involving 1049 consecutive patients undergoing elective major knee surgery. Both treatments were subcutaneous and were initiated postoperatively. The primary efficacy measure was the incidence of venous thromboembolism up to postoperative day 11. Thromboembolism was defined as deep vein thrombosis detected by mandatory bilateral venography, documented symptomatic deep vein thrombosis, or documented pulmonary embolism. Major bleeding was the primary measure of safety.

Results.—Efficacy was assessed in 724 patients. The fondaparinux group had a significantly lower incidence of venous thromboembolism by day 11 compared with the enoxaparin group (12.5% vs 27.8%). Major bleeding was a more frequent occurrence in the fondaparinux group, but there were no significant differences between the 2 groups in the incidence of bleeding leading to death or reoperation or bleeding occurring in a critical organ.

Conclusions.—Postoperative treatment with 2.5 mg of fondaparinux once daily was significantly more effective than 30 mg of enoxaparin twice daily for the prevention of deep vein thrombosis in patients undergoing elective major knee surgery.

▶ Fondaparinux has been termed a "designer heparin." It is a synthetic pentasaccharide structurally similar to the antithrombin-binding site of heparin, and thus acts to inhibit activated factor X (factor Xa). It is sure to be a major competitor of low molecular weight heparin in venous thromboembolism prophylaxis. It has a standard dose that is independent of patient weight, requires no monitoring, is given once daily, and does not appear to react with platelet factor IV, making it unlikely to result in heparin-induced thrombocytopenia. In addition, it appears to be more effective than low molecular weight heparin in reducing venous thrombosis. Of course, the true goals of venous thrombosis prophylaxis are to reduce deaths from pulmonary embolism and reduce the late sequela of venous thrombosis. In this study, both low molecular weight heparin and fondaparinux prevented death from pulmonary embolism, and development of postphlebitic syndrome was not addressed. In my mind, the principle advantages of this drug are ease of administration and apparent lack of heparin-associated thrombocytopenia.

G. L. Moneta, MD

Extended Out-of-Hospital Low-Molecular-Weight Heparin Prophylaxis Against Deep Venous Thrombosis in Patients After Elective Hip Arthroplasty: A Systematic Review
Hull RD, Pineo GF, Stein PD, et al (Univ of Calgary, Alta, Canada; St Joseph Mercy–Oakland, Detroit; Ullevaal Univ Hosp, Oslo, Norway; et al)
Ann Intern Med 135:858-869, 2001   15–6

Background.—The need for in-hospital prophylaxis is well established for deep venous thrombosis in patients who have undergone hip arthroplasty, and evidence-based guidelines derived from venographic end points recommend low molecular weight heparin (LMWH) prophylaxis or warfarin prophylaxis for 7 to 10 days in these patients. European trials indicate the need for extended out-of-hospital prophylaxis in patients who undergo hip arthroplasty, but the risk-benefit ratio for this approach is unclear. To provide a practical pathway for the translation of clinical research into practice, trials that compared extended out-of-hospital LMWH prophylaxis with placebo were systematically reviewed.

Methods.—A search of PubMed, MEDLINE, and the Cochrane Library Database was conducted for randomized controlled trials comparing extended out-of-hospital prophylaxis with LMWH versus placebo in patients undergoing elective hip arthroplasty. References from these articles and abstracts of conference proceedings were reviewed, and pharmaceutical com-

Study	Year	Patients with Events		Relative Risk (95% CI Fixed)	Weight	Relative Risk (95% CI Fixed)	P Value
		LMWH Group	Control Group				
		n/n (%)			%		
Bergqvist et al. (29)	1996	21/117 (17.9)	45/116 (38.8)		28.6	0.46 (0.30–0.73)	0.001
Planes et al. (30)	1996	6/85 (7.1)	17/88 (19.3)		10.6	0.37 (0.15–0.88)	0.025
Dahl et al. (31)	1997	11/93 (11.8)	23/89 (25.8)		14.9	0.46 (0.24–0.88)	0.020
Lassen et al. (32)	1998	5/113 (4.4)	12/102 (11.8)		8.0	0.38 (0.14–1.03)	0.057
Hull et al. (45)	2000	14/291 (4.8)	14/133 (10.5)		12.2	0.46 (0.22–0.93)	0.031
Comp et al. (46)	2001	15/152 (9.9)	39/138 (28.2)		25.9	0.35 (0.20–0.60)	<0.001
Total		72/911 (7.9)	150/666 (22.5)		100.0	0.41 (0.32–0.54)	<0.001

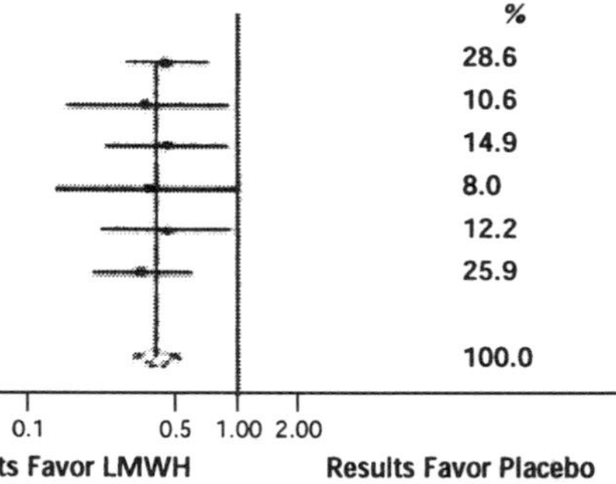

0.1   0.5   1.00 2.00

Results Favor LMWH   Results Favor Placebo

FIGURE 1.—Relative risk for all deep venous thrombosis during the out-of-hospital time interval. Summary and individual study results are shown. *Abbreviation: LMWH,* Low molecular weight heparin; *CI,* confidence interval. (Courtesy of Hull RD, Pineo GF, Stein PD, et al: Extended out-of-hospital low-molecular-weight heparin prophylaxis against deep venous thrombosis in patients after elective hip arthroplasty: A systematic review. *Ann Intern Med* 135:858-869, 2001.)

panies and the investigators of the original reports were contacted. Reviewers evaluated the study quality with a validated 4-item instrument.

Results.—Six double-blind trials were included in the final analysis. Compared with placebo, the use of extended out-of-hospital prophylaxis decreased the frequency of all episodes of deep venous thrombosis, proximal venous thrombosis, and symptomatic venous thromboembolism. The only incident of major bleeding occurred in one patient in the placebo group (Fig 1).

Conclusions.—The use of extended LMWH prophylaxis in an out-of-hospital setting demonstrated a consistent level of effectiveness and safety in the trials for venographic deep venous thrombosis and symptomatic venous thromboembolism in patients undergoing elective hip arthroplasty. These benefits were seen regardless of study variations in clinical practice and length of hospital stay. These findings support the need for extended out-of-hospital prophylaxis in these patients.

▶ I always take what Dr Hull says very seriously. He knows more about low molecular weight heparins than almost anybody. If he says you ought to treat hip surgery patients with additional prophylaxis after they leave the hospital, then you should treat hip patients with additional prophylaxis after they leave the hospital.

G. L. Moneta, MD

Prophylaxis Against Fat and Bone-Marrow Embolism During Total Hip Arthroplasty Reduces the Incidence of Postoperative Deep-Vein Thrombosis: A Controlled, Randomized Clinical Trial

Pitto RP, Hamer H, Fabiani R, et al (Friedrich-Alexander Univ Erlangen-Nuremberg, Erlangen, Germany)

J Bone Joint Surg Am 84-A:39-48, 2002   15-7

Background.—Methods used to prevent deep venous thrombosis, a major complication of total hip arthroplasty, are usually initiated after the procedure, but recent studies suggest that the greatest risk for thrombogenesis occurs during preparation of the femur. The efficacy of an operative technique designed to reduce the increase in intramedullary pressure and to avoid embolization of fat and bone marrow was evaluated prospectively.

Methods.—Study participants were 130 patients with advanced osteoarthritis who were scheduled for primary total hip arthroplasty. Excluded were patients with a history or symptoms of deep vein thrombosis or pulmonary embolism. Sixty-five patients were randomly assigned to have the femoral component inserted with standard cementing technique and 65 to have the femoral component cemented with the use of a bone-vacuum technique (Fig 1). The incidence of intraoperative fat and bone marrow embolism was measured with echocardiography and a transesophageal probe; serial duplex US, performed on the day before surgery and on postoperative days 4, 14, and 45, was used to detect deep vein thrombosis. All patients

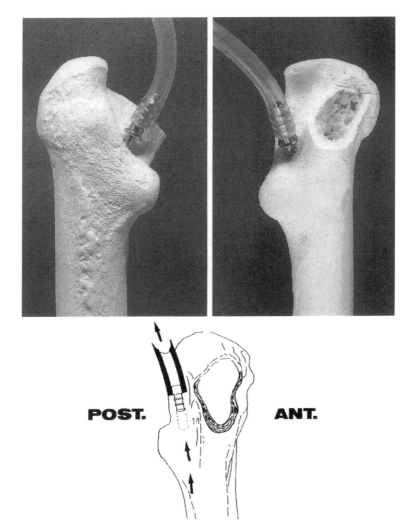

FIGURE 1.—The position of the proximal drainage cannula used for the bone vacuum cementing technique. The cannula is placed between the greater and lesser trochanters, in the trochanteric fossa, along the projection of the linea aspera. Care is taken to avoid intramedullary placement of the 20 mm long cannula. (Courtesy of Pitto RP, Hamer H, Fabiani R, et al: Prophylaxis against fat and bone-marrow embolism during total hip arthroplasty reduced the incidence of postoperative deep-vein thrombosis: A controlled, randomized clinical trial. *J Bone Joint Surg Am* 84-A:39-48, 2002.)

received low molecular weight heparin as prophylaxis against deep vein thrombosis.

Results.—The bone vacuum technique and control groups were similar in patient demographics, duration of surgery and of hospitalization, and American Society of Anesthesiologists physical status. Control subjects had significantly more severe and prolonged echocardiographic embolic events than did patients who underwent the bone vacuum technique. During insertion of the stem, a cascade of fine echogenic particles of embolic masses (≤ 5 mm in diameter) was observed in 91% of control hips versus 15% of hips in which the bone vacuum cementing technique was used. The incidence of deep vein thrombosis detected on postoperative day 4 was significantly greater in the control group (18% vs 3%).

Conclusion.—The use of the bone vacuum technique during total hip arthroplasty with cement prevents fat and bone marrow embolism, an important cause of thrombogenesis. Patients undergoing the procedure with this technique had a significantly lower incidence of postoperative deep vein thrombosis.

▶ In addition to distortion of the femoral pelvic veins during total hip arthroplasty, migration of fat and bone marrow into the venous system during this procedure may help activate the clotting cascade and contribute to the high incidence of venous thromboembolism in total hip arthroplasty patients. The authors describe a technique to reduce fat embolism that was documented to be effective by transesophageal echocardiography and was associated with a lower incidence of venous thromboembolism postoperatively. I continue to be amazed at the number of ways blood can be made to clot, although it is perhaps even more amazing that it usually does not.

G. L. Moneta, MD

A Potentially Expanded Role for Enoxaparin in Preventing Venous Thromboembolism in High Risk Blunt Trauma Patients

Norwood SH, McAuley CE, Berne JD, et al (East Texas Med Ctr, Tyler; Univ of Texas, Tyler)
J Am Coll Surg 192:161-167, 2001   15–8

Introduction.—Venous thromboembolism (VTE) is a common and potentially life-threatening complication in patients with trauma. The effectiveness of enoxaparin in preventing deep vein thrombosis (DVT) and pulmonary embolism (PE) after injury in patients at high risk for developing VTE was examined in a prospective, single-cohort investigational trial.

Methods.—All patients with serious blunt trauma injury admitted to a level I trauma center during a 7-month period were eligible if they were hospitalized for at least 72 hours, their Injury Severity Score (ISS) was 9 or above, enoxaparin was initiated within 24 hours after admission, and one or more of these high-risk criteria were met: age greater than 50 years, ISS of 16 or higher, presence of a femoral vein catheter, Abbreviated Injury Score of 3 or higher for any body region, Glasgow Coma Scale Score of 8 or less, presence of a major pelvic, femoral, or tibial fracture, and presence of direct blunt-mechanism venous injury. Patients with closed head injuries and nonoperatively treated solid abdominal organ injuries were also considered. The main outcome measures were thromboembolic events: either a documented lower extremity DVT by duplex color-flow Doppler US or a PE documented by rapid-infusion CT pulmonary angiography or conventional pulmonary angiography.

Results.—Of 118 patients evaluated, 2 (2%) developed DVT, 1 in the common femoral vein and the other in a peroneal vein at mid-calf level. Eighty percent of the patients had 2 or more risk factors for developing VTE. Two of 12 patients (17%) with splenic injuries failed nonoperative treatment and underwent splenectomy for delayed bleeding on postadmission days 4 and 7. Five patients had rapid-infusion CT pulmonary angiograms for unexplained hypoxemia, and 1 patient had a conventional pulmonary angiogram. None had PE. One patient (1%) died of multiple organ system failure on the 39th hospital day.

Conclusion.—Enoxaparin is practical and effective in reducing the rate of VTE in high-risk, seriously injured patients.

▶ I would not for one moment take this article seriously. There are so many protocol violations and exclusions that only 22% of eligible patients were enrolled in the study, a fact conveniently missing in the abstract. (The authors and the *Journal of the American College of Surgeons* need to be reminded that Doppler is a proper name and should be capitalized.) If John Porter were alive, this would receive a Camel Dung Award with Oak Leaf Cluster.

G. L. Moneta, MD

Pneumatic Compression Versus Low Molecular Weight Heparin in Gynecologic Oncology Surgery: A Randomized Trial

Maxwell GL, Synan I, Dodge R, et al (Duke Univ, Durham, NC)
Obstet Gynecol 98:989-995, 2001   15–9

Introduction.—Thromboembolism occurs in 14% of patients undergoing gynecologic surgery for benign indications and 38% of those undergoing gynecologic oncology surgery. Pulmonary embolism is an important cause of postoperative death in higher-risk patients with uterine and cervical carcinoma. The use of unfractionated heparin as deep venous thrombosis (DVT) prophylaxis in these patients is correlated with a significantly increased transfusion requirement, compared with pneumatic calf compression.

Low molecular weight (LMW) heparin has been associated with less bleeding complications than unfractionated heparin in treatment of venous thromboembolism and may be a good alternative to pneumatic calf compression in gynecologic cancer patients for prevention of venous thromboembolism. The efficacy and treatment-related complications of LMW heparin versus external pneumatic compression were examined in the prevention of venous thromboembolism after major gynecologic oncology surgery in 211 patients aged more than 40 years.

Methods.—Patients were randomly assigned to perioperative thromboembolism prophylaxis with either LMW heparin or external pneumatic compression (105 and 106 patients, respectively). Data were gathered regarding demographics and clinical outcome. All patients underwent bilateral Doppler US of the lower extremities on postoperative day 3 to 5 to determine the presence of occult DVT. Bleeding complications were determined using operative estimated blood loss and number of transfusions needed intraoperatively and postoperatively. A follow-up interview at 30 days after surgery was performed to determine whether DVT or PE developed in any patients after hospital discharge.

Results.—Two patients who received LMW heparin and 1 who received external pneumatic compression were given a diagnosis of DVT. LMW heparin was discontinued postoperatively in 3 patients because of hemorrhage. The frequency of bleeding complications was similar in both groups.

Conclusion.—LMW heparin and external pneumatic compression are similarly effective in the postoperative prophylaxis of thromboembolism. The use of LMW heparin is not correlated with an increased risk of bleeding complications when compared with external pneumatic compression. Both modalities are efficacious in this high-risk group of patients.

▶ LMW heparin and intermediate pneumatic compression both afford good venous thromboembolism prophylaxis in gynecologic oncology patients, at least for the first 3 to 5 days postoperatively. However, one cannot say one method is better, or if they are truly equal, as the study was insufficiently powered to detect a difference between methods. Lacking better data, either method appears appropriate in a gynecologic oncology patient.

G. L. Moneta, MD

Deep Vein Thrombosis: Can a Second Sonographic Examination Be Avoided?

Friera A, Giménez NR, Caballero P, et al (Hosp de la Princesa, Madrid)
AJR 178:1001-1005, 2002   15–10

Introduction.—Sonography has become the method of choice for assessing deep vein thrombosis (DVT). Recent series have considered sonography to be the reference standard. The necessity of repeated sonography for patients with either intermediate or high clinical probability for DVT after an initial examination with negative findings was prospectively assessed in 438 consecutive patients.

Methods.—All patients with clinical suspicion of DVT of the lower limbs were classified according to clinical probability (high, intermediate, low). Sonography with positive findings was considered diagnostic for DVT. Patients with intermediate or high clinical risk whose initial sonographic examination revealed negative findings underwent a repeat examination after 1 week.

Results.—Sonographic findings were positive for 112 (26%) patients and negative for 326 (74%). Of the 202 patients classified as intermediate and high-risk with negative initial sonography, 140 underwent a single follow-up sonographic examination 1 week later. Findings were positive for DVT in

3 patients. Two patients had pulmonary embolism develop. Sonographic follow-up increased the identification of DVT for patients with intermediate or high probability from 23.5% to 33.5%. The incidence of thromboembolic disease was 34%.

Conclusion.—The prevalence of DVT as analyzed by sonographic findings was 33.5% for patients with intermediate or high clinical risk. The initial examination showed a prevalence of 32.5%; a second examination 1 week later identified an additional 1%. Sonography did not identify 0.5% of thromboembolic events. These findings do not justify a routine second scanning at 1 week.

▶ The answer to the question posed in the title of this article is "maybe." There were only 140 follow-up examinations, and the tibial veins were not examined at either the first or second examination. If you are inclined to treat calf vein thrombosis, and I am, this study doesn't begin to answer the question posed. If you don't feel isolated calf vein thrombosis should be treated, the answer is still maybe, because the small number of follow-up examinations included in this study do not allow for definitive conclusions. Finally, if all that matters is death from pulmonary embolism, the study is insufficiently powered to answer the question.

G. L. Moneta, MD

Diagnosis of Lower-Limb Deep Venous Thrombosis: A Prospective Blinded Study of Magnetic Resonance Direct Thrombus Imaging
Fraser DGW, Moody AR, Morgan PS, et al (Univ Hosp, Nottingham, England)
Ann Intern Med 136:89-98, 2002   15–11

Background.—Venography is the reference standard diagnostic test for diagnosis of lower-limb deep venous thrombosis (DVT) but has been largely replaced by noninvasive tests. The current noninvasive methods for assessment of DVT have several disadvantages. MR direct thrombus imaging (MRDTI) has the potential to provide accurate diagnoses of above-the-knee DVT and thrombus below the knee. The reliability of MRDTI as a diagnostic test for suspected acute symptomatic DVT was assessed.

Methods.—This prospective blinded study was conducted in a 1355-bed hospital. The study group included 101 patients with suspected DVT who had undergone routine venography. The patients were recruited by random sequence from a larger cohort of patients with suspected DVT and included all patients with a positive venogram and 25% of patients with a negative venogram. MRDTI was performed within 48 hours of venography and was interpreted by 2 reviewers. The primary outcome measures were overall diagnosis of DVT; isolated calf, femoropopliteal, and iliofemoral DVT; and detection of thrombus in the calf, femoropopliteal, and iliac segments.

Results.—Sensitivities from the 2 readers were 96% and 94%, and specificities were 90% and 92%, respectively, for the diagnosis of DVT. Sensitivities were 92% and 83% for isolated DVT in the calf, 97% and 97% for

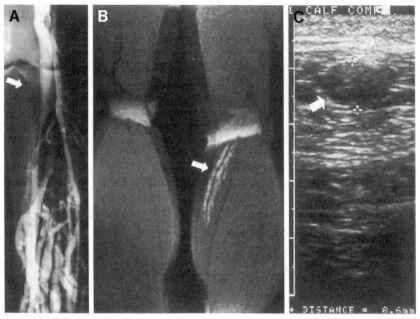

FIGURE 3.—Venography, MRDTI, and US in a patient with gastrocnemius thrombus. A, Venogram. The gastrocnemius veins have not been visualized (*arrow*). B, MRDTI. The technique demonstrates high-signal filling paired gastrocnemius veins (*arrow*). C, US image. This image under compression shows a gastrocnemius vein filled with thrombus (*arrow*). (Courtesy of Fraser DGW, Moody AR, Morgan PS, et al: Diagnosis of lower-limb deep venous thrombosis: A prospective blinded study of magnetic resonance direct thrombus imaging. *Ann Intern Med* 136:89-98, 2002.)

femoropopliteal DVT, and 100% and 100% for iliofemoral DVT. Specificities for isolated calf DVT were 94% and 96%; the specificities for both femoropopliteal and iliofemoral DVT were 100% and 100% (Fig 3). Within each of the venous segments, sensitivity and specificity ranged from 91% to 100%. Interobserver variability ranged from 0.89 to 0.98 for these measures with use of a weighted κ statistic.

Conclusions.—MRDTI is an accurate, noninvasive diagnostic tool for the assessment of DVT both above and below the knee. The results of MRDTI are strongly correlated with venographic findings and are highly reproducible.

▶ It appears MRI can identify DVT even below the knee in England. I wouldn't trust it in Oregon, at least at my university hospital. Keep in mind almost half the patients in this study actually had DVT. Since the usual portion of positive studies in DVT screenings is about 20%, and since sensitivity and specificity can be greatly influenced by the composition of the population studied, this study needs to be repeated in an "all-comers" protocol.

G. L. Moneta, MD

Eligibility for Home Treatment of Deep Vein Thrombosis: A Prospective Study in 202 Consecutive Patients

Schwarz T, Schmidt B, Beyer J, et al (Univ Clinic "Carl Gustav Carus," Dresden, Germany)

J Vasc Surg 34:1065-1070, 2001   15–12

Background.—Until recently, the standard treatment for deep vein thrombosis (DVT) was continuous IV infusion with unfractionated heparin in a hospital for 5 to 7 days, followed by oral anticoagulation with vitamin K antagonists. Recent studies have found home treatment of DVT to be safe and effective. However, these studies were based on predefined patient selection criteria. The study reported here was the first to systematically assess eligibility for home treatment.

Methods.—Possible reasons for hospital treatment were evaluated in consecutive patients with acute DVT over 9 months. The patients were evaluated by means of a check list that included medical reasons, home care situation, preferences, and hospital service logistics. All of the patients were treated with low molecular weight heparin and concomitant oral vitamin K antagonists and compression therapy. A follow-up examination at 3 months included assessment of recurrent venous thromboembolism (VTE), bleeding events, and mortality rate.

Results.—Two hundred two patients were included in the study, 117 (58%) as outpatients and 85 (42%) as patients hospitalized before DVT diagnosis. Of the 117 outpatients, 95 (81%) were considered eligible for home treatment. Only 2 patients (1.7%) were admitted to the hospital for DVT-related morbidity. One patient (0.85%) was admitted for comorbidity, 11 (9.4%) for home care reasons, and 8(6.83%) because of hospital service logistics. Among the hospitalized patients, 79 (93%) remained inpatients, and 6 (7%) were discharged within 48 hours. Pre-existing comorbidity was the only reason for hospitalization in these patients. Outcomes after 3 months in outpatients showed a 4% rate of recurrent VTE, no major bleeding, and an 8% mortality rate. Cancer accounted for 75% of the deaths. There were no deaths from VTE. Inpatients had a statistically significant higher mortality rate (8% vs 19%).

Conclusions.—Among patients with DVT who were outpatients, fewer than 3% had to be hospitalized because of DVT morbidity. For the entire DVT population, comorbidity, rather than management issues or DVT morbidity, was the primary reason for hospital treatment.

▶ It is utterly ridiculous that the insurance programs of some patients in the United States will pay for inpatient but not outpatient treatment of deep venous thrombosis. DVT patients do not need bedrest, and they do not always need hospitalization. While outpatient treatment requires an appropriate infrastructure, as far as I am aware every study addressing this issue suggests outpatient DVT treatment is safe, effective, and cost-effective. These results, however, should not be extrapolated to outpatient treatment of pulmonary embolism or massive DVT with associated phlegmasia. Until further data are forthcoming on these issues, I would still treat such patients in the hospital.

G. L. Moneta, MD

Venous Thromboembolism During Pregnancy: A Retrospective Study of Enoxaparin Safety in 624 Pregnancies

Lepercq J, Conard J, Borel-Derlon A, et al (Hôpital Saint Vincent-de-Paul, Paris; Hôtel Dieu, Paris; CHRU, Caen, France; et al)
Br J Obstet Gynaecol 108:1134-1140, 2001   15–13

Background.—Venous thromboembolism during pregnancy, a leading cause of maternal morbidity and mortality, has presented a management dilemma because of the risk of anticoagulation for mother and fetus and the resulting possibility of teratogenic effects. Unfractionated heparin does not cross the placenta and has been used more safely in pregnant patients. Low molecular weight heparins have higher bioavailability, longer half-life, and more-predictable responses than unfractionated heparins and are standard therapy in preventing and treating venous thromboembolism in nonpregnant patients. The maternal, fetal, and neonatal safety of the low molecular weight heparin enoxaparin was assessed retrospectively in cases from 55 French perinatal centers.

Methods.—The case reports of 604 women who experienced 624 pregnancies from 1988 to 1997 were reviewed, with particular attention paid to the indication and regimen for enoxaparin plus outcome measures. The main outcome measures were the incidence, severity, and cause of maternal, fetal, and neonatal adverse events, the outcome of pregnancy, and the incidence of venous thromboembolism.

Results.—In 92.0% of cases, enoxaparin was used for prophylaxis of venous thromboembolism, and in 7.8% of cases to treat an acute venous thromboembolic event; in 1 case, information was missing. The prophylaxis was chosen based on previous venous thromboembolism in 29.8% of cases, thrombophilia in 15.2%, and family history of venous thromboembolism and/or additional risks in 55%. During pregnancy, 1.8% of women suffered serious maternal hemorrhage; 1 case was connected to enoxaparin. Nine women had serious hemorrhages at delivery, but these were not related to enoxaparin. None of the 10 cases of thrombocytopenia were related to enoxaparin. The rate of stillbirth was 1.1%, and these cases were not related to enoxaparin. In 2.5% of patients, major congenital abnormalities developed, and 1.4% of patients suffered serious neonatal hemorrhages, but none of these was linked to enoxaparin. Overall, the rate of venous thromboembolic events was 1.3%, with 5 cases before delivery and 3 during the postpartum period. All the venous thromboembolic events that occurred before delivery took place despite prophylactic treatment with enoxaparin in women whose first deep vein thrombosis took place during the current pregnancy.

Conclusions.—The incidence of venous thromboembolic events was higher than is usually reported during pregnancy, but it is close to the incidence reported for women who are at high risk of thromboembolic complications and are receiving low molecular weight or unfractionated heparin. It appears that enoxaparin is well tolerated during pregnancy and that the occurrence of adverse events reflects the high risk profile of the women studied.

▶ This study from France is the largest study to date to examine the use of low molecular weight heparin as prophylaxis for venous thromboembolism in pregnancy. Like unfractionated heparin, low molecular weight heparin does not cross the placenta and therefore is potentially desirable as an anticoagulant during pregnancy. The incidence of adverse events in this study was acceptable, given the high-risk patient population. Low molecular weight heparin therefore appears to be a reasonable alternative to unfractionated heparin in women who require long-term anticoagulation during pregnancy. As a precaution, some consideration should be given to the fact that low molecular weight heparins have longer half-lives than unfractionated heparin; therefore, as delivery becomes eminent, it may be prudent to switch from low molecular weight to unfractionated heparin to prevent potential hemorrhagic complications at the time of delivery. It is noted, however, that there was no significant increase in hemorrhagic complications attributed to low molecular weight heparins in this study.

G. L. Moneta, MD

A 16-Year Haemodynamic Follow-up of Women With Pregnancy-Related Medically Treated Iliofemoral Deep Venous Thrombosis
Rosfors S, Norén A, Hjertberg R, et al (Karolinska Institutet, Stockholm)
Eur J Vasc Endovasc Surg 22:448-455, 2001   15–14

Background.—The risk of iliofemoral deep venous thrombosis (DVT) is increased during the third trimester of pregnancy and shortly after delivery. In an earlier study, these authors followed up women with pregnancy-related iliofemoral DVT for 9 years and reported that these patients had few lingering functional abnormalities or postthrombotic signs. The authors have now expanded their follow-up to 16 years to investigate longer-term clinical and functional results after medically treated pregnancy-related ileofemoral DVT.

Methods.—Between 1978 and 1989, 37 women received aggressive medical management for pregnancy-related iliofemoral DVT. Of these, 25 patients could be contacted and agreed to participate in follow-up studies a mean of 9 years later (1992-1994; patient age, 25-48 years; mean age, 37 years) and a mean of 16 years later (2000; patient age, 32-55 years; mean age, 43 years). All patients underwent clinical examinations, color duplex US, and computerized strain-gauge plethysmography at both follow-up visits. Additionally, at the 16-year follow-up, clinical and functional results were examined in light of the extent of the initial thrombus as follows: group

1, initial thrombus from iliac vein to groin; group 2, from iliac vein to femoral vein; and group 3, from iliac vein to below the knee.

Results.—At the 16-year follow-up, 10 patients (40%) were completely asymptomatic and 13 (52%) had no clinical signs of venous disease. The most common symptoms were leg swelling (13 patients, or 52%) and venous claudication (8 patients, or 32%). Six patients (24%) had mild or moderate symptoms and 6 patients (24%) had varicose veins of greater than 4 mm. Two patients had been treated for ipsilateral DVT in the calf (both in group 3), 4 had been treated for contralateral DVT, and 3 had undergone surgery for varicose veins. None of the 25 patients had trophic skin changes or ulcers.

Disability scores were low; 21 patients were able to perform activities of daily living without the need for a support device, but the other 4 patients required stockings for support. Neither signs, symptoms, nor disability scores differed significantly according to the extent of the initial thrombus. Color duplex US indicated that all deep veins were normal in 6 of the 25 patients (24%), but the remaining 19 patients (76%) had postthrombotic changes. One patient (group 3) had an occluded iliac vein at the 16-year follow-up, and 9 patients (36%) had deep venous reflux.

Deep venous reflux was significantly associated with the presence of leg pain, but there was no clear relationship between deep venous reflux and the extent of the initial thrombus. Plethysmography did not identify any outflow obstruction in any patient. These results at 16 years were virtually identical to those at the 9-year follow-up, except that the number of patients with reflux in the posterior tibial vein increased significantly (from 1 limb in follow-up 1 to 8 limbs in follow-up 2), as did venous volume and venous emptying.

Conclusion.—After 16 years of follow-up, these 25 women with medically treated pregnancy-related ileofemoral DVT still had relatively mild symptoms and signs of venous disease. The extent of initial thrombus did not appear to be associated with long-term outcomes. Thus, this population does not appear to be at increased risk for development of postthrombotic syndrome.

▶ In this study, patients with pregnancy-related iliofemoral DVT did well long-term with medical treatment only of their iliofemoral DVT. This certainly is a kick in the teeth to those who advocate thrombolytic therapy for DVT or surgical thrombectomy for iliofemoral DVT. However, it is admittedly a small kick, as patients with pregnancy-related DVT would not, I hope, be considered for thrombolytic therapy. The main point is that patients with pregnancy-related iliofemoral DVT probably will do just fine with medical treatment only. While it is tempting to extrapolate this to all iliofemoral DVT, that is probably a bit of a reach.

G. L. Moneta, MD

Prognosis After Percutaneous Closure of Patent Foramen Ovale for Paradoxical Embolism
Wahl A, Meier B, Haxel B, et al (Univ Hosp Bern, Switzerland)
Neurology 57:1330-1332, 2001   15–15

Background.—A recent meta-analysis has confirmed the association between a patent foramen ovale (PFO) with or without atrial septal aneurysm and cryptogenic stroke in young adults. Percutaneous PFO closure has been shown to be feasible for the treatment of these patients in previous studies. The long-term outcome and risk factors for recurrent paradoxical embolism after percutaneous PFO closure were assessed.

Methods.—Percutaneous PFO closure was performed on 152 consecutive patients with PFO who had at least 1 embolic event. All patients underwent contrast transesophageal echocardiography, color Doppler and duplex examination of the extracranial carotid and vertebral arteries, transcranial Doppler, and an ECG. The PFO procedure was performed with the patient under local anesthesia, and 6 different devices were used during the 6 years of the study. Patients were treated with 100 mg of acetylsalicylic acid once daily for 6 months to provide antithrombotic protection until full device endothelialization. Patients were followed up prospectively for up to 6.5 years, and follow-up was complete in all but 3 patients.

Results.—Complete closure of the PFO was achieved in 79% of patients, whereas a minimal, moderate, or large shunt persisted in 11%, 6%, or 4% of patients. The actuarial freedom from recurrent embolism was 95.1% at 1 year and 90.6% at 2 and 6 years. A residual shunt was present in 5 of 9 patients, with recurrence at follow-up contrast transesophageal echocardiography. A residual shunt was found to be predictive of recurrence.

Conclusions.—Percutaneous PFO closure was performed safely with a high rate of success by using a variety of devices. Morbidity was low and there was no mortality. All the complications were without long-term sequelae. Until the results of randomized trials comparing medical treatment with interventional PFO closure are available, the implantation of PFO occlusion devices is feasible but should be considered investigational.

▶ It is hard to know what to make of this study. No information is given as to whether the patients had deep venous thrombosis or were treated with anticoagulation. It seems this information would be important to truly know whether closure of the PFO adds anything to anticoagulation or antiplatelet therapy, or if closure of the PFO can allow discontinuation of all forms of anticoagulation. The randomized trials comparing medical treatment to percutaneous closure of PFO noted at the end of the article are obviously years away from completion.

G. L. Moneta, MD

Severe Pulmonary Embolism Associated With Air Travel

Lapostolle F, Surget V, Borron SW, et al (Université Paris XIII; George Washington Univ, Washington, DC)
N Engl J Med 345:779-783, 2001   15–16

Background.—Air travel is considered a risk factor for pulmoanry embolism. However, no one has documented the association between pulmonary embolism and distance flown. Whether air travel duration is associated with the risk of pulmonary embolism was investigated.

Methods and Findings.—All cases of pulmonary embolism necessitating medical attention on arrival at the Charles de Gaulle Airport, the busiest airport in France, between 1993 and 2000 were reviewed. Data on 56 passengers with confirmed pulmonary embolism were analyzed. Passengers traveling more than 3100 miles had a much greater incidence of pulmonary embolism than those traveling a shorter distance. (Fig 1). These incidences were 1.5 and 0.01 cases per million, respectively. Those traveling more than 6200 miles had an incidence of 4.8 cases per million.

Conclusions.—These data strongly suggest an association between air travel duration and the risk of pulmonary embolism. A greater distance traveled significantly contributes to pulmonary embolism risk.

▶ Air travel-related pulmonary embolism has probably been the subject of more discussions among professors of surgery than patients afflicted with the disease. I reviewed this article on United flight 170 from San Francisco to Boston, and I breathed a sigh of relief when I realized I had none of the factors that may have increased my risk of pulmonary embolism. My flight was less than

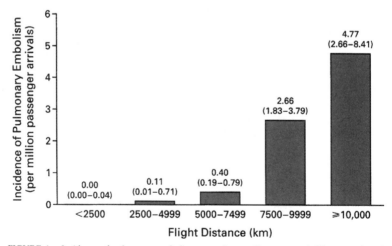

FIGURE 1.—Incidence of pulmonary embolism according to distance traveled by air. Values shown above the bars are numbers of cases per million passenger arrivals, with 95% confidence intervals. To convert kilometers to miles, multiply by 0.62. (Reprinted by permission of *The New England Journal of Medicine* from Lapostolle F, Surget V, Borron S, et al: Severe pulmonary embolism associated with air travel. *N Engl J Med* 345:779-783. Copyright 2001, Massachusetts Medical Society. All rights reserved.)

3000 miles, I was in first class, I got up during the flight, I have no risk factors for DVT that I know of, and I am younger than the mean age of the pulmonary embolism patients described in this study. I am also male, and 75% of the air travel pulmonary embolism patients in this study were female. The main point is, the longer the trip, the greater the risk, but the risk is very low.

G. L. Moneta, MD

Seasonal Variations in Hospital Admission for Deep Vein Thrombosis and Pulmonary Embolism: Analysis of Discharge Data
Boulay F, Berthier F, Schoukroun G, et al (Nice Teaching Hosp, France)
BMJ 323:601-602, 2001   15–17

Background.—The occurrence of fatal pulmonary embolism has been shown to vary according to season. However, seasonal variation in occurrence has not been established for deep vein thrombosis. Whether a relationship between deep vein thrombosis and the seasons exists was determined by analyzing French hospital admission data from the national hospital discharge register.

Methods.—Cases occurring between 1995 and 1998 with a discharge diagnosis of pulmonary embolism or deep vein thrombosis were included for

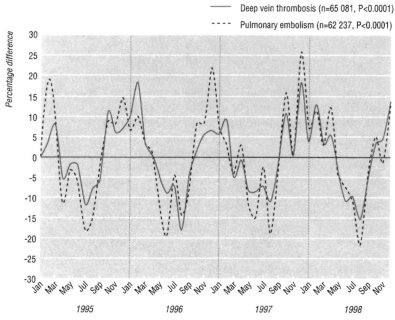

FIGURE 1.—Monthly percentage variations in French hospital admissions for deep vein thrombosis and pulmonary embolism (0 represents the sum of monthly variations). (Courtesy of Boulay F, Berthier F, Schoukroun G, et al: Seasonal variations in hospital admission for deep vein thrombosis and pulmonary embolism: Analysis of discharge data. *BMJ* 323:601-602, 2001. Reprinted with permission from the BMJ Publishing Group.)

analysis. Monthly percentage variations in admission data were compared with the sum of monthly variations (set at zero) for pulmonary embolism (n = 62,237; median age, 68 years; 57% women) and deep vein thrombosis (n = 65,081; median age, 69 years, 58% women) (Fig 1).

Results.—The number of admissions per month for both deep vein thrombosis and pulmonary embolism was higher in the winter than in the summer (Roger's test: $P < .0001$). For deep vein thrombosis, the mean monthly admissions ranged from 18% below average (August 1996) to 18% above average (February 1996 and December 1997). For pulmonary embolism, the mean monthly admissions ranged from 22% below average (August 1998) to 26% above average (December 1997).

Conclusion.—Admissions to hospitals for pulmonary embolism and deep vein thrombosis clearly increase during the winter months, showing a seasonal variation.

▶ More people in France get deep venous thrombosis and pulmonary embolism in winter than in summer. Perhaps the French are less active in winter, or perhaps there is a seasonal variation coagulation status. The observation of this article is interesting but without obvious explanation.

G. L. Moneta, MD

Systematic Study of Occult Pulmonary Thromboembolism in Patients With Deep Venous Thrombosis

López-Beret P, Pinto JM, Romero A, et al (Cardiovascular Inst, Toledo, Spain)
J Vasc Surg 33:515-521, 2001   15–18

Background.—Pulmonary thromboembolism (PTE) continues to be underdiagnosed. The prevalence and extension of PTE in asymptomatic patients with symptomatic deep vein thrombosis (DVT) in the lower limbs were determined, along with their possible implications in the treatment of thromboembolic disease.

Methods.—One hundred fifty-nine patients with acute DVT, as confirmed by duplex scanning, but no symptoms of PTE were examined. Pulmonary spiral CT angiography was performed. At 30 days, CT was repeated to assess the evolution of these clinically occult PTEs.

Findings.—Silent PTE was detected in 41% of the patients at all levels of lower limb venous thrombosis. The prevalence of PTE was associated significantly with male sex and previously diagnosed heart disease. The level of DVT was unassociated with the presence of PTE, and the DVT side was unrelated to thromboembolic pulmonary localization. Fifty-two of the 65 patients with positive CT findings had features of acute PTE, 10 had chronic PTE, and 3 had both. Chronic PTE was more common in patients with previous DVT episodes. One hundred sixty-five pulmonary artery–affected segments were identified at several locations. Fifty-nine percent of the patients had multiple affected segments. In 90.6% of the 53 patients undergoing repeat CT examinations after initial positive CT findings, PTE was completely resolved.

Conclusion.—Silent PTE is commonly associated with lower-limb clots. CT is a readily available, cost-effective modality for identifying underestimated PTE. The use of CT in the systematic diagnostic strategy of most patients with DVT may be useful for establishing the extension of thromboembolic disease at diagnosis.

▶ Sometimes all you can say is "wow." Forty percent of patients with DVT, regardless of location, above- or below-knee, iliofemoral or femoropopliteal, and without symptoms of pulmonary embolism actually had pulmonary embolism by CT scanning. Since CT scanning can miss small distal pulmonary emboli, the true incidence is probably higher. I think the data on all fronts are accumulating that most of us undertreat DVT.

G. L. Moneta, MD

Clinical Outcome of Patients With Suspected Pulmonary Embolism: A Follow-up Study of 588 Consecutive Patients

Hvitfeldt Poulsen S, Noer I, Møller JE, et al (Randers Hosp, Denmark; Svendborg Hosp, Randers, Denmark)
J Intern Med 250:137-143, 2001   15–19

Background.—Pulmonary embolism is a common and potentially fatal cardiovascular condition often occurring in the setting of an additional illness. In this study, the clinical outcome was investigated in patients with clinically suspected pulmonary embolism and compared between patients in which pulmonary embolism was confirmed and patients whose pulmonary embolism was excluded.

Methods.—This retrospective study looked at 588 consecutive patients with suspected pulmonary embolism who were referred for lung scintigraphy from 1995 to 1998. The mean follow-up time was 653 ± 424 days.

Results.—The diagnosis of pulmonary embolism was excluded in 394 patients and confirmed in 194, for an overall prevalence of 33%. Among clinical and paraclinical variables, age, chronic obstructive pulmonary disease, heart rate, pleuritic pain, deep venous thrombosis, and ECG signs of right ventricular strain were all identified as independent predictors of a diagnosis of pulmonary embolism. Anticoagulation was given to 96% of patients with pulmonary embolism for at least 3 months, and 13% of patients received thrombolytic therapy. Pulmonary embolism recurred in 6% of patients, while no patients in whom it was not diagnosed experienced pulmonary embolism during follow-up. For patients with pulmonary embolism, the 1-year mortality rate was 18%, compared with 15% among those with no diagnosis of pulmonary embolism (Fig 1). Among patients with pulmonary embolism, the cause of death was cancer in 42% and pulmonary embolism in 28%; the excess mortality among patients with no diagnosis of pulmonary

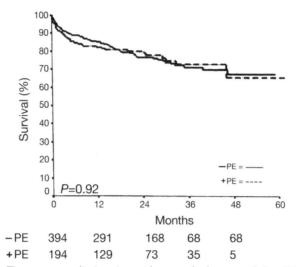

FIGURE 1.—Time course mortality in patients with suspected pulmonary embolism (PE). (Courtesy of Hvitfeldt Poulsen S, Noer I, Møller JE, et al: Clinical outcome of patients with suspected pulmonary embolism. A follow-up study of 588 consecutive patients. *J Intern Med* 250:137-143, 2001. Reprinted by permission of Blackwell Science, Inc.)

embolism was caused by cancer, chronic obstructive pulmonary disease, acute myocardial infarction, and heart failure.

Conclusions.—The risk of adverse clinical outcome is increased in patients admitted to a hospital with suspicion of pulmonary embolism regardless of whether that diagnosis is confirmed or excluded. Patients in whom the diagnosis is excluded often have other serious illnesses that mandate further evaluation.

▶ If you are sick enough to require a lung scan to rule out pulmonary embolism, you don't do well regardless of whether you actually have a pulmonary embolism or not. In fact, patients suspected of pulmonary embolism with negative lung scans had the same 1-year mortality as those with positive lung scans (see Fig 1).

G. L. Moneta, MD

Pulmonary Embolism and Stroke in Relation to Pregnancy: How Can High-Risk Women Be Identified?
Ros HS, Lichtenstein P, Bellocco R, et al (Karolinska Institutet, Stockholm)
Am J Obstet Gynecol 186:198-203, 2002   15–20

Introduction.—Pregnancy and puerperium are characterized by hypercoagulability and an increased risk of thromboembolism. The risk is particularly increased during late pregnancy and around time of delivery. Preeclampsia, multiple birth, and cesarean delivery were analyzed to determine whether they could account for the increased risk of pulmonary embolism and stroke in late pregnancy, around and after delivery.

Methods.—A population-based cohort of 1,003,489 deliveries were evaluated through cross-linking of the nation-wide Swedish Inpatient and Birth Registers of the National Board of Health and Welfare. The relative risks of both pulmonary embolism and stroke were modeled by means of a Poisson regression.

Results.—Pre-eclampsia was correlated with a 3- to 12-fold increase in the risk of pulmonary embolism and stroke during late pregnancy, at delivery, and in the puerperium. Similar increases in risks were seen for multiple pregnancies and cesarean delivery. These strong correlations, however, could not explain the overall pregnancy-associated risks of pulmonary embolism and stroke.

Conclusion.—Pre-eclampsia and cesarean delivery are important risk factors for both pulmonary embolism and stroke. They do not, however, explain most of the excess risks correlated with pregnancy.

▶ It is interesting that established risk factors for pulmonary embolism such as preeclampsia, multiple births, and cesarean delivery do not account for the increased risk of pulmonary embolism in pregnant women. The only possible conclusion is that pregnancy itself is the etiology of the increased risk. The data also indicate the risk is by far the most pronounced at the time of delivery. Just another thing for your mother to remind you about.

G. L. Moneta, MD

16 Chronic Venous and Lymphatic Disease

Validation of Venous Leg Ulcer Guidelines in the United States and United Kingdom
McGuckin M, Waterman R, Brooks J, et al (Univ of Pennsylvania, Philadelphia; Oxfordshire Community (NHS) Trust, Oxon, England; Churchill Hosp, Oxford, England; et al)
Am J Surg 183:132-137, 2002   16–1

Background.—Venous leg ulcers account for treatment costs in the billions of dollars and lost work days in the millions each year. Multidisciplinary guidelines to diagnose and treat such ulcers have been developed in the United States and United Kingdom. The US guideline had been accepted for inclusion in the National Guideline Clearinghouse of the federal Agency for Healthcare Research and Quality. Validation through a prospective evaluation for clinical efficacy and effect on cost is presented to provide a standard of care for the diagnosis and treatment of venous leg ulcers.

Methods.—Forty retrospective patients (treated before the guideline was developed) and 40 prospective patients (treated after it was in place) from the United States and United Kingdom were enrolled. The median age of retrospective patients was 78 years (UK) and 71 years (US); the median ages of prospective patients was 77 years (UK) and 74 years (US). Women accounted for 86% of the UK retrospective patients and 68% of the UK prospective patients; these numbers were 55% and 43% for US patients.

Results.—A significant effect attributed to the guideline was noted on performance of the ankle-brachial index, with an increase from the retrospective performance of 36% (UK) and 8% (US) to the prospective performance of 93% (UK) and 96% (US). Compression, used in 55% of retrospective UK patients and 27% of US patients, was used in 100% of all patients prospectively in both countries. Time to healing declined significantly, as did number of visits, which produced a significant fall in the cost per patient in both countries. Healing rates increased after the guideline was implemented, with patients having a higher probability of being healed at a given date after the guideline went into effect than before.

Conclusions.—Diagnostic aspects, healing time, and healing rates all improved dramatically with the guideline, producing lower costs.

▶ I suspect the improvement in healing of venous ulcers after implementation of the guidelines described in this paper had little to do with measuring ankle/brachial indexes, dressing changes, wound tracings, etc, and everything to do with 100% compliance with the use of compression therapy in the treatment of venous ulcers. If guidelines can get people to use compression effectively, I am all for them.

G. L. Moneta, MD

Pentoxifylline for Treatment of Venous Leg Ulcers: A Systematic Review
Jull A, Waters J, Arroll B (Auckland Hosp, New Zealand; Univ of Auckland, New Zealand)
Lancet 359:1550-1554, 2002   16–2

Introduction.—High compression therapy is effective in the treatment of venous ulcers. Adjuvant therapy may be helpful for patients with ulcers refractory to compression treatment. Randomized controlled trials that compared pentoxifylline (with and without compression therapy) with placebo or other treatments for patients with venous leg ulcers were reviewed.

Methods.—The CENTRAL registers of the Cochrane Wounds Group and the Cochrane Peripheral Vascular Diseases Group were reviewed back to September 2000. These registers differ from the Cochrane Controlled Trials Register in that they include references that have not been verified as controlled trials or trials that have not yet been forwarded for inclusion in the Cochrane register. Trials were included if they reported an objective outcome measure, such as percentage change in ulcer area, proportion of healed

	Treatment n/N	Control n/N	Relative risk (95% CI)	Weight (%)	Relative risk (95% CI)
Barbarino[9]	4/6	1/6		1·0	4·00 (0·61–26·12)
Colgan[5]	23/38	12/42		10·9	2·12 (1·23–3·65)
Dale[6]	65/101	52/99		50·2	1·23 (0·97–1·55)
Falanga[10]	61/86	28/45		35·1	1·14 (0·87–1·49)
Schürmann[12]	2/12	3/12		2·9	0·67 (0·13–3·30)
Total (95% CI)	155/243	96/204		100·0	1·30 (1·10–1·54)
Test for heterogeneity		p=0·17			

0·1 0·2   1·0   5·0 10·0
Favours control   Favours treatment

FIGURE 1.—Relative risk of healing associated with pentoxifylline compared with placebo (with compression therapy as standard treatment) in patients with venous leg ulcers. (Courtesy of Jull A, Waters A, Arroll B: Pentoxifylline for treatment of venous leg ulcers: A systematic review. *Lancet* 359:1550-1554, 2002. Copyright by The Lancet Ltd, 2002.)

ulcers, or any other measure indicating substantial improvement. Eight trials (547 adults) were identified. Of these, 5 (445 patients) compared pentoxifylline and compression with placebo and compression. Three trials compared pentoxifylline alone with placebo (102 patients).

Results.—Pentoxifylline was more effective than placebo in complete healing or significant improvement of venous leg ulcers (relative risk [RR], 1.49; 95% confidence interval [CI], 1.11-2.01). Pentoxifylline with compression was more effective than placebo and compression in complete healing (RR, 1.30; CI, 1.10-1.54) (Fig 1). Patients who received pentoxifylline had no more adverse events than those who received placebo (RR, 1.25; CI, 0.87-1.80). The most common adverse effect was mild gastrointestinal disturbance (43%).

Conclusion.—Pentoxifylline provided additional benefit to compression in the treatment of venous leg ulcers. It may be effective for patients not receiving compression.

▶ This is a well-done meta-analysis that suggests pentoxifylline provides a small incremental benefit to compression in healing venous leg ulcers. While the drug may have an effect independent of compression, it seems to work best as an adjunct to compressive therapy. The evidence is not so convincing that pentoxifylline can be recommended for all venous ulcers, but it certainly should be considered in ulcers that are likely to be difficult to heal, such as large ulcers and/or longstanding ulcers.

G. L. Moneta, MD

Randomized Clinical Trial Comparing the Efficacy of Two Bandaging Regimens in the Treatment of Venous Leg Ulcers
Meyer FJ, Burnand KG, Lagattolla RF, et al (St Thomas' Hosp, London)
Br J Surg 89:40-44, 2002   16–3

Background.—For centuries, compression bandaging has been used to treat leg ulcerations caused by venous disease. Elastic compression has been used since the 1930s. More recently the Unna boot was developed and provided rigid encasement of the limb, which produced compression only when the leg altered its profile during exercise. Advocates of this type of inelastic compression believe that it is safer and more effective than elastic compression. The time to total healing in patients treated with an elastic regimen using Tensopress bandages and in patients treated with an inelastic regimen using Elastocrepe bandages was compared.

Methods.—A total of 112 patients were enrolled in the study and treated with a zinc-impregnated paste bandage that was applied directly to the ulcer. In 57 patients, the paste was covered with Tensopress bandages; in 55 patients, the paste was covered with Elastocrepe bandages. In both groups, tubular bandages were then applied over the tops of the bandages to hold them in place. All of the ulcers were stratified and randomized within 1 of 3 size groups and an intention-to-treat analysis was performed. The venous cause of the ulcer was confirmed on completion by ascending phlebography, foot volumetry, or venous duplex imaging.

Results.—At 26 weeks, healing had occurred in 58% of the ulcers covered with Tensopress bandages and in 62% of ulcers treated with Elastocrepe bandages. The median healing time for patients in the Tensopress group was 6 weeks, compared with 9.5 weeks for patients in the Elastocrepe group. Large ulcers took significantly longer to heal than small ulcers.

Conclusions.—The use of higher-compression elastic bandages did not result in a significant improvement in healing of venous ulcers.

▶ I think it is difficult to know what levels of sustained compression were achieved in this study, as pressures under the dressings were apparently not measured and clearly can degrade with time. What is clear is that compression does matter, but the degree of optimal compression is unknown. However, a reasonable suggestion is that in legs with normal circulation, the bandage should be wrapped sufficiently tight that when the patient returns for dressing changes there is no edema at the level of the ankle.

G. L. Moneta, MD

Reproducibility of Ultrasound Scan in the Assessment of Volume Flow in the Veins of the Lower Extremities

Ogawa T, Lurie F, Kistner RL, et al (Univ of Hawaii, Honolulu; Straub Found, Honolulu, Hawaii)
J Vasc Surg 35:527-531, 2002   16–4

Background.—A noninvasive method is needed to quantify venous flow. The optimal settings of US scan flow measurement were studied in the veins and assessed as to whether the standardization of these settings provides acceptable reproducibility of the venous flow measures in individual segments of the lower extremity veins.

Methods.—Twelve healthy volunteers were evaluated with duplex US scanning. Venous cross-sectional area, time average mean velocity, and venous flow were studied. Different measurement settings were assessed to determine reproducibility. Doppler scan sample volume size, US scan beam incident angle, and time interval of measurement varied across a spectrum. Test-retest venous flow measure reproducibility was then studied with optimized settings.

Findings.—The best volume flow measure repeatability was obtained when the full lumen of the vein was insonated, the US scan beam incident angle equaled 60 degrees, and the measurement time exceeded 40 seconds. The mean volume flow values in the common femoral vein, superficial femoral vein, profunda femoral vein, and greater saphenous vein were 360, 147, 86, and 38 mL/min, respectively. Test-retest repeatability coefficients for the common femoral vein, superficial femoral vein, profundus femoral vein, and greater saphenous vein were 96.9, 70.2, 40.8, and 16.8 mL/min, respectively.

Conclusions.—The use of sampling volumes that cover the entire venous lumen, an incident angle of 60 degrees, and measurement for 40 seconds or longer optimize the reproducibility of US scan measures of volume flow in veins. The repeatability of volumetric measurements is acceptable with these parameters. The values of flow volume determined with duplex US scanning were similar to those with thermodilution methods reported previously.

▶ Volume flow measurements in the venous system using ultrasound techniques have been previously relegated to the Journal of Unreproducible Results. In this article, the authors have described a technique to optimize measurements of venous volume flow in normal veins. They have taken a systematic approach to determine the optimal technique to measure venous volume flow. This is the first logical look at this problem that I am aware of. Volume of reflux flow ought to be important in patients with chronic venous insufficiency. It is hoped that the authors' techniques will be applicable to diseased as well as normal veins.

G. L. Moneta, MD

Hemodynamic Effects of Supervised Calf Muscle Exercise in Patients With Venous Leg Ulceration: A Prospective Controlled Study
Kan YM, Delis KT (Imperial College School of Medicine, London)
Arch Surg 136:1364-1369, 2001   16–5

Background.—A supervised exercise program is a well-established treatment for patients with intermittent claudication and is a standard therapeutic regimen for the rehabilitation of patients who have undergone cardiac surgery. More than two thirds of patients with venous ulcer have an impaired calf muscle pump. Physical training through supervised exercise may enhance the ejecting ability of this pump and improve the hemodynamic environment sufficiently to promote healing of the ulcer. The effects of short-term supervised calf exercise on the function of the calf muscle pump and on venous hemodynamics in limbs with venous ulceration were evaluated.

Methods.—This prospective controlled study was conducted at a university-associated tertiary care hospital. The study group consisted of 10 patients assigned to supervised isotonic calf muscle exercise for 7 consecutive days, and a control group of 11 patients matched with the exercise group for age, sex, ulcer size, and ulcer duration. Both exercise subjects and the study subjects had perimalleolar venous leg ulcers, impaired calf muscle function, and full movement of the ankle joint. Both groups provided a complete clinical history and then underwent a physical examination, venous duplex scanning, and air plethysmography. Hemodynamic parameters were measured with plethysmography at baseline and on day 8, and calf muscle endurance was determined by the maximal number of plantar flexions performed against a fixed 4-kg resistance during 6 minutes. The exercise group performed active plantar flexions with a standardized 4-kg resistance pedal ergometer. The main outcome measures were the ejected venous volume and ejection fraction in both groups at baseline and on day 8.

Results.—Hemodynamic performance at baseline was similar in both groups. After 7 days of exercise, patients in the exercise group improved a mean 67.5% in their ejected venous volume, with an improved ejection fraction of 62.5%, improved residual venous volume by 25%, and improvement of 28.6% in their residual volume fraction. Small changes were noted in the control group. No change was seen in venous filling index and venous volume in either group. The exercise group posted a 135% increase in muscular endurance from a median of 153 plantar flexions at baseline to 360 on day 7.

Conclusions.—Isotonic exercise increases muscular endurance, efficacy, and power in the calf muscle, all of which improve the ejecting ability of the calf and the global hemodynamic function of limbs with venous ulcerations.

▶ I have always wondered how much of the impairment in ejection fraction as determined by air plethysmography in patients with chronic venous insufficiency was due to pure calf muscle dysfunction, and how much was secondary to the presence of reflux and/or obstruction. It appears that ejection fraction can be improved with training, as can residual volume fraction, an air plethysmography calculated value that correlates with ambulatory venous pressure, which we know correlates with the severity of chronic venous insufficiency and the likelihood of venous ulceration. It is therefore reasonable that improvements in ejection fraction should correlate with clinical improvements of chronic venous insufficiency. Of course, we don't know that, as no clinical end points were assessed in this study, and it is unclear if improvements in ejection fraction in the lab translate to improvements in ejection fraction in daily life.

G. L. Moneta, MD

Effect of Healing on the Expression of Transforming Growth Factor βs and Their Receptors in Chronic Venous Leg Ulcers

Cowin AJ, Hatzirodos N, Holding CA, et al (Women's and Children's Hosp, North Adelaide, South Australia; Univ of Adelaide, South Australia; Royal Adelaide Hosp, South Australia; et al)
J Invest Dermatol 117:1282-1289, 2001   16–6

Background.—Venous ulceration results from chronic venous insufficiency. It is possible increased pressure in the venous system, which reduces the perfusion pressure and capillary flow rate, may result in the trapping of white blood cells in distal leg capillaries. It has been postulated that these trapped leukocytes become activated and release toxic metabolites, enzymes, and cytokines, damaging endothelial cells and allowing the passage of plasma proteins. These trapped leukocytes may also cause local areas of ischemia. Transforming growth factor β is part of the wound repair process. However, no previous studies have investigated the role of the transforming growth factor β receptors in chronic venous leg ulcers.

Methods.—Immunofluorescent analysis and quantitative competitive reverse transcription–polymerase chain reaction were used to identify protein and mRNA expression in biopsy samples from wounds in 12 patients with chronic venous leg ulcers and normal skin from 3 patients undergoing reconstructive surgery. Four of the patients with chronic leg ulcers had a second biopsy performed at 2 to 8 weeks after the first biopsy, when the wounds had entered the healing phase. The excised tissue included the surrounding intact skin, the ulcer edge, and the ulcer base.

Results.—Immunofluorescent staining for transforming growth factors β1, β2, and β3 was observed within the epidermis of skin that surrounded the chronic venous ulcers, as well as in fibroblasts and inflammatory cells of the dermis. However, this staining was not as strong as the staining observed in normal, unwounded skin. There was very little staining observed in the ulcers for any of the ligands. Transforming growth factor β type I receptor was observed throughout the ulcers and the unwounded skin biopsies, particularly in the basal epidermal cells. Immunofluorescence for type II transforming growth factor β receptor was not observed in any of the ulcer biopsy specimens but was seen throughout the epidermis and in fibroblasts and inflammatory cells in the surrounding skin.

Conclusions.—Transforming growth factor β1 and transforming growth factor β receptor II mRNA were expressed in all the chronic nonhealing ulcers, although the levels for the type II receptor were very low. These findings suggest that the absence of a viable receptor complex for the transforming growth factor βs in nonhealing chronic venous ulcers may be a contributing factor to wound chronicity.

▶ There are undoubtedly many factors that contribute to the chronicity of a venous ulcer. Since ultimately everything is basically chemistry, it is gratifying to see biochemical and genetic questions being addressed in venous disease. Research such as described here and in the following article (Abstract 16–7) is therefore important. I have no idea if the authors are barking up the right tree, but at least they are in the hunt.

G. L. Moneta, MD

Expression of Cyclooxygenase Isoforms in Normal Human Skin and Chronic Venous Ulcers
Abd-El-Aleem SA, Ferguson MWJ, Appleton I, et al (Univ of Manchester, England; Univ Hosp of South Manchester, England)
J Pathol 195:616-623, 2001   16–7

Background.—The persistence of inflammation may be one of the major factors delaying healing in chronic venous leg ulcers. Prostaglandins are significant mediators of inflammation and have proinflammatory effects, mediated mainly by affecting the vasculature. Cyclooxygenase (COX) is the rate-limiting enzyme in prostanoid synthesis and is present in 2 forms, COX-1 and COX-2. COX-1 is a factor in the maintenance of normal hemo-

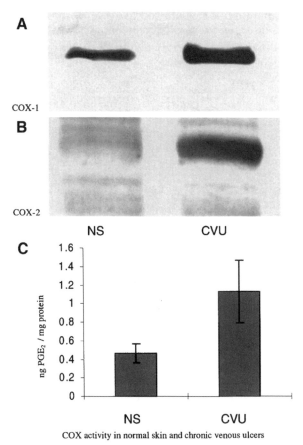

FIGURE 3.—Western blot analysis for COX-1 and COX-2 both in normal skin (*NS*) and in chronic venous ulcer (*CVU*). An equal amount of protein from both normal skin and chronic venous ulcer biopsies was loaded in each lane. The proteins were transferred to a blotting membrane and then stained using COX-1 and COX-2 antibodies. Both COX-1 and COX-2 bands were detected at approximate molecular weights 70 kD. **A,** The COX-1 band was present both in the normal skin and in the chronic venous ulcer biopsies, but it was denser and thicker in the latter. **B,** Chronic venous ulcer biopsies showed expression of COX-2 as indicated by the appearance of a band at approximate molecular weight 70 kD. This was not present in the lane containing normal skin. **C,** The activity of COX in normal human skin and chronic venous ulcer biopsies was measured as the ability of the homogenized tissues to metabolize arachidonic acid into prostaglandin E_2. There was a significant increase of COX-2 activity in chronic venous ulcer biopsies ($P < .05$) when compared with normal human skin. In both cases, the number of samples was 7. (Courtesy of Abd-El-Aleem S, Ferguson MWJ, Appleton I, et al: Expression of cyclooxygenase isoforms in normal human skin and chronic venous ulcers. *J Pathol* 195:616-623, 2001. Reprinted by permission of John Wiley & Sons, Ltd.)

static functions, and COX-2 is induced during inflammation in response to cytokines. The expression of COX-1 and COX-2 in normal skin and chronic venous ulcers was investigated.

Methods.—Sixteen normal skin and 14 long-standing nonhealing chronic venous ulcer biopsy specimens were used from patients with a mean age of 55 years. The patients were not taking steroids, nonsteroidal anti-inflammatory drugs (NSAIDs), or antibiotics, and none had evidence of diabetes, diabetic ulcers, or clinical evidence of infection. Samples were investigated with immunoenzymatic labeling and Western blot analysis.

Results.—Both COX-1 and COX-2 were upregulated in chronic venous leg ulcers in comparison with normal human skin (Fig 3). Macrophages and endothelial cells were the main cellular sources of both COX isoforms, but COX-2 was also produced by mast cells and fibroblasts. A COX radioimmunoassay showed upregulation of COX activity in chronic venous leg ulcers compared with normal skin.

Conclusions.—Upregulation of COX-1 in chronic venous leg ulcers could produce prostacyclin, which contributes to angiogenesis; therefore, inhibition of COX-1 by NSAIDs could increase the local ischemia and hypoxia associated with chronic venous ulcers. The upregulation of COX-2, however, is probably responsible for the persistent inflammation in chronic venous ulcers. Selective inhibitors of COX-2 could therefore show efficacy in the treatment of chronic venous ulcers.

▶ There are enough "could bes" and "maybes" in this article to choke a horse (and I have a few that I would like to choke). However, it is clear venous stasis disease has an inflammatory component, and the authors' hypothesis that COX-2, but not COX-1, inhibitors may be useful in the treatment of venous ulcers deserves consideration, although probably not a recommendation at this time.

G. L. Moneta, MD

Prospective Evaluation of Endoluminal Venous Stents in the Treatment of the May-Thurner Syndrome
Lamont JP, Pearl GJ, Patetsios P, et al (Baylor Univ, Dallas)
Ann Vasc Surg 16:61-64, 2002   16–8

Introduction.—The May-Thurner syndrome is pain, edema, or deep venous thrombosis (DVT) resulting from an acquired stenosis of the left common iliac vein. The patency and efficacy of endoluminal venous stents for treatment of May-Thurner syndrome in all patients seen between 1995 and 2000 were prospectively investigated.

Methods.—The study included 12 women and 3 men ages 23 to 72 years (median age, 43 years). The characteristic May-Thurner syndrome lesion was diagnosed with the use of venography after thrombus clearance (Fig 1). Patients underwent angioplasty, then stenting. Self-expanding Wallstents or Smart stents were used for stenting. The number of stents placed was individualized to allow a wide patent lumen (Fig 2). Stent patency was assessed with the use of a duplex US unit with a 5-mHz linear array probe with multihertz capability. All patients underwent anticoagulation with warfarin for a minimum of 6 months. Follow-up protocol included a complete physical examination and duplex US at 3 months, then at 6-month intervals thereafter.

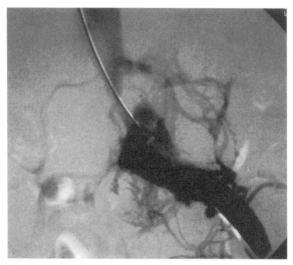

FIGURE 1.—Characteristic May-Thurner lesion. (Courtesy of Lamont JP, Pearl GJ, Patetsios P, et al: Prospective evaluation of endoluminal venous stents in the treatment of the May-Thurner syndrome. *Ann Vasc Surg* 16:61-64, 2002.)

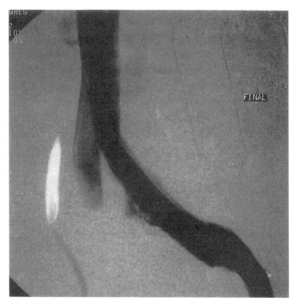

FIGURE 2.—Post-stent appearance showing widely patent lumen. (Courtesy of Lamont JP, Pearl GJ, Patetsios P, et al: Prospective evaluation of endoluminal venous stents in the treatment of the May-Thurner syndrome. *Ann Vasc Surg* 16:61-64, 2002.)

Results.—Fourteen Wallstents and 1 Smart stent were placed into the left common iliac. Complications were minor hematomas at the venous access site in 2 patients and hematuria related to thrombolytics in 1 patient. Fourteen patients (93%) had primary patency; 15 (100%) had assisted primary patency. One patient experienced an immediate stent thrombosis necessitating further thrombolytic therapy. The "CEAP" classification system showed 12 patients with C_0, 2 patients with $C_{1(s)}E_sA_DP_O$, and 1 patient with $C_{3(s)}E_s$-A_DP_O. The symptoms were mild in all 3 patients who were symptomatic. Duplex US revealed patent stents in 13 patients (87%). Two patients had stent occlusion at 14 and 41 months, respectively, which were treated conservatively. No patients had stent embolization or migration.

Conclusion.—Treatment of the May-Thurner syndrome using endoluminal stenting was correlated with low morbidity and high patency rates.

▶ Studies such as this and the next (Abstract 16–9) confirm stents can be placed in the iliac vein, and that many stay open in the short-term. Objective follow-up is crucial, as we all know collateral development in the venous system can very well compensate for a segmental venous occlusion. The word on venous stents is to be cautious. We didn't use them before, and patients seemed to do pretty well. (See Abstract 15–14.)

G. L. Moneta, MD

Incidence and Pattern of Long Saphenous Vein Duplication and Its Possible Implications for Recurrence After Varicose Vein Surgery
Corrales NE, Irvine A, McGuinness CL, et al (St Thomas' Hosp, London)
Br J Surg 89:323-326, 2002   16–9

Background.—Long saphenous vein (LSV) duplication may have implications for recurrence after varicose vein surgery. The incidence of this anomaly has not been definitively established. A consecutive cohort of saphenograms was reviewed to describe the pattern and incidence of LSV duplications and perforator vein connections.

Methods.—Eighty-five patients being evaluated for peripheral arterial bypass surgery were included in the study. A total of 103 saphenograms were obtained after nonionic contrast medium injection directly into the vein or its tributaries at the ankle. Two independent examiners assessed duplications of the LSV and their relation to thigh and calf perforator veins.

Findings.—Forty-nine percent of the saphenograms showed evidence of LSV duplication. Eighty-eight percent of the duplications were observed in the thigh. The most common pattern, present in 54%, was a closed loop. Perforator veins were connected to one branch of the duplication in 42% of the legs. In half, the perforator vein was attached to the nondominant branch of the duplication. Of 18 patients with bilateral saphenograms, only 10 had duplications in both legs. Only 1 had the same pattern of duplication on both sides.

Conclusions.—The incidence of venous duplication may be greater than previously believed. If left intact during LSV stripping, either limb of a duplication is a potential source of recurrent varicose veins.

▶ The authors' findings, although not new, are important in that they serve to remind us of the variability of the venous system and how it may influence venous surgery. Most surgeons are aware of duplications of the greater saphenous vein, as described in this article. The most useful information here is a description of connections of the duplicated veins to perforating veins. Precise mapping of the saphenous vein before venous surgery may allow preservation of 1 duplication if only part of the saphenous vein is malfunctioning. The anatomic data presented in this article suggest that we should not be routinely removing saphenous veins in patients undergoing varicose vein surgery. They should be removed only if the vein or a portion of the vein is found to be incompetent.

G. L. Moneta, MD

Endothelin Receptors in the Aetiology and Pathophysiology of Varicose Veins

Agu O, Hamilton G, Baker DM, et al (Royal Free and Univ College Med School, London)
Eur J Vasc Endovasc Surg 23:165-171, 2002   16–10

Background.—Varicose veins affect 10% to 45% of the adult population in Western societies. The primary cause of venodilatation, poor contractility, and recurrence after treatment of varicose veins remains unclear. Often the etiology, diagnosis, and treatment of varicose veins are explained on the basis of valvular insufficiency. However, the primary etiology of varicosis in the lower limb may lie in the inherent venous wall weakness. Smooth muscle maintenance of venous tone is achieved in part by the local effect of endogenous vasoconstrictor agents, of which endothelin (ET-1) is the most potent. The hypothesis that endothelial cells and endothelin receptor density and distribution may play a role in the development of varicose veins was investigated.

Methods.—Saphenous vein segments in 9 patients with varicose veins were compared with vein segments in 6 control subjects. Slide-mounted sections were incubated in radioactive-labeled ET-1, and autoradiography was used to assess receptor subtype-selective ligands and binding sites. Endothelial cells and ET-1 cells were identified by immunohistochemistry, and CD31-positive staining cells were counted.

Results.—There was a reduction in radioactive-labeled ET-1 and ET-B receptor binding in the varicose veins compared with control veins. ET-A receptor binding was diffuse, however, with no difference in density in both groups. ET-B receptor binding was diffuse, with superimposed clusters. The density of medial ET-B receptor binding was reduced in the varicose vein group, but more clusters were identified in these veins compared with control veins. These clusters were identified as endothelial cells through CD-31 staining.

Conclusions.—A reduction in ET-1 binding and ET-B receptor density may be partially responsible for the reduced vasocontractility in varicose veins. It is speculated that the increase in ET-B receptor binding CD31-positive endothelial cells in varicose veins may spur mitogenesis and migration, resulting in the formation of new vessels.

▶ The 2 primary theories of the etiology of varicose veins are valve dysfunction and inherent vessel wall weakness. Both mechanisms may play a role, but only inherent wall weakness could explain late development of valve dysfunction. The etiology of "weakness" of the venous wall is currently unknown. The evidence presented in this article that endothelin is the culprit is really quite weak. However, it is gratifying research is focusing on the biochemistry of the varicose vein wall. Hopefully, funding agencies will start tossing a few bones toward basic science venous research.

G. L. Moneta, MD

Varicose Veins: Loss of Release of Vascular Endothelial Growth Factor and Reduced Plasma Nitric Oxide
Hollingsworth SJ, Tang CB, Dialynas M, et al (London Med School)
Eur J Vasc Endovasc Surg 22:551-556, 2001   16–11

Background.—Vessel wall reactivity is maintained by the production and release of mediators of constricting and dilatory responses. Whether varicose veins (VVs) are the product of a central defect in the balance between these agents or of another pathologic condition is unclear. Experiments have been done with "ring" sections of veins used to evaluate the vein's ability to respond to exogenous doses of the agents that mediate venous constriction and dilatation. Patients with primary VVs have higher plasma levels of endothelin-1, which functions as a principal constrictor. Yet the veins remain dilated in these cases, suggesting an imbalance between contraction and dilatation that is caused by an aberrant or continued stimulus to dilate. Primary VVs were assessed for their ability to release vascular endothelial growth factor (VEGF), a principal factor in maintaining vascular reactivity and integrity, and nitric oxide (NO), a mediator of vasopermeability and dilatory response, in response to induced venous stasis.

Methods.—Twenty-one patients with primary VVs (age range, 21 to 78 years; median, 46 years) and 11 control subjects (age range, 22 to 55 years; median, 32 years) rested supine for 15 minutes during which blood samples were taken from an arm and a foot vein. Next, a below-the-knee cuff was inflated to 90 to 95 mm Hg for 10 minutes to produce venous stasis. The foot vein was sampled again and levels of plasma VEGF and NO assessed.

Results.—Baseline values for VEGF were similar in the 2 groups, but after the cuff was applied, the control subjects showed an increase in mean plasma VEGF of 8.5%, whereas those with VVs showed a change of only 4.2%.

Similar findings were found for NO at baseline, but neither group showed a significant effect after application of the cuff. The NO levels of patients with primary VVs were lower than those of control individuals in all samples.

Conclusions.—The development of primary VVs may be related to the loss of VEGF release and reduced plasma levels of NO when compared with normal healthy subjects.

▶ More biochemistry of the venous wall, with hopefully more to come.

G. L. Moneta, MD

Comparison of Clinical Outcome of Stripping and CHIVA for Treatment of Varicose Veins in the Lower Extremities
Maeso J, Juan J, Escribano JM, et al (Vall d'Hebron Gen Hosp, Barcelona)
Ann Vasc Surg 15:661-665, 2001   16–12

Background.—The latest in a series of innovations in the treatment of varicose veins is the conservative hemodynamic cure of venous insufficiency, which is known by its French acronym, CHIVA. CHIVA was designed to allow the treatment of varicose veins without sacrificing the entire superficial vein network. The only standard treatment for venous insufficiency is stripping of the saphenous veins with or without extirpation or sclerosis of varices. The outcome of stripping versus CHIVA for the treatment of varicose veins in the lower extremities were compared in a nonrandomized case-review study.

Methods.—Saphenous vein stripping with phlebectomy was performed in 85 patients, and CHIVA was performed in 90 patients. All the patients were followed up for 3 years.

Results.—The presence of varicose veins as a cause of failure occurred in 1.1% of the CHIVA group versus 15.3% in the stripping group. Telangiectasia developed in 8.95% of patients in the CHIVA group compared with 65.9% of patients in the stripping group, and the patient dissatisfaction rate was 3.3% for CHIVA versus 16.5% in the stripping group. Postoperative symptoms were a cause of failure in 1.1% of patients in the CHIVA group compared with 21.2% of patients in the stripping group. One patient in the CHIVA group and 16 patients in the stripping group had saphenous nerve injury.

Conclusions.—For the 5 criteria examined, patients who underwent CHIVA fared significantly better than did patients who underwent saphenous vein stripping with phlebectomy. Clinical results at 3 years were better for the CHIVA patients in terms of the presence of varicose veins, clinical symptoms, presence of telangiectasia, cosmetic satisfaction, and neurologic complications. Findings in this series are comparable to findings in the literature, and better than findings in 3 previous studies of stripping procedures with 3 years of follow-up.

▶ CHIVA is a French acronym for Conservative Hemodynamic Cure of Venous Insufficiency. It is designed as an alternative to stripping and is based on the use of Doppler US to map specific areas of hemodynamic incompetence in the superficial veins. It has some standing in Europe but is not widely practiced in North America. Indeed, it is not mentioned in most textbooks of venous surgery. I have no personal experience with this technique, and to me it seems unnecessarily complicated. The authors are correct in that the nonrandomized case review nature of this study does not allow one to determine if the CHIVA technique is superior to stripping. However, the results in this study do justify the conclusion that it does not appear to be terribly worse than stripping either.

G. L. Moneta, MD

Percutaneous Bioprosthetic Venous Valve: A Long-term Study in Sheep
Pavcnik D, Uchida BT, Timmermans HA, et al (Oregon Health Sciences Univ, Portland; Portland VA Med Ctr, Ore)
J Vasc Surg 35:598-602, 2002   16–13

Background.—Previously developed percutaneously placed prosthetic and bioprosthetic venous valves (BVVs) have been somewhat successful in the short term. However, they have not been assessed over the long term. A long-term experimental study of a new percutaneously placed square stent-based BVV was reported.

Methods.—Twelve sheep were included in the study. The new BVV was a bioprosthetic consisting of a square stent and small intestinal submucosa (SIS) covering. Twenty-six BVVs were placed into the jugular veins. Gross and histologic examinations were performed after the sheep were killed. Two were killed at 1 month and 5 were killed at 3 and 6 months.

Findings.—Twenty-five BVVs exhibited good valve function on immediate venography and 22 on venograms obtained before the animals were killed. Examination showed incorporation of remodeled and endothelialized SIS BVVs into the vein wall. Slight to moderate leaflet thickening, mostly at their bases, was observed.

Conclusions.—The percutaneously placed SIS BVV tested in this study is promising. It provides a 1-way, competent valve that resists venous backpressure while allowing forward flow. A trial in human beings is now warranted.

▶ The search for an implantable venous valve continues. This one seems to work in the short term in sheep jugular veins. Clinical trials in human beings are starting at this time.

G. L. Moneta, MD

Management of Congenital Venous Malformations of the Vulva

Marrocco-Trischitta MM, Nicodemi EM, Nater C, et al ("Istituto Dermopatico dell'Immacolata," Rome; Baylor College of Medicine, Houston)
Obstet Gynecol 98:789-793, 2001   16–14

Background.—The classification of congenital vascular anomalies is based on the endothelial characteristics that correlate with the clinical features and natural history of these lesions. Vascular anomalies can be grouped into 2 major categories, hemangiomas and vascular malformations. Vascular malformations can be further classified on the basis of the predominant channel type and flow characteristics. Slow-flow lesions include capillary, lymphatic, and venous malformations, and fast-flow lesions include arterial malformations, arteriovenous fistula, and arteriovenous malformations. Venous malformations are the most common and account for two thirds of all congenital vascular malformations. The differential diagnosis and management of venous malformations of the vulva were discussed.

Methods.—The experiences with treatment of 5 symptomatic patients were reported. The patients provided self-assessments of pain and discomfort by using a horizontal visual analog scale before and after treatment. All patients underwent preoperative evaluation with Doppler US, and 1 patient underwent MRI. All the patients also had direct-injection venography and sclerotherapy. Follow-up was accomplished with Doppler US scanning and clinical examinations.

Results.—All the patients had significant swelling after the injections, and cutaneous necrosis developed in 1 patient, which healed within 2 weeks. Transient hemoglobinuria developed in 2 patients. There were no early or late complications. At a mean follow-up of 23 months, all patients had complete relief from symptoms and currently have normal vulvar sensation. Complete ablation of the treated lesion was obtained in 4 patients. In 1 patient, there was a significant but incomplete occlusion of the lesion, and no additional treatment was necessary. Both patients and physicians considered the results successful from a cosmetic standpoint.

Conclusions.—Vulvar venous malformations should be distinguished from vulvar varicosities, hematomas, soft tissue neoplasms, and other vascular anomalies (Table 1). The most accurate diagnostic modalities are Doppler US, MRI, and direct-injection venography. Sclerotherapy is a successful therapeutic modality in patients with vulvar venous malformations. Direct-injection venography with digital subtraction serial imaging is preferred for monitoring this procedure.

▶ It appears selective sclerotherapy of primary venous malformations can be effective. In this case, vulvar lesions were treated. Note that the volume of sclerosant used and the sensitivity of the vulvar area necessitate an anesthetic for performance of this procedure. Ouch!

G. L. Moneta, MD

TABLE 1.—Distinguishing Criteria Between Vulvar Varicosities and Venous Malformations of the Vulva

	Vulvar Varicosities	Vulvar Venous Malformations
Natural history	Typical complication of pregnancy Usually shrink and disappear spontaneously within 6 wk after delivery	Present at birth, although not always evident Slowly worsen and grow during the lifeteime of the patient and, by definition, do not regress
Morbidity	Rarely symptomatic Complications such as intralesional thrombosis, ulceration, and hemorrhage are extremely rare	Often symptomatic and functionally disabling Spontaneous intralesional thromboses frequently occur
Gross appearance	Grapelike cluster of veins on the vulva	Bluish masses that may extensively involve the subcutaneous subfacial tissue
Histologic pattern	Veins with a greater cross-sectional area than normal vessels but without wall thinning Venous walls with considerable disrupted elastic tissue and endothelial-cell packing that increase proportionately with severity of the disease	Dysmorphic vessels composed of thin-walled channels, deficient in muscle cells and pericites, and lined by a single layer of flat, quiescent endothelium

(Reprinted with permission from The American College of Obstetricians and Gynecologists from Marrocco-Trischitta MM, Nicodemi EM, Nater C, et al: Management of congenital venous malformations of the vulva. *Obstet Gynecol* 98:789-793, 2001.)

Value of Isotope Lymphography in the Diagnosis of Lymphoedema of the Leg

Burnand KG, McGuinness CL, Lagattolla NRF, et al (St Thomas' Hosp, London; Sal Manyia Med Centre, Manama, Bahrain)
Br J Surg 89:74-78, 2002   16–15

Introduction.—Isotope lymphography has been reported to have good sensitivity and specificity in diagnosing lymphedema of the leg and has nearly replaced lymphography in the diagnosis of lymphedema. Its accuracy has only been evaluated in small trials. It is not known whether isotope lymphography can identify patients with proximal lymphatic obstructions who may be appropriate candidates for lymphatic bypass surgery. The accuracy of isotope lymphography in diagnosing lymphedema and the presence and level of proximal lymphatic obstructions in the leg were determined.

Methods.—Three hundred ninety-five patients with suspected lymphedema underwent isotope lymphography between 1985 and 1995. Contrast lymphography was also performed in 29 patients in this cohort when the isotope results were thought to be misleading or when lymphatic bypass surgery was a possibility.

Results.—For the 29 patients who underwent both investigations, isotope lymphography identified 20 (83.3%) of 24 abnormal lymphatic systems. Four legs with obstructed groin lymphatics were reported as normal by isotope lymphography. Lymphoedema was incorrectly diagnosed in 2 legs with normal contrast lymphograms. Detectable groin nodes on the scintigrams were suggestive of either normal lymphatics or proximal lymphatic obstruction. An increase of less than 50% in isotope uptake during 30 to 60 minutes or a total absence of isotope within groin nodes were sensitive indicators that lymphatic bypass surgery was not appropriate.

Conclusion.—Isotope lymphography is moderately sensitive in the assessment of lymphedema, which means that it will mistakenly classify some normal legs as lymphedematous. This method usually correctly identifies patients who are suitable for undergoing lymphatic bypass surgery.

▶ There are little hot beds of lymphatic surgery here and there, and there appears to still be one at St Thomas'. I have very rarely (this means never) found it necessary to perform lymphography in patients with suspected lymphedema. Of course, I think the large majority (this means all) of lymphatic procedures are a waste of time, energy, and money.

G. L. Moneta, MD

17 Portal Hypertension

The Hemodynamic Response to Medical Treatment of Portal Hypertension as a Predictor of Clinical Effectiveness in the Primary Prophylaxis of Variceal Bleeding in Cirrhosis
Merkel C, Bolognesi M, Sacerdoti D, et al (Univ of Padua, Italy)
Hepatology 32:930-934, 2000
17–1

Background.—Hemodynamic response to drug treatment predicts clinical efficacy in the prevention of variceal rebleeding. The role of the hemodynamic response to β-blockers or β-blockers plus nitrates in predicting the clinical efficacy of prophylaxis was investigated.

Methods.—Forty-nine cirrhotic patients with varices at risk for bleeding and without previous variceal bleeding underwent hepatic vein catheterization before and after 1 to 3 months of treatment with nadolol or nadolol plus isosorbide mononitrate. The patients were followed up for up to 5 years.

Findings.—Thirty patients (61%) responded well hemodynamically. In this group, the hepatic venous pressure gradient (HVPG) was 12 mm or less in 24%. Nine patients had variceal bleeding during treatment; 7 of these

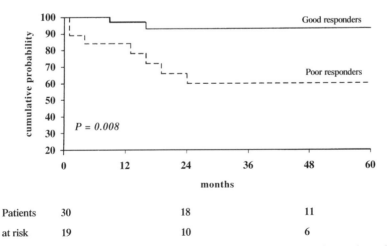

FIGURE 1.—Cumulative probability of being free of a first variceal bleeding in good responders (*solid line*) and poor responders (*dashed line*) according to hemodynamic criteria. (Courtesy of Merkel C, Bolognesi M, Sacerdoti D, et al: The hemodynamic response to medical treatment of portal hypertension as a predictor of clinical effectiveness in the primary prophylaxis of variceal bleeding in cirrhosis. *Hepatology* 32:930-934, 2000.)

were poor responders and 2 were good responders. After 3 years of follow-up, the probability of bleeding was significantly greater in poor responders than in good responders (41% and 7%, respectively) (Fig 1). None of the patients with an HVPG of 12 mm Hg or less during treatment had variceal bleeding during follow-up. In a Cox regression analysis, poor hemodynamic response was the main predictor of bleeding. Eleven patients died from hepatic causes during follow-up. Survival correlated with Child-Pugh class and initial HVPG value.

Conclusion.—In patients with cirrhosis treated with β-blockers with or without nitrates, the best predictor of the efficacy of prophylaxis of bleeding from esophageal varices is the hemodynamic response to medical treatment of portal hypertension. Such response is reflected in an HVPG reduction to 12 mm Hg or less or by a decrease of more than 20% of the initial value.

▶ Patients with varices and cirrhosis treated with β-blockers and who had a decrease in their hepatic venous pressure gradient to 12 mm Hg, or a decrease greater than 20% from baseline, suffered virtually no variceal bleeding during follow-up. β-blockers were given to reduce the heart rate to 75% of baseline. The results imply that β-blockers in such patients should be pushed as much as possible to decrease the hepatic vein pressure gradient to 12 mmHg or less, as long as the patient can tolerate the cardiac and side effects of the β-blocker.

G. L. Moneta, MD

Efficacy of Irbesartan, a Receptor Selective Antagonist of Angiotensin II, in Reducing Portal Hypertension

Debernardi-Venon W, Barletti C, Alessandria C, et al (Molinette Hosp, Turin, Italy)
Dig Dis Sci 47:401-404, 2002   17–2

Background.—Portal hypertension is characterized by a pathologic increase in hepatic venous pressure and is most frequently caused by cirrhosis of the liver. This risk of variceal bleeding becomes significant when the hepatic venous pressure, as measured by the hepatic venous pressure gradient (HVPG), increases above 12 mm Hg. The use of a receptor-selective antagonist of angiotensin II has been proposed for the treatment of portal hypertension. The effect of irbesartan on portal pressure was assessed and its safety in cirrhotic patients with portal hypertension evaluated.

Methods.—In this pilot study, 25 patients (18 men, 7 women; mean age, 55 years) with cirrhosis of the liver and portal hypertension were treated with irbesartan, 300 mg orally once daily for 60 days. Hemodynamic evaluations and biochemical tests were performed before therapy and after 2 months of treatment.

Results.—Three patients discontinued treatment after developing symptomatic arterial hypotension about 10 days from the start of therapy. In 4 of the long-term treated patients (18%), therapy did not modify HVPG. In the rest of the patients who responded to therapy, treatment with irbesartan

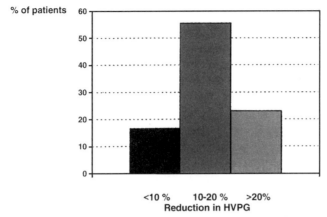

FIGURE 2.—The magnitude of the reduction in the hepatic venous pressure gradient (*HVPG*) after 60 days of therapy with irbesartan. (Courtesy of Debernardi-Venon W, Barletti C, Alessandria C, et al: Efficacy of irbesartan, a receptor selective antagonist of angiotensin II, in reducing portal hypertension. *Dig Dis Sci* 47:401-404, 2002. Copyright 2002, Plenum Publishing Corporation.)

yielded a mean reduction in HVPG from 18.1 ± 3.5 mm Hg to 14.9 ± 4.2 mm Hg (Fig 2). This reduction was related both to a reduction in wedged hepatic venous pressure and to an increase in free hepatic venous pressure. The mean arterial pressure declined significantly during therapy, from 109 ± 25 mm Hg to 92 ± 7 mm Hg.

Conclusions.—Irbesartan therapy can produce a marginal reduction in portal pressure. However, there are significant side effects that may limit the utility of this drug.

▶ β-blockers may have a favorable effect on portal hypertension and variceal bleeding. Angiotensin-converting enzyme inhibitors, at least irbesartan, appear to be less effective.

G. L. Moneta, MD

Preliminary Results of a New Expanded-Polytetrafluoroethylene–covered Stent-Graft for Transjugular Intrahepatic Portosystemic Shunt Procedures

Otal P, Smayra T, Bureau C, et al (Rangueil Hosp, Toulouse, France; Purpan Hosp, Toulouse, France)
AJR 178:141-147, 2002 17–3

Background.—For more than a decade, transjugular intrahepatic portosystemic shunts (TIPS) have been used to treat variceal bleeding or refractory ascites from portal hypertension. However, the primary patency rate is only about 50% at 1 year. Delayed dysfunction is usually the result of pseudointimal hyperplasia that may be caused by biliary leaks of transected bile ducts into the shunt lumen or by hepatic vein stenosis from

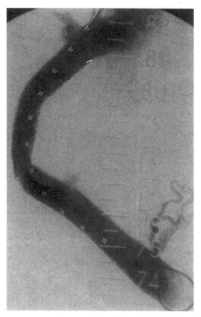

FIGURE 3.—Follow-up venogram at 6 months in 47-year-old woman with variceal bleeding shows patent, stenosis-free transjugular portosystemic shunt. Portosystemic pressure gradient is 2 mm Hg. (Courtesy of Otal P, Smayra T, Bureau C, et al: Preliminary results of a new expanded-polytetrafluoroethylene-covered stent-graft for transjugular intrahepatic portosystemic shunt procedures. *AJR* 178:141-147, 2002.)

intimal hyperplasia. The safety and feasibility of TIPS with a new expanded-polytetrafluoroethylene–covered stent were investigated.

Methods.—Twenty cirrhotic patients hospitalized with a history of esophageal variceal bleeding or refractory ascites were studied. Five patients needed treatment for TIPS revision. Doppler US was performed at discharge and periodically for up to 15 months. Venography with a portosystemic pressure gradient was measured at 6 months and when needed (Fig 3).

Findings.—Complications included 3 TIPS restenoses and 1 recurrent ascites treated successfully by balloon dilation. Segmentary liver ischemia occurred in 2 patients and encephalopathy requiring shunt reduction in 1. The mean portosystemic pressure gradient declined from 18 to 5 mm Hg after TIPS placement. At 387 days, primary and secondary patency rates were 80% and 100%, respectively.

Conclusion.—Placement of the Gore (W L Gore, Flagstaff, Ariz) TIPS endoprosthesis stent-graft is feasible, with improved patency. Further research is needed to compare the efficacy of covered and noncovered TIPS stents.

▶ Covering a TIPS shunt with polytetrafluoroethylene (PTFE) theoretically obviates what is felt to be a major contributor to TIPS failure; leakage of bile into the shunt tract. Whatever the mechanism of failure, the PTFE-covered stents in this series appear to perform much better than the usual bare metal stents. If these results hold up in larger trials, perhaps TIPS will move from a bridge to transplantation to first-line treatment for variceal bleeding. No one, save for a few dinosaurs, will miss the days of portocaval shunts.

G. L. Moneta, MD

Extrahepatic Portal Vein Aneurysm: A Case Report and Review of the Literature
Lau H, Chew DK, Belkin M (Harvard Med School, Boston)
Cardiovasc Surg 10:58-61, 2002   17–4

Background.—Ultrasonographic studies have evaluated the normal dimensions of the portal vein, but there is significant variation in the reports of mean portal vein diameter. In cirrhotic patients, the maximal diameter of the vein was reported as approaching 19 mm. A diameter greater than 2 cm is therefore considered aneurysmal. Portal vein aneurysm is the most common type of visceral venous aneurysm. The increasing number of case reports of portal vein aneurysm is attributable to the increasing use of radiologic imaging for the diagnosis and screening of abdominal disorders. A woman was described who had an extrahepatic portal vein aneurysm that was an incidental finding during a workup for dyspepsia. In addition, the literature was reviewed regarding the etiology, clinical significance, and management of portal vein aneurysm.

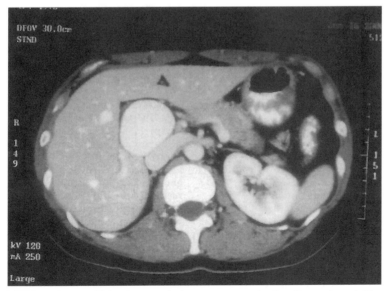

FIGURE 1.—Contrast CT showing a portal vein aneurysm measuring 4 cm diameter (*arrow*). (Courtesy of Lau H, Chew DK, Belkin M: Extrahepatic portal vein aneurysm: A case report and review of the literature. *Cardiovasc Surg* 10:58-61, 2002. Copyright 2002, The International Society for Cardiovascular Surgery. Published by Elsevier Science Ltd. All rights reserved.)

Case Report.—Asian woman, 30, complained of dyspepsia for 3 months. She was previously well and had no history of liver disease. The physical examination revealed no stigmata of chronic liver disease or signs of portal hypertension. Peripheral arterial and venous examinations were normal. Her abdomen was soft and nontender with no palpable masses. There was no bruit on auscultation. Abdominal US showed dilatation of the portal vein with a diameter of 4 cm. The gallbladder was normal. CT showed a homogenous contrast-enhancing lesion over the hilum of the liver, a finding compatible with an extrahepatic portal vein aneurysm (Fig 1). There was no intramural thrombus, and laboratory studies and a liver function test were normal. Because this patient's symptoms were minimal, an expectant management strategy was adopted, with serial imaging to monitor the size of the aneurysm. The patient was subsequently lost to follow-up.

Conclusions.—Extrahepatic portal vein aneurysm is a rare condition that is increasingly recognized. In asymptomatic patients without portal hypertension, expectant treatment appears to be justified until the natural history of the aneurysm is determined. Regular surveillance with duplex imaging is advised, and surgery should be considered if the patient develops symptoms or if the aneurysm enlarges.

▶ When one is unclear what to do, a reasonable plan is to do nothing . . . too bad we haven't adopted the same approach for neurogenic thoracic outlet syndrome.

G. L. Moneta, MD

18 Technical Notes

External Carotid Artery Reconstruction Performed Using an Autologous Internal Carotid Artery Patch
Pritz MB (Indiana Univ, Indianapolis)
J Neurosurg 94:996-998, 2001

18–1

Background.—At times, the obliteration of a residual stump of an occluded cervical internal carotid artery (ICA) is indicated. There may also be a need for reconstruction of an external carotid artery (ECA). Several procedures for obliteration of the ICA and ECA reconstruction are described in the literature, including patching with a variety of synthetic and autologous materials. A procedure was described in which the cervical ICA is obliterated and used as a graft to patch the ECA.

Methods.—In this procedure, positioning of the patient and exposure of the carotid arteries are performed in the standard fashion. The patient is given an infusion of sodium heparin, 100 U/kg, and 5 minutes after the infusion has been completed, the relevant vessels are occluded. An arteriotomy is made in the ICA first, and a separate incision is then made in the common carotid artery (CCA), extending distally to just proximal to the branching of the ECA (Fig 1, a). If indicated, an endarterectomy of the ICA, ECA, and proximal CCA is carried out (Fig 1, b). The stump of the ICA is excised (Fig 1, c and d), a diamond-shaped patch is formed, and the distal ICA is ligated (Fig 1, e). The orifice of the ICA is obliterated, and the ICA patch is sewn in place by using standard techniques (Fig 1, f). The ECA is backbled after reconstruction is complete (Fig 1, g). The clip leading to the superior thyroid artery is removed, and the CCA clamp released, and after 30 seconds the ECA clip is removed. Heparin therapy is not reversed. The incision is closed after placement of a drain in the carotid artery bed, and the drain is removed the next day.

Results.—This procedure was performed in 3 patients before extracranial-intracranial bypass. ICA obliteration and ECA reconstruction were satisfactory in all 3 patients. There were no perioperative complications and no postoperative morbidity at 30 days.

Conclusions.—This technique for obliteration of the ICA and reconstruction of the ECA may be more difficult and time-consuming than some other procedures, but it offers 2 advantages: the smooth obliteration of the ICA, and the precise placement of the patch graft by the use of autologous artery.

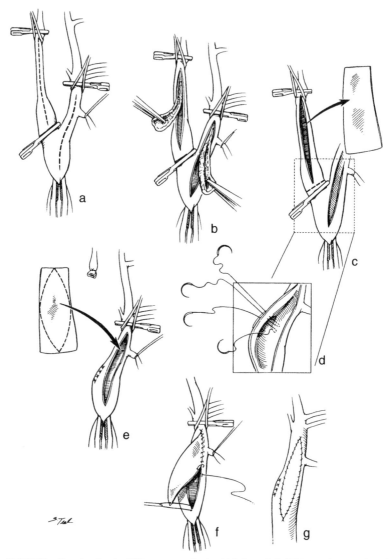

FIGURE 1.—Drawing showing ECA reconstruction in which the occluded ICA is used as a patch graft for angioplasty. See text for explanation. (Courtesy of Pritz MB: External carotid artery reconstruction performed using an autologous internal carotid artery patch. *J Neurosurg* 94:996-998, 2001.)

▶ The neurosurgeons have discovered the fact that an endarterectomized vessel can be used as a patch graft. Seems to me this is Vascular Surgery 101.

G. L. Moneta, MD

Anteposition of the Internal Carotid Artery for Surgical Treatment of Kinking
Székely G, Csécsei GI (Univ of Debrecen, Hungary)
Surg Neurol 56:124-126, 2001   18–2

Background.—When kinking of the extracranial portion of the internal carotid artery (ICA) causes neurologic symptoms, surgical reconstruction is needed. A simple surgical procedure without arteriotomy was presented.

Methods and Outcomes.—Three patients (age, 45-54 years) underwent the procedure. All had vertigo, and 2 had amaurosis fugax and sensorimotor transient ischemic attacks. Duplex US revealed a tortuous ICA course at the extracranial portion. Angiography showed double kinking with stenosis of greater than 60% at the bends.

The procedure involved carefully exposing the carotid bifurcation and anterior part of the digastric muscle along the medial aspect of the sternocleidomastoid muscle. The ventral and lateral bends disappeared after the ICA was mobilized. The surgeon then sectioned the tendon of the digastric muscle next to the hyoid bone. The ICA was positioned lateral to the muscle and the digastric muscle repaired with sutures behind the vessel. This fixed the ICA in the optimal position without kinking. After this procedure, all patients were clinically and radiologically improved.

Conclusion.—Anteposition of the ICA ventral to the digastric muscle was performed successfully in 3 patients. With this technique, arteriotomy and its complications can be avoided.

▶ The authors describe dividing the gastric muscle and then re-approximating it behind the ICA as a means of eliminating a distal internal carotid artery kink. While I do not believe that carotid kinks deserve treatment on their own merit, the authors do describe an interesting technique of eliminating distal kinking of the carotid artery. This may be useful in some cases of bifurcation endarterectomy, where otherwise a surgeon would need to extend the endarterectomy onto the area of the kink in order to avoid postoperative thrombosis of the vessel. With the use of the authors' technique, the arteriotomy perhaps could be limited to the bifurcation and the distal kink eliminated without the use of an extended arteriotomy.

G. L. Moneta, MD

The Bridge Graft: A New Concept for Infrapopliteal Surgery

Deutsch M, Meinhart J, Howanietz N, et al (Lainz Hosp, Vienna; Ludwig Boltzmann Inst for Applied Cardiovascular Biology, Vienna; Univ of Cape Town, South Africa)

Eur J Vasc Endovasc Surg 21:508-512, 2001

18–3

Background.—The long-term results of ePTFE (expanded polytetrafluoroethylene) prostheses are disappointing in crural reconstructions. It is believed that surface thrombogenicity and a mismatch of anastomotic compliance are contributing factors to the poorer performance of prosthetic graft material. In femorocrural bypass grafts, however, additional factors such as distinct diameter mismatches and particularly low-flow conditions aggravate thrombogenicity. The results of ePTFE grafts can be significantly improved by reducing the impact of anastomotic size and compliance mismatch through sleeves such as the Linton and Taylor patch, the St Mary's boot, and the Millar collar. A surgical technique that addresses both anastomotic mismatch and poor run-off was developed. The results of this technique were evaluated in the first group of patients in which it was used.

Methods.—The study group comprised 45 patients. Short segments of vein grafts measuring 5 to 15 cm were used to bridge 2 crural artery segments (Fig 2). A femorodistal ePTFE graft was then anastomosed to the bridge graft. Venous valves were rendered incompetent to allow bidirectional flow. Twelve of the patients were in stage III and 33 patients were in stage IV. The reconstruction was the first procedure in 18 patients, and the first or second reoperation in the remaining 28 patients.

Results.—The primary patency rates at 1, 2, 3, and 4 years were 53%, 44%, 35%, and 26%, respectively. The corresponding rates of limb salvage were 70%, 61%, 56%, and 45%. Among the patients in whom the crural bridge was the first reconstructive procedure, the primary patency rate was 76% at 1 year and 64% at 4 years.

Conclusion.—Crural bridge-graft reconstruction is an effective new tool for distal reconstructions.

▶ This technique essentially attempts to increase runoff for a PTFE lower extremity bypass graft by using a short segment of vein to connect 2 tibial arteries. Theoretically, this sounds appealing as "2-vessel" runoff is to be preferred over "1-vessel" runoff. I am unsure, however, if theory matches fact and total flow within the PTFE graft is actually increased by this procedure. In addition, it has always been my impression that revascularization of a single tibial artery is sufficient for treatment of lower extremity ischemia.

G. L. Moneta, MD

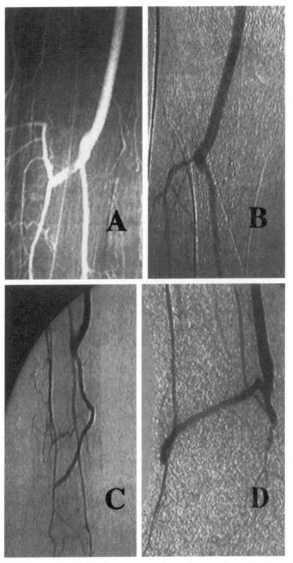

FIGURE 2.—A, Short proximal bridge between posterior and peroneal artery. **B**, Long bridge from the tractus to the distal posterior tibial artery. **C**, Bridge from the posterior tibial to the anterior tibial artery. **D**, Bridge from the posterior tibial (retromalleolar) artery to the dorsal pedal artery. (Courtesy of Deutsch M, Meinhart J, Howanietz N, et al: The bridge graft: A new concept for infrapopliteal surgery. *Eur J Vasc Endovasc Surg* 21:508-512, 2001. Copyright 2001, by permission of Harcourt Publishers Ltd.)

Renal Autotransplantation for Renovascular Hypertension: Extraperitoneal Renal Approach and Use of the Ovarian Vein for Vascular Reconstruction

Johnston WK III, London ET, Perez RV (Univ of California, Davis, Sacramento)
J Am Coll Surg 194:88-92, 2002   18–4

Background.—Renovascular hypertension caused by arteriosclerosis, aneurysms, and intimal or medial fibroplasia is a common cause of secondary hypertension. Autotransplantation is considered for patients in whom in situ repair is difficult, extensive reconstruction is expected, or where there is distal or intrarenal vascular disease requiring multiple small anastomoses. A patient with fibromuscular hyperplasia extending into both primary and secondary renal arterial branches with refractory hypertension after failed angioplastic intervention is described. In this case, a novel surgical approach was used for autotransplantation into the pelvis with the use of an extraperitoneal approach for nephrectomy and ex vivo renal arterial reconstruction with the ovarian vein.

Case Report.—Woman, 34, had severe hypertension. US examination after unsuccessful medical management revealed renal artery stenosis. Renal angiography suggested fibromuscular dysplasia. Angioplasty initially obtained a good response, but the hypertension returned, and a repeat angiogram demonstrated lesions extending into the primary and secondary branches of the renal artery. Surgical intervention involved harvesting of the right kidney through a paramedian incision and a retroperitoneal approach. Reconstruction was completed ex vivo under hypothermic conditions, after perfusion of the kidney with standard preservation solution. The entire renal arterial system was dissected to identify a markedly stenotic secondary branch, which was excised and replaced with an ovarian vein interposition graft. Autotransplantation was performed through a separate lower-quadrant incision with vascular anastomosis with a cold perfusion time of 70 minutes. By the second postoperative day, the peripheral vein renin level had decreased to 0.6 ng/mL, and the patient remained normotensive without medications. Technetium-99m MAG 3 nuclear scan at 6 months demonstrated normal flow and uptake in the repaired kidney. The patient continued to be free of symptoms and free of medication at 2-year follow-up.

Conclusions.—This is apparently the first report of nephrectomy through an extra-abdominal approach using the ovarian vein for ex vivo renal artery reconstruction and subsequent autotransplantation. Autotransplantation is a viable option in patients in whom in situ repair is difficult or in patients with distal or intrarenal vascular disease that requires multiple small anastomoses.

▶ Another source of vein I had previously not thought of.

G. L. Moneta, MD

Is There a Place for External Mesh Wrapping of Abdominal Aortic Aneurysms in the Modern Endovascular Era?
Karkos CD, Kenshil AY, Bruce IA, et al (Blackpool Victoria Hosp, England)
Eur J Vasc Endovasc Surg 23:172-174, 2002   18–5

Background.—Vascular surgeons sometimes must treat patients unfit for open repair and with aneurysms unsuitable for endovascular repair. In such cases, surgeons must decide between not operating and less invasive options. One experience with external mesh wrapping of abdominal aortic aneurysms (AAAs) was reported.

Patients.—From 1988 to 1999, 10 patients underwent mesh wrapping (external grafting) of their AAAs. The mean patient age was 74 years. None of the patients were candidates for endovascular repair. Eight had a suprarenal extension. One hundred forty underwent conventional open repair during that time.

Findings.—The mean operating time was about 1 hour, and the mean blood loss was 150 mL. No blood transfusions were needed. The mean length of hospitalization was 8 days. One patient died of rupture on postoperative day 4. Another 8 patients died during follow-up, 7 of rupture of their AAAs at between 5 weeks and 48 months. The eighth patient died 5 years postoperatively of rupture of the left iliac aneurysm, which was not present at initial surgery. One patient is alive 54 months after surgery.

Conclusion.—Circumferential wrapping of the aorta (external grafting), with or without preservation of the lumbar and inferior mesenteric vessels, reinforces the aortic wall by circumferential synthetic prosthesis, but the procedure is technically demanding and time consuming. Patients who are not fit for standard graft repair of AAAs are probably also unfit for external grafting.

▶ In my opinion, the answer to the question posed in the title is no! Wrapping clearly did not prevent rupture in this study. The suggestion that wrapping may delay rupture is clearly an attempt to put a shine on a buffalo turd.

G. L. Moneta, MD

Ureteral Injury During Aortic Aneurysm Repair by the Retroperitoneal Approach
Sheehan MK, Shireman PK, Littooy FN, et al (Loyola Univ, Maywood, Ill; Hines Veterans Affairs Hosp, Ill)
Ann Vasc Surg 15:481-484, 2001   18–6

Background.—Ureteral injury is known to occur rarely in vascular reconstructive surgery, with an incidence of 0.8% to 2.2% and direct injury occurring in 0.67% to 0.85% of cases. Vascular surgery accounts for up to 8% of all iatrogenic ureteral injuries, but that number increases to 43.8% of all ureteral injuries among men. Three cases of traction-associated ureteral injury after abdominal aortic aneurysm (AAA) repair with the retroperitoneal approach were reported.

Case 1.—Man, 64, had an aneurysm discovered during exploration for an iatrogenic injury of the colon. Colostomy and subsequent takedown were performed, and 4 months later the patient underwent an uneventful aortic aneurysm repair with tube graft placement by means of a left retroperitoneal approach. Retraction was maintained by a self-retaining instrument attached to the operating room table. He was seen in the emergency department on postoperative day 13 complaining of left flank and back pain. Abdominal CT revealed a large retroperitoneal fluid collection. After the patient continued to experience increasing abdominal girth and pain, a drain was placed under CT guidance on postoperative day 21, and approximately 4 L of clear fluid was removed.

Case 2.—Man, 65, was found to have a 5-cm infrarenal AAA, which was replaced with a Dacron tube graft via a left retroperitoneal approach. The patient was seen in the emergency department 2 weeks later with left flank and back pain and abdominal distension. A CT showed a retroperitoneal fluid collection.

Case 3.—Man, 64, with an asymptomatic AAA underwent repair through a left retroperitoneal approach. On the fifth postoperative day, the patient had serous drainage through the wound site, although the wound was still well approximated. Drainage continued until the 20th postoperative day, when CT revealed a fluid collection in the posterior perirenal space and mild hydronephrosis of the left kidney and poor visualization of the left ureter.

Conclusions.—All the patients underwent a percutaneous nephrostomy tube placement in response to ureteral injury. Ureteral repair was not possible because extensive fibrosis was present in each patent, necessitating a left nephrectomy in all 3 patients. It is likely that all 3 injuries were caused by traction on the ureter in a setting in which the kidney was not fully mobilized from the posterior and lateral position.

▶ The retroperitoneal approach for a large aneurysm with kidney up can clearly result in significant traction on the left ureter. I think with careful placement of retractors there really does not need to be stretching of the ureter when the kidney is left down.

G. L. Moneta, MD

External Iliac Artery–to–Internal Iliac Artery Endograft: A Novel Approach to Preserve Pelvic Inflow in Aortoiliac Stent Grafting
Bergamini TM, Rachel ES, Kinney EV, et al (Surgical Care Associates, Louisville, Ky)
J Vasc Surg 35:120-124, 2002   18–7

Introduction.—Adjuvant open and endovascular techniques have been developed to facilitate endovascular repair of abdominal aortic aneurysms (AAAs) associated with common iliac artery aneurysms that extend to the iliac bifurcation. Interruption of 1 and sometimes both internal iliac arteries can usually be performed safely, but it is prudent to preserve at least 1 internal iliac artery if at all feasible. A novel approach to preserving pelvic perfusion during endovascular AAA repair in patients with bilateral common iliac artery aneurysms extending to the iliac bifurcation is presented.

Methods.—The study included 4 patients (ages 70-79 years) who had multiple risk factors, an AAA with a mean diameter of 6.6 cm, and bilateral common iliac artery aneurysm. They underwent contrast-enhanced CT, arteriography, and intravascular US. Aortobiiliac endovascular AAA was not possible because the common iliac artery aneurysms extended to the iliac bifurcation bilaterally.

Results.—The AAAs were repaired by means of an aortouniiliac graft and a femoral-femoral graft. The ipsilateral internal iliac artery was treated with coil embolization and extension of the endograft to the external iliac artery. The contralateral common iliac artery aneurysms were excluded (with a custom-made stent graft in 2 patients or a commercial stent graft in the remaining 2 patients) from the external iliac artery to the internal iliac artery, preserving pelvic inflow by retrograde perfusion from the femorofemoral bypass (Fig 2). The mean length of hospital stay was 3.5 days. One patient

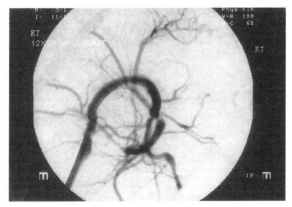

FIGURE 2.—Intraoperative arteriogram, obtained retrograde through the femoral sheath, of Wallgraft external iliac artery-to-internal iliac artery endograft with intimal irregularity of external iliac artery and internal iliac artery. Anterior and posterior trunks of internal iliac artery are patent. No endoleak or filling of common iliac artery aneurysm was seen. (Courtesy of Bergamini TM, Rachel ES, Kiney EV, et al: External iliac artery-to-internal iliac artery endograft: A novel approach to preserve pelvic inflow in aortoiliac stent grafting. *J Vasc Surg* 35:120-124, 2002.)

experienced hip claudication. At a mean follow-up of 10 months (range, 6-17 months), color-flow duplex scanning and contrast-enhanced CT revealed that all 4 external iliac artery-to-internal iliac artery endografts remained patent. No endoleaks or deaths occurred.

Conclusion.—Patients with bilateral common iliac artery aneurysms that extend to the iliac bifurcation may be excluded from endovascular AAA repair because of concerns about pelvic ischemia after occlusion of both internal iliac arteries. External iliac-to-internal iliac artery endografting is a possible alternative to maintain pelvic perfusion and still permit endograft repair of the AAA.

▶ There have been increasing reports of hip claudication associated with hypogastric ablation performed to facilitate aortic endografting. This is a clever endovascular method to maintain patency of the internal iliac artery with aortoiliac stent grafting when common iliac artery aneurysms extend to the iliac bifurcation.

G. L. Moneta, MD

Successful Endografting With Simultaneous Visceral Artery Bypass Grafting for Severely Calcified Thoracoabdominal Aortic Aneurysm
Watanabe Y, Ishimaru S, Kawaguchi S, et al (Tokyo Med Univ)
J Vasc Surg 35:397-399, 2002   18–8

Introduction.—The inability to reattach the intercostal arteries is a serious disadvantage of endografting for patients with thoracoabdominal aortic aneurysm (TAAA). Severe calcification of the distal thoracic aorta can pre-

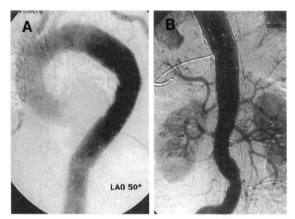

FIGURE 3.—Digital subtraction angiography after endografting. Endografts were interplaced from the proximal descending aorta to just above the renal arteries. No endoleaks or collateral perfusion within the aneurysmal sac were observed. The CA and SMA were well enhanced through the bifurcated prosthetic graft. A, case 1; B, case 2. *Abbreviations: CA,* Celiac axis; *SMA,* superior mesenteric artery. (Courtesy of Watanabe Y, Ishimaru S, Kawaguchi S, et al: Successful endografting with simultaneous visceral artery bypass grafting for severely calcified thoracoabdominal aortic aneurysm. *J Vasc Surg* 35:397-399, 2002.)

clude endografting of the thoracic aorta. Successful endografting procedures with simultaneous visceral artery bypass used in 2 patients with severely calcified TAAA are described.

Procedure.—Both patients had an aneurysm in the descending aorta and severe calcification of the descending thoracic aortic wall. Stent grafts were constructed with the use of a self-expanding Gianturco Z stent that was covered with polyester graft fabric. Potential spinal cord ischemia was determined by an occlusion test of the intercostal arteries with a retrievable stentgraft ("Retriever") while monitoring evoked spinal cord potential (ESP). The Retriever is composed of self-expanding stents connected with longitudinal stents. Each stent is placed in a bundle fixed to a pushing rod. Endografting was divided into 2 stages because a long Retriever is difficult to withdraw. During endografting, the Retriever was inserted into the target region and expanded. If no changes in amplitude or latency of evoked spinal cord potential are seen, the Retriever is withdrawn and the permanent stent graft is placed. In these 2 patients, a calcified aorta necessitated landing the distal graft in the visceral aorta, thereby requiring surgical stent revascularization. No changes in evoked spinal cord potential and no endoleaks or complications were noted in these 2 patients who underwent endografting with simultaneous visceral artery bypass grafting (Fig 3).

Conclusion.—This approach is feasible and less invasive in the treatment of severely calcified TAAAs.

▶ The authors describe combining thoracic aorta stent grafting using the celiac and superior mesenteric arteries as landing zones, and then performing a retrograde infrarenal aorta-to-superior mesenteric artery bypass to restore visceral circulation. In addition, they advocate placement of a retrievable stent graft in the thoracic aorta and following with a permanent graft if there are no changes in evoked spinal cord potentials. With this technique, no paraplegia has resulted in their thoracic aortic stent graft patients. This latter technique appears interesting, but I wonder if paraplegia will eventually be observed. Delayed paraplegia is well-known after thoracic and thoracoabdominal aneurysm repair.

G. L. Moneta, MD

Sloughing of the Scrotal Skin and Impotence Subsequent to Bilateral Hypogastric Artery Embolization for Endovascular Aortoiliac Aneurysm Repair

Lin PH, Bush RL, Lumsden AB (Emory Univ, Atlanta, Ga)
J Vasc Surg 34:748-750, 2001   18–9

Background.—Endoluminal stent-graft placement for infrarenal aortic aneursyms is an alternative treatment for patients at high risk for conventional surgery. When the aneurysm extends distally to the hypogastric artery, selective coil occlusion of the hypogastric artery may be needed to prevent retrograde flow into the anuerysm and allow the stent-graft to be positioned in the disease-free iliac artery. Unilateral ligation or embolization of the hypogastric artery can usually be performed without significant risk of complications. However, bilateral hypogastric artery ligation or embolization may result in pelvic ischemic symptoms, the 2 most common being buttock claudication and colonic ischemia. A patient was described who had an extremely unusual complication of bilateral hypogastric artery embolization—sloughing of the scrotal skin and impotence.

Case Report.—Man, 71, with a 5.8-cm infrarenal aortic aneurysm and bilateral common iliac artery aneurysms underwent bilateral hypogastric artery embolization for endoluminal aortoiliac aneurysm repair. A repeat penile plethysmography assessment 2 days after surgery demonstrated a flattened waveform and a 75% reduction in the preoperative penile brachial index (Fig 2). The patient complained of

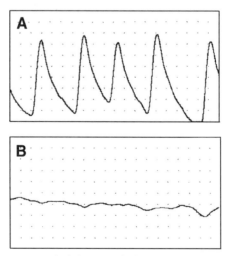

FIGURE 2.—A, Preoperative penile plethysmography demonstrated biphasic waveform with penile brachial index (PBI) of 0.93. B, Postoperative penile plethysmography demonstrated flattened waveform with PBI of 0.20. (Courtesy of Lin PH, Bush RL, Lumsden AB: Sloughing of the scrotal skin and impotence subsequent to bilateral hypogastric artery embolization for endovascular aortoiliac aneurysm repair. *J Vasc Surg* 34:748-750, 2001.)

severe scrotal pain the following day, and the physical examination demonstrated patchy dermal sloughing of the right scrotal skin. The sloughing was consistent with an ischemic rather than an infectious cause. The scrotal area was treated daily with topical silver sulfadiazine ointment, and the pain was controlled with analgesics. The patient was discharged home on the fifth postoperative day. Follow-up evaluation showed that the patient had impotence, which did not respond to sildenafil. The scrotal skin improved slowly, with minimal granulation tissue coverage 3 months later.

Conclusions.—This case report highlights the importance of maintaining pelvic collateral circulation in endovascular aortoiliac aneurysm repair; pelvic ischemia appeared to be the primary cause of this complication.

▶ Please refer to Abstract 18–7 as a potential means to avoid this complication.

G. L. Moneta, MD

Colonic Necrosis Subsequent to Catheter-Directed Thrombin Embolization of the Inferior Mesenteric Artery Via the Superior Mesenteric Artery: A Complication in the Management of a Type II Endoleak
Bush RL, Lin PH, Ronson RS, et al (Emory Univ, Atlanta, Ga)
J Vasc Surg 34:1119-1122, 2001   18–10

Background.—Endovascular abdominal aortic aneurysm (AAA) repair is performed to prevent aneurysm rupture by exclusion of the aneurysm from the aortic circulation by using a stent-graft device. Several reports have noted that 8% to 44% of patients have a persistent flow within the aortic aneurysm sac, or endoleak, despite a technically successful repair. The presence of an endoleak implies the potential pressurization of the AAA, which may lead to aneurysm enlargement and subsequent rupture if left untreated. A type II endoleak is characterized by the persistent flow of side-branch vessels that perfuse the aneurysm sac. The inferior mesenteric artery (IMA) and lumbar arteries are the most common side-branch vessels. A patient with a type II endoleak 1 year after endovascular AAA was described. The patient underwent a transcatheter embolization of the aneurysm sac and the IMA to eliminate the endoleak, resulting in colonic necrosis.

Case Report.—Man, 78, with a diagnosis of a 3.6-cm AAA 3 years earlier, was found to have an enlarging aneurysm of 4.8 cm on a surveillance US scan. The aneurysm was confirmed by CT. The patient was evaluated for an endovascular AAA repair and deemed a suitable candidate for aortic endograft placement. He underwent an uneventful endovascular grafting with a modular bifurcated stent-graft device. CT scans at 1, 6, and 12 months showed contrast extravasation into the AAA sac with no increase in aneurysm diameter.

The patient underwent a diagnostic and therapeutic aortogram to seal an endoleak involving the IMA because of the persistent endoleak 13 months after the stent-grafting procedure. Completion angiography demonstrated no flow into either the aneurysm sac or the IMA, but the sigmoidal arteries were noted to be thrombosed. The patient had back pain and mild lower abdominal pain 6 hours after the procedure, progressing to severe guarding with mild rebound tenderness. The patient also had a fever (temperature, 102.2°F) and a leukocytosis of 30,000. Diagnostic laparoscopy showed a necrotic sigmoid colon. A left hemicolectomy and transverse colostomy were performed. The patient's recovery was uneventful. Abdominal CT scan 3 months later showed no evidence of an endoleak, and the diameter of the aneurysm was unchanged.

Conclusions.—This case highlights the devastating complication of colonic ischemia that can result from catheter-directed embolization of the IMA in the management of an endoleak.

▶ Dr Lumsden reports another complication of aortic endografting (see Abstract 18–9). Ligation of the IMA during open AAA surgery should be at its origin to avoid interrupting IMA collaterals and increasing the risk of colon necrosis. Interrupting this circulation with embolization agents, perhaps not surprisingly, can also produce colonic necrosis. Obviously, attempts at embolization of the IMA should probably concentrate on occlusive devices at the very origin of the vessel.

G. L. Moneta, MD

Use of the Percutaneous Vascular Surgery Device for Closure of Femoral Access Sites During Endovascular Aneurysm Repair: Lessons From Our Experience

Teh LG, Sieunarine K, van Schie G, et al (Royal Perth Hosp, Australia)
Eur J Vasc Endovasc Surg 22:418-423, 2001   18–11

Introduction.—The usual approach for access to the femoral artery in endoluminal repairs has been an open femoral incision. Yet the trend to minimize the extent of the open incision with the expected benefit of further decreases in morbidity (especially local complications such as seromas and lymphoceles) has led to the trial use of percutaneous closure devices that allow the entire procedure to be performed without an open component. Described are the early results with a percutaneous vascular surgery device and recommendations based on experience.

Methods.—Between February 2000 and January 2001, 44 patients underwent percutaneous repair of aortic aneurysms (Fig 1). The 10F Prostar XL percutaneous vascular surgery device was used for the repair of 1 iliac, 1 thoracic, and 42 abdominal aortic aneurysms. Eighty-two groins in 44 patients were closed percutaneously.

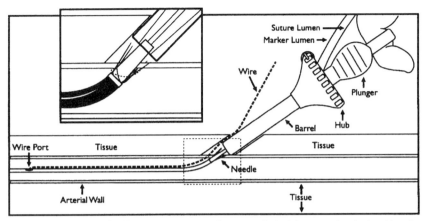

FIGURE 1.—Side profile of the percutaneous vascular surgery device in its correct (marker) position. *Inset* demonstrates needle deployment toward barrel. (Courtesy of Teh LG, Sieunarine K, van Schie G, et al: Use of the percutaneous vascular device for closure of femoral access sites during endovascular aneurysm repair: Lessons from our experience. *Eur J Vasc Endovasc Surg* 22:418-423, 2001. Copyright 2001 by permission of the publisher.)

Results.—Closure was successful in 70 access sites (85%). Twelve sites required conversion to an open groin incision. The reasons for failure were difficult device introduction because of a tortuous iliac, deflection of needles because of previous scar, femoral artery occlusion, and failure of the device to close the arteriotomy. There was 1 intraoperative death from retroperitoneal hemorrhage. One patient had a pseudoaneurysm at the cannulation site.

Conclusion.—Careful patient selection is crucial with use of the percutaneous vascular surgery device. Preoperative radiologic evaluation of the iliofemoral vessels is important in determining calcification and tortuosity. High device failure rates are more likely in obese patients and those with scarred groins. In the presence of difficulty during the procedure, there should be a low threshold for conversion to an open groin incision.

▶ Percutaneous delivery of stent grafts has been made possible with the introduction and now widespread use of "closure" devices. This article details technical and patient-related factors that are likely to result in failure of a percutaneous approach for stent graft placement. These investigators from Perth are very experienced endografters. The article should be reviewed carefully by those wishing to move to a totally percutaneous approach for stent grafts. Clearly, it can work in some patients.

G. L. Moneta, MD

Percutaneous Endovascular Abdominal Aortic Aneurysm Repair

Rachel ES, Bergamini TM, Kinney EV, et al (Baptist Hosp East, Louisville, Ky)
Ann Vasc Surg 16:43-49, 2002   18–12

Introduction.—The currently approved devices for endovascular abdominal aortic aneurysm (AAA) repair are delivered via large sheaths that range between 22F and 24F. Percutaneous endovascular aneurysm repair is technically possible using a modification of the currently available Federal Drug Administration-approved femoral closure device, the Prostar XL (Perclose). The Perclose Prostar XL device is placed before percutaneous passage of the large delivery sheaths and vascular intervention is performed to provide sufficient purchase of the artery wall. The clinical outcome of endovascular aortic aneurysm repair with the use of open femoral arteriotomy was compared with percutaneous closure of large-bore femoral access.

Methods.—Between January 1999 and August 2000, aortic aneurysm repair was performed in 150 patients. Patients who underwent open aneurysm repair (n = 38) and thoracic aneurysm repair (n = 2) were excluded. The devices were introduced by means of 22F and/or 16F sheaths in 95 patients who underwent endovascular AAA repair. The 8 Fr/10 Fr Perclose devices were used for an off-label "preclose technique." Thirty-three patients underwent bilateral open femoral arteriotomies, 44 underwent bilateral attempted percutaneous closure, and 18 had open femoral arteriotomy on 1 side and attempted percutaneous closure on the other side.

Results.—Percutaneous closure was successful in 85% (47/55) and 64% (28/44) of 16F and 22F sheaths, respectively. Twenty-four of 106 percutaneous attempts resulted in conversion to open femoral arteriotomy because of bleeding. No dissections, arterial thromboses, or pseudoaneurysms related to percutaneous arterial closure occurred. Wound complications occurred in 3.6% (3/84) open arteriotomies and 0.9% (1/106) of all percutaneous attempts and arterial closures ($P < .05$). Sex, prior femoral access, obesity, and iliac occlusive disease were not predictive of percutaneous failure.

Conclusion.—The procedural success for percutaneous AAA repair is dependent on sheath size. Devices delivered through 16F or smaller sheaths will yield successful femoral artery closure rates of at least 85%.

▶ This article is similar to the previous study (Abstract 18–11) from Australia. As the devices to deliver AAA stent grafts come down in size, so will the possibilities increase for making AAA repair an entirely percutaneous procedure.

G. L. Moneta, MD

Femoral Artery Infections Associated With Percutaneous Arterial Closure Devices

Johanning JM, Franklin DP, Elmore JR, et al (Geisinger Med Ctr, Danville, Pa)
J Vasc Surg 34:983-985, 2001   18–13

Background.—The traditional approach for achieving hemostasis after femoral artery catheterization for angiography has been manual compression, which results in consistently low rates of major complications requiring surgical repair. Septic endarteritis is a rare complication of femoral artery catheterization, and there are only 20 case reports documenting this complication. In all of these cases, septic endarteritis developed after coronary angioplasty with risk factors including repeat ipsilateral puncture and long sheath times. Septic endarteritis has not previously been reported to occur after diagnostic angiography. Two cases were reported in which infection of the femoral artery occurred after diagnostic cardiac catheterization in non-immunocompromised men, both of whom had arterial access controlled with the Perclose percutaneous closure device.

Case 1.—Man, 50, with hypertension was admitted for exertional chest pain relieved by nitroglycerin. After standard povidone-iodine skin preparation, he underwent left heart catheterization via the right common femoral artery with a 6F catheter sheath. There was no evidence of significant coronary artery disease. The patient was seen in the emergency department 19 days after catheterization and was found to have a possible groin hematoma with overlying erythema and scattered red macules on the distal right leg. He was discharged but returned the next day complaining of increasing right leg pain, hemorrhage from the catheter site, and increasing macules at the ankle. Septic endarteritis was diagnosed. Operative findings included gross purulent fluid and a necrotic anterior wall of the common femoral artery. The patient recovered uneventfully after 6 weeks of IV cefazolin for a methicillin-sensitive *Staphylococcus aureus* infection.

Case 2.—Man, 55, was evaluated for chest pain syndrome and an abnormal thallium stress test. He underwent cardiac catheterization via the right femoral artery with a 6F catheter sheath, revealing normal coronary anatomy. Hemostasis was controlled with a Perclose device. The patient went to a second facility 4 days after catheterization complaining of right groin pain and a fever (temperature, 104°F). A duplex scan demonstrated a common femoral artery pseudoaneurysm. The infected aneurysm was drained and the closure suture removed and a saphenous vein patch placed. The methicillin-sensitive *S aureus* infection was treated with ampicillin/sulbactam and vancomycin. Arterial hemorrhage from the incision developed 5 days later, and the patient was transferred to the authors' institution. An incomplete suture line was noted. The existing vein patch was used, and a simple revision of the femoral artery vein patch angioplasty was placed with a running suture. The patient recovered uneventfully after 4 weeks of IV cefazolin.

Conclusions.—These reports suggest that the use of Perclose in femoral artery catheterization is associated with a risk of severe arterial infection. Surgeons should be aware of this potential for septic endarteritis associated with Perclose use and the need for aggressive management of any such infections.

▶ We also have dealt with a number of arterial infections in the groin associated with percutaneous arterial closure devices. No limbs have been lost, but these infections can be very significant and require extensive debridement, autogenous repair, and occasional muscle flap coverage of the repaired artery.

G. L. Moneta, MD

BioGlue Surgical Adhesive for Thoracic Aortic Repair During Coagulopathy: Efficacy and Histopathology

Hewitt CW, Marra SW, Kann BR, et al (Univ of Medicine and Dentistry of New Jersey, Camden; Auburn Univ, Ala)
Ann Thorac Surg 71:1609-1612, 2001   18–14

Background.—Coagulopathy is often a complication of thoracic aortic operation for the repair of aneurysms, tissue injury, or other disorders. There are several possible factors involved in this dilemma, including dysfunction of the normal coagulation mechanisms resulting from excessive hemorrhage, hypothermia, multiple blood transfusions, acidosis, or aortic cross-clamping. Coagulopathy can then lead to increased morbidity and mortality. A number of surgical tissue adhesives have been investigated to control bleeding from suture lines and needle holes. A new tissue bioadhesive (Bio-Glue) was investigated in a sheep model of surgical repair of the thoracic aorta.

Methods.—Anticoagulation was induced in sheep with aspirin and heparin. A bypass was constructed with end-to-side anastomoses of a graft to a partially occluded descending thoracic aorta. Nine experimental anastomoses were then treated with BioGlue, while 5 control anastomoses were treated with Surgicel to gain intraoperative hemostasis.

Results.—Animals in the experimental group showed significantly less postsurgical bleeding, a reduced rate of blood loss in the first 2 hours postoperatively as well as over the entire recovery period, and reduced total blood loss compared with the control animals. Histologic examination of tissues explanted after 3 months showed that BioGlue was relatively inert and induced only a minimal inflammatory response.

Conclusions.—In a sheep model of coagulopathy, a tissue bioadhesive (BioGlue) provided a significantly reduced rate and volume of postsurgical bleeding during thoracic aortic surgery with only a minimal inflammatory response. This new surgical bioadhesive could be beneficial for use in coagulopathic patients who are undergoing such procedures.

▶ The surgical adhesives appear to work. To me, they are most useful in controlling suture line bleeding when 2 pieces of polytetrafluoroethylene are sewn together.

G. L. Moneta, MD

Subject Index

A

Author Index